Current Topics in Microbiology and Immunology

176

AF826035

Editors

Genetic Diversity of RNA Viruses

Edited by J. J. Holland

With 34 Figures and 14 Tables

Springer-Verlag
Berlin Heidelberg NewYork
London Paris Tokyo
Hong Kong Barcelona
Budapest

JOHN J. HOLLAND, Ph.D.

Professor of Biology and Molecular Genetics
Department of Biology, C-016
University of California
San Diego
La Jolla, CA 92093
USA

ISBN 3-540-54652-9 Springer-Verlag Berlin Heidelberg New York
ISBN 0-387-54652-9 Springer-Verlag New York Berlin Heidelberg

Library of Congress Catalog Card Number 15-12910
Printed in Germany

Typesetting: Thomson Press (India) Ltd, New Delhi;
Offsetprinting: Saladruck, Berlin; Bookbinding: Lüderitz & Bauer, Berlin
23/3020-5 4 3 2 1 0 – Printed on acid-free paper.

Preface

Many RNA viruses have been known for decades to be genetically and biologically quite variable. Some well-known examples are influenza viruses, foot and mouth disease viruses, and Newcastle disease virus. During the past decade, it has become clear that most, it not all, RNA viruses (riboviruses and retroviruses) are much more mutable than was recognized previously, and that this great mutability generates extremely complex populations consisting of indeterminate mixtures of related variants (i.e., "mutant swarms" or "quasispecies" populations). This is also true of DNA viruses (such as hepatitis B virus) which replicate their DNA genomes via RNA transcripts that are reverse-transcribed back to DNA. This hypermutability of RNA replicons provides great biological adaptability for RNA virus genomes. It also allows (but does not necessitate) extremely rapid evolution of RNA viruses, so that they can evolve over a million times more quickly than their eukaryotic DNA-based hosts.

The genetics of RNA replicons is so unusual (and often counterintuitive) that it has many important biological consequences which are neither readily apparent nor widely understood. Failure to understand the distinctive aspects of RNA genetics frequently generates confusion and controversy and can adversely impact vaccine and antiviral drug programs and other applications of medical virology. The 14 chapters in this volume describe advances in a number of significant areas of RNA virus genetics and evolution. The authors provide clear, concise reviews of RNA replicase error frequencies and quasispecies genome populations; rapid evolution of RNA genomes in vitro and in natural hosts in vivo as contrasted to RNA virus population equilibrium and relative genome stasis; the role of environmental selection pressures in driving the evolution of complex RNA populations; the role and mechanisms of RNA recombination; RNA genome hypermutations and defective genomes in persistent infections; the rapid emergence of drug-resistant virus genomes during prophylaxis/therapy in humans, and the conditions favoring transmission of drug-resistant viruses. Also presented are an analysis of the origins and evolutionary relationships of retroviruses; the replication and evolution of small circular viroid-like RNA pathogens, and analysis of the possible involvement of such small,self-replicating circular RNAs as early primitive molecular life forms which evolved to conjoined RNA molecules, and then to RNAs and DNA based genetic systems; and a number of other topics.

The editor wishes to thank all of the contributors to this volume for having taken time from their busy schedules to prepare these concise and interesting reviews.

J. J. HOLLAND

List of Contents

List of Contributors

(Their addresses can be found at the beginning of the respective chapters.)

RNA Virus Populations as Quasispecies

J. J. HOLLAND[1], J. C. DE LA TORRE[2], and D. A. STEINHAUER[3]

1 Introduction

This chapter discusses the high mutation frequencies and rapid evolution potential of RNA viruses. The concepts discussed are applicable to all "ordinary" RNA viruses (riboviruses), viroids and satellite RNAs; to retroviruses; and to viruses (such as the hepadnaviruses) with DNA genomes which replicate via RNA transcripts. Because DNA virus polymerases can have proofreading (KORNBERG 1974), their mutation frequencies can be much lower than those of RNA viruses. For example, the mutation rate of bacteriophage T4 approximates 10^{-8} per base pair per replication (DRAKE 1969). However, some DNA viruses may avoid high-fidelity replication mechanisms (DRAKE et al. 1969; HALL et al. 1984) to

[1] Department of Biology and Institute of Molecular Genetics, University of California at San Diego, La Jolla, California 92093-0116, USA
[2] Department of Neuropharmacology, Research Institute of Scripps Clinic, La Jolla, California 92037, USA
[3] National Institute for Medical Research, The Ridgeway, Mill Hill, London NW7 1AA, England

Current Topics in Microbiology and Immunology, Vol. 176

gain the evolutionary advantages of high mutation frequencies (SMITH and INGLIS 1987).

1.1 Mutation Frequencies and Rates of Evolution of RNA Viruses Are Generally Very High

Recent evidence indicates that most RNA viruses form complex "quasispecies" populations which can evolve very rapidly, due to extremely high mutation frequencies per site in RNA virus genomes (ranging between 10^{-3} and 10^{-6} and usually of the order of 10^{-4}–10^{-5}). This evidence has been reviewed extensively and referenced in the following reviews and recent articles (HOLLAND et al. 1982, 1989, 1990, 1991; DOMINGO et al. 1985; SMITH and INGLIS 1987; ZIMMERN 1988; DOMINGO and HOLLAND 1988; COFFIN 1986, 1990; TEMIN 1989; PATHAK and TEMIN 1990; DE LA TORRE et al. 1990; DOMINGO 1989; EIGEN and BIEBRICHER 1988; CHAO 1990; MYERHANS et al. 1989; GROENINK et al. 1991; DOUGHERTY and TEMIN 1988; KEW et al. 1990; KINNUNEN et al. 1990; SMITH and PALESE 1988; STEINHAUER and HOLLAND 1987; STEINHAUER et al. 1989a, b; BILSEL and NICHOL 1990; BALFE et al. 1990; VARTANIAN et al. 1991; SKEHEL and WILEY 1988; BOEGE et al. 1991; IMAZEKI et al. 1990; HEINZ et al. 1989; STRAUSS and STRAUSS 1988; GEBAUER et al. 1988; VILLAVERDE et al. 1991; HAHN et al. 1989a, b; BURNS and DESROSIERS 1991; WARD et al. 1988).

1.2 RNA Virus Clones are Quasispecies Populations

Obviously if mutation frequencies usually exceed 10^{-5} at most sites in RNA virus genomes that average about 10 kb in size, then even clones of such viruses will inevitably consist of a complex mixture of different but related genomes, all of which must compete during replication of the clone and its progeny. Eigen, Schuster and their colleagues (EIGEN and SCHUSTER 1979; EIGEN et al. 1981; EIGEN and BIEBRICHER 1988) introduced the term "quasispecies" to refer to the diverse, rapidly evolving and competing RNA populations postulated as earliest life forms on earth, and the principles they have elaborated for quasispecies evolution apply well to RNA virus populations today (see for example DOMINGO et al. 1985; DOMINGO and HOLLAND 1988; GEBAUER et al. 1988; HOLLAND et al. 1989, 1990, 1991; PATHAK and TEMIN 1990; COFFIN 1990; DE LA TORRE et al. 1990; KURATH and PALUKAITIS 1990; GROENINK et al. 1991; BURNS and DESROSIERS 1991). For the discussion below, the term "consensus sequence" refers to the (average) sequence actually observed when aggregate genomes of a clonal (or non-clonal) virus population are sequenced. "Master sequence" refers to the most fit genome sequence (or sequences) within a complex quasispecies population replicating in a defined environment. "Mutant spectrum" refers to all of those competing virus variants which differ from the master sequence(s) and/or from the single genome which generated a quasispecies clone. Quasispecies populations are not hypothetical abstractions. They exist in animals and humans infected by RNA viruses such as vesicular stomatitis virus (VSV), foot-

and-mouth disease virus, poliovirus, human immunodeficiency virus (HIV)-1, influenza viruses, etc. as reviewed in the following chapters of this volume. Quasispecies populations also exist in clones of RNA viruses (including retroviruses) as shown by extreme mutation frequencies in clones and by rapid selection of mutants with increased fitness in the presence of antibody, drugs, new host cell types, etc. (See the following chapters, and the references cited above.)

The concept that RNA viruses are highly mutable and adaptable is not new. Very high mutation frequencies for phenotypes such as temperature sensitivity, pathogenicity, or plaque size mutants were reported decades ago (see for example GRANOFF 1961, 1964; FIELDS and JOKLIK 1969; EGGERS and TAMM 1965; PRINGLE 1970; KUNKEL 1947; THEILER and SMITH 1939). Indeed, the great adaptability of RNA viruses was utilized to prepare attenuated vaccines even before the genetic and biochemical nature of viruses was understood. More than 100 years ago Pasteur and his colleagues prepared the "fixed" vaccine strain of rabies virus by repeated passage of wild-type "street" virus intracerebrally in rabbits until it was no longer virulent for dogs by the subcutaneous route. Subsequently, a number of successful human attenuated virus vaccines have been prepared by multiple adaptive passages of virulent virus in new host cell types in vitro (THEILER and SMITH 1937; SABIN and BOULGER 1973; ENDERS et al. 1960). Despite this general knowledge that RNA viruses are quite mutable and adaptable, their extreme mutation frequencies have been documented only recently with the advent of rapid techniques for genome sequencing and mapping. Although many virologists are now aware of the quasispecies nature of populations of RNA viruses, their many biological implications are probably not generally appreciated. A number of authors have reported a quite low mutation frequency for some RNA viruses or some genome sites or genome regions of certain RNA viruses, and some examples of these will be discussed below following the general review of polymerase misincorporation frequencies. If it eventually can be rigorously proved that certain sites (or segments) of some RNA virus have very low mutation frequencies, this would not negate the quasispecies nature of populations of that virus if most other nucleotide sites (and segments) undergo mutation frequencies between 10^{-4} and 10^{-5}. As discussed below, polymerase error of the order of 10^{-4}–10^{-5} is generally to be expected in the absence of proofreading and repair functions.

2 Base Misinsertion Frequencies of Polymerases in the Absence of Proofreading and Repair Mechanisms

2.1 Tautomeric Equilibrium Constants and Polymerase Misinsertion Error

The relative contributions of various mechanisms to DNA and RNA polymerase mutation frequencies are not completely established, and they clearly vary with different polymerases. Most investigations have been done using DNA polymerases. The most elemental basis for inevitable polymerase errors is quantum mechanical. The Watson–Crick base pairing rules apply to the bases in their most favored tautomeric form, but shifts to rare tautomeric forms make mutations unavoidable during replication of both DNA and RNA. WATSON and CRICK (1953), in their original papers on the structure of DNA, suggested that base substitution mutations could be caused by the presence of minor tautomeric forms — for example, a shift of the hydrogen atom from the 6 amino position of adenine to the N1 position causing a mismatched pairing with cytosine. Quantum mechanical, spectral, thermodynamic, and kinetic analyses of various tautomeric forms of the bases and their tautomeric equilibria in aqueous solution have been laborious (see for example DANIELS 1972; KENNER et al. 1955; WOLFENDEN 1969; KWIATKOWSKI and PULLMAN 1975; DREYFUS et al. 1976), and are subject to uncertainties regarding the state of (and the effects of) base solvation or desolvation within the active sites of various polymerases (CULLIS and WOLFENDEN 1981). However, estimates of rare tautomer equilibrium constants of the order of 10^{-4}–10^{-5} suggest a lower limit of about the same order of magnitude for base substitution frequencies at most sites in DNA and RNA. The classical paper by TOPAL and FRESCO (1976) utilized estimates of rare tautomer equilibria together with modeling of steric fit within a double helix to determine those rare tautomers able to be accommodated within a double helix in alternative base-pairing alignments. On this basis, they calculated likely base-mispairing frequencies, and compared their results with data available at that time. They proposed that rare tautomer mispairing (particularly of pyrimidine rare tautomers) should dictate transition frequencies at a level approximating 10^{-4}–10^{-5} per site. However, transversions were suggested to require anti→syn isomerization together with minor tautomeric forms to allow mispairing of purines, and hence were estimated to be about an order of magnitude less frequent than transitions. Because their model agreed well with transition and transversion frequencies of the mutD5 mutator strain of *Escherichia coli* they predicted that the mutD5 mutation probably eliminated the proofreading function of the DNA polymerase (TOPAL and FRESCO 1976). ECHOLS et al. (1983) later confirmed that mutD does lack the 3′-→5′-exonucleolytic editing function (which is on the ε subunit of the DNA polymerase III holoenzyme), so the observed mutD5 mutation frequency is the basic unedited polymerase misinsertion frequency. Kinetic analyses of *E. coli* DNA polymerase I base misinsertion transitions in vitro (FERSHT et al. 1982, 1983) also generally agreed with the 10^{-4}–10^{-5} frequencies predicted from tautomerization constant by TOPAL and FRESCO (1976). Their kinetic analysis also suggested that the polymerase does not greatly affect the tautomerization constant of active site-bound deoxynucleotide triphosphate (dNTP, as opposed to bases in the template). Specific misinsertions by some eukaryotic DNA polymerases such as chick γ polymerase are so low ($<10^{-5}$) that these polymerases might be affecting tautomeric equilibria of some bases (KUNKEL and ALEXANDER 1986). Desolvation within the active site could be a factor. Also, protein complexes or DNA binding proteins might enhance polymerase fidelity, perhaps by stabilizing templates (KUNKEL et al. 1979). Tautomer equilibrium constants provide only one of the reasons why minimal polymerase error frequency (in the absence of proofreading and repair) will generally exceed 10^{-5}.

2.2 Thermodynamic Constraints on Base Pair Discrimination

The pioneering studies of Kornberg and colleagues (KORNBERG 1974) demonstrated that there is a single active site in DNA polymerase at which all four dNTPs must compete for incorporation. This likely precludes the best possibility for extreme fidelity in which each specific dNTP in solution is bound to one of four specific sites and its major tautomeric form "confirmed" by steric fit before insertion opposite the one correct template base, the major tautomer of which was similarly confirmed. Early mutagenesis studies with base analogs demonstrated that base pairing is critical for much polymerase insertional specificity. This has been highlighted by the recent work of PICCIRILLI et al. (1990). They designed and synthesized two new " bases" designated kappa and pi. Although chemically distinct from natural bases, these were designed to form hydrogen-bonded base pairs in a DNA double helix. Kappa, which base pairs with xanthosine was able to direct incorporation of xanthosine opposite itself into both DNA and RNA. This exhibited approximately normal DNA and RNA polymerase misincorporation frequencies. It is clear here that base-pairing steric fit, rather than accurate base (and major tautomer) identification by polymerases is the chief mechanism for insertional specificity. However, base-pairing discrimination in aqueous solution involves major thermodynamic problems for polymerase fidelity as pointed out by LOEB and KUNKEL (1982). Free energy differences ($\Delta\Delta G$) between matched and mismatched base pairs in aqueous solution are estimated at no better than about 1–2 kcal/mol. This small difference in $\Delta\Delta G$ values cannot provide adequate base pair discrimination in solution to maintain base misinsertion frequencies per site better than about 10^{-1}–10^{-2}. Nevertheless, as will be discussed below, unedited in vitro polymerase misincorporation frequencies per site generally average about 10^{-4}–10^{-5}, and range between 10^{-3} to less than 10^{-5} (PRESTON et al. 1988). In contrast, a primitive lead-catalyzed, nonenzymatic polymerization of polyguanylate directed by a poly C template did exhibit the expected error levels, approximating 10^{-2} per site (LOHRMANN and ORGEL 1980). PETRUSKA et al. (1986, 1988) suggested that the $\Delta\Delta G$s between matched and mismatched nucleotides are magnified at polymerase active sites by exclusion of water. Their studies suggested that *Drosophila* polymerase γ in vitro can amplify $\Delta\Delta G$ values more than ten fold (to approximately those expected in vacuo) by reducing entropy differences and increasing enthalpy differences. In this way, polymerase misincorporation frequencies can be lowered to about 10^{-4}–10^{-5} per site, which is the level generally observed in vitro. Thus, for basic thermodynamic and quantum mechanical reasons, unedited polymerase mutation frequencies cannot ordinarily be expected to be much lower than about 10^{-4}–10^{-5} per site. Many other factors can also contribute to elevate base misinsertion frequencies above absolute minimal levels. Prominent among these are polymerase effects. Some polymerases exhibit generally high fidelity and others are more error prone. The latter are clearly not genetically designed to achieve the maximum possible base insertion fidelity, and their misinsertions are often favored at certain template sites.

2.3 Polymerase Misinsertion Frequencies In Vitro

It is not possible in this short chapter to review the extensive literature on mutagenesis. The reader is referred to the excellent recent reviews edited by MOSES and SUMMERS (1988). However, several important points relevant to this volume are outlined below.

In the absence of a proofreading function (or when the 3′-→5′-exonuclease editing function is suppressed) in vitro polymerase error frequencies vary from as high as approximately 10^{-3} or 10^{-4} to as low as about 6×10^{-6} (LOEB and KUNKEL 1982; PRESTON et al. 1988). The latter value was obtained only with the four-subunit complex of calf thymus polymerase α-primase whereas homopolymeric preparations of the same polymerase α exhibited a misincorporation frequency between 10^{-4} and 10^{-5}. Therefore the presence of an undetected 3′-→5′-exonuclease editing function could not be ruled out. Editing nucleases are often absent from polymerases of eukaryotic cells, but in some cases exogenous 3′-→5′-exonuclease proteins may associate with these polymerase molecules in vivo, so the absence of editing functions on polymerases in vitro cannot disprove a role in vivo. Not only do different polymerases exhibit varying error rates in vitro, but they also can exhibit bias toward certain types of mismatch and preferentially misincorporate at or near certain template sequences. They also differentially incorporate certain base analogs, so template sequences and steric considerations at or near the active site are clearly important (LOEB and KUNKEL 1982; PRESTON et al. 1988; KUNKEL and ALEXANDER 1986; see also the chapter by WILLIAMS and LOEB).

Recent studies by KUNKEL and his colleages (KUNKEL 1986; BEBENEK and KUNKEL 1990) suggest that base substitutions may often result from transient misalignment of the primer (nascent) strand on the template, and that base substitutions may, in a similar manner, initiate frameshift errors. There are many other factors which influence mutation frequencies and specificities. These include NTP substrate concentrations, metal ion variations, thermal effects on polymerase, base damage by oxidation, UV light, etc. Regardless of the multiplicity of factors which can be involved in mutagenesis, base misinsertion is an inevitable process with frequencies varying from about 10^{-3} to less than 10^{-5} and averaging about 10^{-4}–10^{-5}. Editing and/or mismatch repair are required to achieve significantly higher fidelities.

3 Editing and Mismatch Repair: Do They Occur for RNA Molecules or for RNA Virus Genomes?

Proofreading (KORNBERG 1974) and mismatch repair are important processes in achieving fidelity in bacterial and phage DNA replication, but related processes are not presently as well characterized for eukaryotic cells (RADMAN and WAGNER 1986; LAHUE et al. 1989; MOSES and SUMMERS 1988). In eukaryotic systems, editing functions may be less tightly coupled with DNA polymerase than for bacteria and phages (i.e., they may be part of accessory proteins or protein complexes) and may therefore be more elusive. This makes it difficult to rule out their presence and function wherever they may not exist. Proofreading can improve DNA fidelity by orders of magnitude, and mismatch repair has the potential to achieve extreme fidelity via repeated scanning and repairing of DNA.

Mismatch repair is not possible for any RNA (or DNA) virus genomes if they are replicated and packaged as single-stranded molecules. This includes the vast majority of RNA viruses. Nor has proofreading yet been rigorously documented for any RNA molecules, viral or nonviral. There is no evidence to suggest the existence of 3'-→5'-exonuclease editing functions acting during synthesis of any RNA molecules. However it is difficult to disprove that they might exist on accessory protein molecules or complexes. Nevertheless, editing entails significant energy costs (FERSHT et al. 1982) and the expenditure of considerable energy to achieve high-fidelity RNA molecules should generally be counterproductive. The maximum error frequency of protein synthesis has been estimated to be between 10^{-3} and 10^{-4} (LOTFIELD and VANDERJAGT 1972; EDELMANN and GALLANT 1977; ELLIS and GALLANT 1982). This is a rather high fidelity in the complex process of translation. Apparently it includes kinetic proofreading by transfer RNA (tRNA) synthetases in aminoacylation (YAMANE and HOPFIELD 1977; JAKUBOWSKI 1990). With error frequencies exceeding 10^{-4} for translation, messenger RNA (mRNA) transcription fidelities need not exceed the usual fidelity levels observed for DNA polymerase insertions. In fact, measurements of RNA polymerase error frequencies (ROSENBERGER and HILTON 1983; BLANK et al. 1986) suggest RNA base misinsertion frequencies between 10^{-4} and 10^{-5}. The most careful measurements for wild-type *E. coli* RNA polymerase approximate 10^{-5} (BLANK et al. 1986) which exceeds by an order of magnitude the fidelity of translation. A mutant of *E. coli* RNA polymerase exhibited a lower fidelity (BLANK et al. 1986), but if any editing function is involved in *E. coli* polymerase transcription, it does not approach the high fidelity that can be provided by DNA polymerases with 3'-→5'-exonuclease. For example, the editing function associated with the ε subunit of the *pol* III DNA polymerase of *E. coli* can improve fidelity by up to 10^4-fold (ECHOLS et al. 1983). It is not possible to exclude some low-fidelity proofreading in RNA synthesis such as the kinetic proofreading postulated by HOPFIELD (1974) (e.g., selective pyrophosphorolysis of mismatched bases). Pyrophosphorolysis does occur at significant levels during RNA transcription (KASSAVETIS et al. 1986).

One might argue that a structural (ribosomal) RNA could require higher fidelity. However, we have recently examined in vivo base misincorporation frequencies in ribosomal RNAs of mouse, hamster, and human cells, and base substitution frequencies greater than 10^{-4} per site were observed (STEINHAUER and HOLLAND, unpublished data). We have also been examining the virion-associated replicase of VSV and have as yet observed no evidence for any proofreading (STEINHAUER, DOMINGO, and HOLLAND, unpublished data). The only report of a proofreading-like activity for RNA is that of ISHIHAMA et al. (1986) for influenza virus RNA polymerase. However, this "editing" involved only removal of excess G residues added to cannibalized capped host cell mRNA primers. This was not inhibited by incorporation of 1-thiotriphosphates into RNA. Such inhibition is a hallmark of exonucleases of the 3'→5' DNA proofreading (LOEB and KUNKEL 1982). All evidence presently available suggests that base misinsertion frequencies of RNA polymerases are similar for DNA polymerases. Proofreading is apparently absent or inefficient for most (or all) RNA synthesis, including viral RNA replication and reverse transcription by retroviruses (see the chapters by DOMINGO et al., COFFIN, WILLIAMS and LOEB, and WAIN HOBSON).

4 Do Most (or All) RNA Viruses Produce Quasispecies Populations?

Not all riboviruses nor retroviruses have yet been examined carefully to determine mutation frequencies and population heterogeneity. The great majority of presently available evidence suggests high mutation frequencies at most sites examined, so that even clonal populations must have heterogeneous quasispecies distributions.

Despite generally high mutation frequencies in most RNA viruses, it is important to remember that polymerase frequencies are known to vary, that for each polymerase there can be template sites at which misincorporation frequencies are considerably higher or lower than average, and that certain polymerase can favor certain specific mispairs. For example, eukaryotic polymerase β produces T·G mispairs at several orders of magnitude higher frequencies than does polymerase γ (KUNKEL and ALEXANDER 1986). Because RNA virus replicases and reverse transcriptases also exhibit preferences and variabilities there can be confusion regarding overall viral mutation frequencies. The following points should be emphasized:

1. Documentation of a low mutation frequency at a particular genome site of an RNA virus does *not* contradict evidence for high frequencies overall. For example, DURBIN and STOLLAR (1986) and HAHN et al. (1989a, b) reported three different specific site reversion frequencies in the Sindbis virus genome exhibiting mutation frequencies of the order of 10^{-7} to less than 10^{-8} yet HAHN

et al. (1989a, b and back references) also observed many other Sindbis virus mutations occurring at frequencies between 10^{-3} and 10^{-5} suggesting that the three low-frequency reversion sites are rather unique, perhaps due to the sequence context in which they are located. Stec et al. (1986) likewise reported spontaneous mutation frequencies for Sindbis virus resistance to neutralizing monoclonal antibodies to be of the order of $10^{-3.5}$–10^{-5}. With poliovirus, Sedivy et al. (1987) reported reversion frequencies for an amber mutant to be of the order of 10^{-6} whereas De La Torre et al. (1990) reported specific single site mutation frequencies for poliovirus of the order of 10^{-4}.

2. Low mutation frequencies in only a few genome sites would not greatly alter population heterogeneity. In fact, if half of the sites in an RNA virus genome could be shown to have very low mutation frequencies, high frequencies at the other sites would still generate quasispecies populations.
3. Extremely low mutation frequencies at a large number of genome sites in any RNA virus (i.e., frequencies of the order of 10^{-7}–10^{-8}) should arouse suspicion of, and a search for, a proofreading function. As mentioned above, such a proofreading function need not necessarily be a part of the virus replicase, but could be due to an accessory protein or protein complex.
4. Low mutation frequencies requiring a specific mismatch at a particular virus genome site do not even dictate a low *overall* mutation frequency at *that* site. For example, a phenotypic reversion requiring a T·T mispair transversion at a site during genome replication might be of low frequency, but the same site could have very high transition frequencies. Also some low frequency (e.g., T·T) mispairing during genome replication might be increased considerably by a more favored (e.g., A·A) mispairing during antigenome replication (or vice versa). Strand replication asymmetry will increase or decrease such compensatory effects.
5. RNA virus mutation frequencies of the order of 10^{-8} or less at any site are extremely unlikely to be due to high polymerase insertion fidelity. Frequencies this low are evidence either for an editing function, or for less interesting causes (e.g., the mutation or reversion requires several base substitutions—one at the site being examined and a necessary compensatory base substitution elsewhere; or the mutation assay allows negative selective forces to skew the observed frequency).
6. If editing functions do exist which can reduce RNA replicase or reverse transcriptase mutation frequencies to 10^{-8} per site or lower, these have profound biological implications. Such editing functions, if they exist, are deserving of considerable effort toward purification and characterization.
7. The RNA virus mutation frequencies observed (between 10^{-3} and 10^{-5}) at most RNA genome sites are so extreme that they approach the error threshold beyond which higher frequencies will lead to irreversible information loss and genome "error catastrophe" (Eigen and Biebricher 1988). In fact, chemical mutagenesis was unable to increase defined single site mutation frequencies in VSV and poliovirus more than 1.1^{-} to 2.8^{-} fold at any level of mutagenesis or virus survival level (Holland et al. 1990). Clearly, RNA virus replicases and

reverse transcriptases can evolve to reduce their fidelity (and enhance their biological adaptability), but only to a limited extent compatible with viability and fitness; VSV mutants described by PRINGLE et al. (1981) and retrovirus "provirus hypermutants" described by PATHAK and TEMIN (1990) are examples.

8. Defective or partially defective (nonmaturing) viruses and, to a limited extent, infectious RNA viruses can exhibit specific biased "hypermutations" (CATTANEO et al. 1988; O'HARA et al. 1984; also see the chapters by CATTANEO and BILLETER). Such hypermutations may occur by various forms of RNA editing (SIMPSON 1990; LAMB and DREYFUSS 1989) such as the cellular unwinding activity of BASS et al. (1989) or less frequently by repetitious replicase errors (PATHAK and TEMIN 1990; BILSEL and NICHOL 1990; VARTANIAN et al. 1991).
9. Whenever sites in RNA virus genomes appear to have low mutation frequencies of the order of 10^{-6}–10^{-8}, chemical mutagenesis should be able to increase greatly the mutation frequencies at such sites. This should occur without massive lethality due to error catastrophe (EIGEN and BIEBRICHER 1988; HOLLAND et al. 1990).

5 Population Biology and Evolution of RNA Virus Quasispecies

Because the mutation frequencies of RNA viruses exceed by more than a millionfold those of their eukaryotic hosts, extremely rapid virus evolution is anticipated and frequently observed (see reviews referenced in Sect. 1). A well-known example is the rapid continuous evolution of HIV-1 in infected humans (see the chapters by COFFIN, WILLIAMS and LOOB, WAIN-HOBSON, and DOOLITTLE and FENG. HIV is, of course, not unique in this respect since similar rapid evolution occurs in animals or humans naturally infected with foot- and-mouth disease virus (DOMINGO et al.), influenza virus (GORMAN et al.), poliovirus (KINNUNEN et al.), measles virus, (CATTANEO and BILLETER) and other viruses. However, relative long-term stasis of virus genomes can be observed in nature and in laboratory experiments. Such relative stasis does not imply that populations of these RNA viruses are not quasispecies, nor that their mutation frequencies are lower, nor that they are incapable of rapid evolution under different circumstances. For example, the genomes of eastern equine encephalitis virus in North America have exhibited relative stasis for the last half century while South American strains have apparently been evolving more rapidly (see chapter by WEAVER et al.). Some plant viruses also exhibit population stability (RODRIGUEZ-CEREZO et al. 1989). Likewise, influenza A virus, despite its obvious capacity for rapid evolution, can exhibit relative stasis of some genes (GORMAN et al. 1990; see chapter by GORMAN et al.). Finally, human T-cell lymphotrophic virus (HTLV) appears to be evolving relatively slowly (INA and GOJOBORI 1990). Clones of VSV under laboratory conditions can exhibit relative population stasis or extremely rapid evolution depending on passage conditions. Rapid evolution is promoted by conditions which lead to loss of population equilibrium (i.e., loss of dominance by previously most fit master sequences, and rise to dominance of new master sequences). Obviously, repeated environmental changes readily promote disequilibrium whether these changes are external (such as sequential infection of new hosts or host cell types) or internal (such as sequential interference due to the generation of changing populations of defective interfering virus particles in persistently infected cells). This is reviewed in HOLLAND et al. 1982; DOMINGO et al. 1985; DOMINGO and HOLLAND 1988; STEINHAUER et al. 1989).

It might seem paradoxical that heterogeneous quasispecies populations of RNA viruses can exhibit slow evolution or periods of stasis despite extreme mutation frequencies and rapid replication. However this can be explained by selection for fit master sequences in rather constant environments (EIGEN and BIEBRICHER 1988). The classical population biology theories of WRIGHT (1977, 1982) provide a useful mathematical paradigm for visualizing evolution of rather small populations (demes) in "adaptive landscapes." Random genetic variation coupled with environmental selection leads to random drift in an adaptive landscape (schematized in Fig. 1). Quantitative polygenic phenotypic characteristics are plotted on the Y and Z axes. Each combination of genetic characters has a mean fitness in a given environment, and this is plotted on the X, or fitness axis to provide an adaptive landscape. Small isolated, related populations can be represented as points on this landscape, and they will tend to spend a large fraction of evolutionary time near peaks of high fitness rather than less adaptive or nonadaptive ridges or valleys. Genetic variation and selection would tend to move a small population up a peak. With continuous selection, a population might become isolated on a peak even if there were much more highly adaptive peaks nearby representing better combinations of characters. However, WRIGHT (1977, 1982) envisioned landscapes with numerous peaks connected by

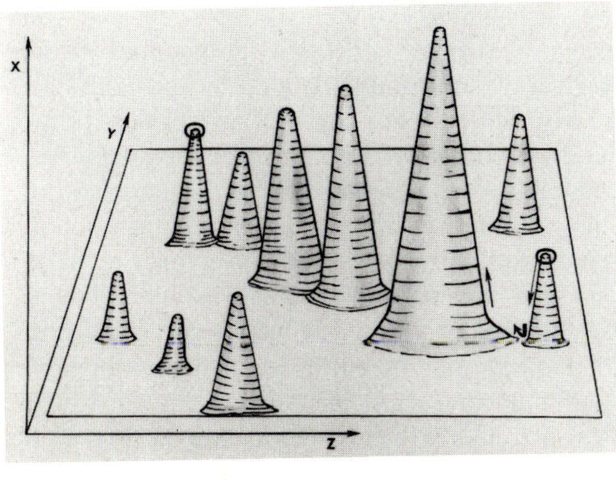

Fig. 1. Hypothetical adaptive landscape for RNA virus evolution in a constant adaptive environment. See text and WRIGHT (1977, 1982)

adaptive valleys so that random genetic drift could allow populations to move to other peaks. Once a population ascended to a very high fitness peak, gene flow would spread adaptive genes to other populations. WRIGHT (1982) suggested that his theories were relevant to recent paleobiological evidence for punctuated equilibrium (GOULD and ELDRIDGE 1977).

LANDE (1985) and NEWMAN et al. (1985) elegantly elaborated the applicability of WRIGHTS theories to punctuated equilibria during evolution. They showed that in a fixed, unchanging landscape, the expected time for population transitions between peaks should be extremely short. In contrast, the time spent near locally optimal peaks is long and increases approximately exponentially with effective population size (LANDE 1985). The timescale during transitions between peaks is short even though random genetic variations are small, and despite initial movement against selection during the transitions from one peak to another (NEWMAN et al. 1985). Thus, punctuated equilibria are explained even in a rather constant environment. Whenever the adaptive landscape changes abruptly as a result of a major environmental change, new selective forces will punctuate the equilibrium.

These theories are applicable to RNA virus populations even though virus populations can be extremely large, and virus mutation rates and evolution rates extremely high. In fact, these characteristics of RNA viruses should make them very useful for studies of population biology. Consider a quasispecies population of an RNA virus in the adaptive landscape of Fig. 1 to have ascended the lower right adaptive peak. The population may remain in equilibrium around the top of this peak even though there is a much higher adaptive optimum nearby. This will occur particularly when the local virus population remains large. Very high mutation frequencies can counter this by accumulating a small proportion of variants having numerous mutations so that there can be movement down the peak (against selection), but the more fit variants near the top (close to the master sequences [s]) will dominate. Thus, population equilibrium might be maintained for relatively long periods of time despite high mutation frequencies. In fact, DE LA TORRE et al. (1990) observed that a mutant of VSV of vastly superior fitness could not rise to dominate its diverse quasispecies progenitor population of lower mean fitness unless it was seeded above a critical threshold level,*and* unless at least some intracellular replication occurred in the absence of competitor variants (by carrying out dilute passages during competition).

Thus, in a constant environment, a quasispecies variant swarm might hover for a relatively long period near the moderately adaptive peak depicted at the lower right hand of Fig. 1. Eventually, when a low probability accumulation of many appropriate mutations moves a subset of the quasispecies population down the peak (against selection) and across a nonadaptive valley or ridge (arrows in Fig. 1), strong positive selection should quickly move the population up the adjacent highly adaptive peak to produce new, highly fit master (and consensus) sequences together with a mutant spectrum of higher average fitness. This movement to the new peak must occur *rapidly*, and *only* when virus transmission leads to a rather low population (LANDE 1985; NEWMAN et al. 1985).

Virus transmission from host to host, or from one area to another within a host, often involves small virus populations or even a single virus particle (genetic bottleneck transmission).

Finally, the fastest way to disrupt a stable virus equilibrium near a highly adaptive peak is to change the adaptive landscape. This happens frequently with viruses (e.g., during immune responses; changes of host species or of cell type within a single host; interference by defective viruses, inflammatory responses, etc.). Hence, rapid evolution of RNA viruses is often more evident than is relative evolutionary stasis, but both do occur (see the chapters by DOMINGO et al., GORMAN et al., WEAVER et al., COFFIN, and DOOLITTLE and FENG). WRIGHTS two-dimensional combinations of characters are of course an oversimplification for viruses which, intracellularly, compete (and interact) with the countless mutants (and mutant gene products) which they regularly generate. Still this paradigm can give useful insights into the complexities of RNA virus evolution. RNA viruses should provide good laboratory models for evolution and evolutionary theories.

6 Implications of RNA Virus Quasispecies Populations for Pathogenesis and Disease

Many of the consequences of RNA virus quasispecies virus populations are rather obvious. For example, RNA genome population diversity can allow rapid evolution, antigenic change and immune system evasion, and rapid development of effective resistance to antiviral drugs (see the chapters by ; DOMINGO 1990). Such diversity also facilitates and complicates the establishment and progression of chronic infections such as acquired immunodeficiency syndrome (AIDS) or SSPE. The presence of a dynamic quasispecies population of RNA genomes in infected individuals can make it difficult to explore fully the pathogenesis of infections. This is fairly obvious in the case of AIDS syndromes (see below), but it is true to some extent for all RNA virus infections. A heterogeneous swarm of RNA genomes in an infected tissue or organ renders it impossible to assign specific pathological significance to any consensus sequence recovered from the diseased tissue, and, of course, the master sequences and consensus sequences continuously evolve during disease progression and/or recovery. For example, in mice infected with the Armstrong strain of lymphocytic choriomeningitis virus (LCMV), variants arise at high frequency which cause selective immunosuppression of those T cells designed to recognize and reject LCMV (AHMED et al. 1984). BOZZOW and OLDSTONE (personal communication) also observed a high frequency of LCMV variants with differing interactions with cellular receptors. Finally, OLDSTONE (personal communication) recently found a high frequency of clones capable of causing the mouse growth hormone "stunting" syndrome within the wild-type quasispecies population of the WE strain of LCMV. Since this wild-type WE strain of LCMV does not cause the growth hormone syndrome in persistently infected mice, it is clear that the complex quasispecies population of WE strain LCMV suppresses and Masks an important disease potential of genomes buried within its mutant spectrum. Quasispecies populations inevitably dictate a certain degree of uncertainty regarding the biology of all RNA virus diseases. In most cases, this should pose no practical problems for diagnosis, treatment, vaccination, etc., but in many cases it will. There is an unspoken assumption among many physicians and scientists that *a particular RNA* virus will generally cause *a particular disease*. This assumption may be true in a very broad practical sense, but it is important to understand that it can never be true in a formal scientific sense. Because *a particular RNA* virus simply does not exist, *a particular RNA virus disease* does not exist either. The science of infectious diseases is still in its infancy because we still understand so little of the fine details of host-pathogen interactions.

Any quasispecies swarm of RNA virus genomes in an infected human creates a quasispecies swarm of virus-encoded proteins, both intracellularly and extracellularly. As was discussed previously, all human (and other) protein pools must contain amino acid misincorporations at a level greater than 10^{-4}, so these could be considered to have a quasispecies type distribution. However, this should not be confused with the *replicating* quasispecies mutant swarms of RNA viruses. The latter selectively replicate and *amplify* certain subsets of their (nonmaster sequence) mutant spectrum in a completely unpredictable manner, thereby creating significant levels of many nonmaster, nonconsensus sequence proteins. During an influenza A virus, or measles virus or rhinovirus outbreak, for example, no two infected humans will encounter the same array of foreign virus-encoded proteins. Therefore, the acute effects and subtle chronic effects of infections will differ not only because we all vary genetically, physiologically and immunologically, but also because we all experience a different array of quasispecies challenges. These facts are easily overlooked by clinicians and scientists because disease syndromes are often grossly similar for each type of virus, and because it would appear to make no difference in a practical sense. However, for the person who develops Guillain–Barré syndrome following a common cold, or for the individual who remains healthy despite many years of HIV-1 infection, for example, it may make all the difference in the world.

The extent to which chronic degenerative diseases and autoimmune diseases of man are triggered by exogenous pathogens is still unknown. It is clear that virus proteins can exhibit molecular mimicry (FUJINAMI and OLDSTONE 1989) and can induce cell-mediated autoimmunity (TER MEULEN 1989; KYUWA et al. 1991). In the case of RNA virus infections, there is no reason to expect that the ability to trigger degenerative and autoimmune diseases of man will be confined solely to those proteins or protein domains encoded by master sequence or consensus sequence genomes. The former may often represent a small percentage of total virus encoded proteins and the latter often be vanishingly small. The consensus sequence is an average of the most abundant nucleotide present at each position of all genomes in the quasispecies swarm and it need not necessarily even exist in any one genome present.

Similar arguments apply to viral cell tropisms, and to cell and tissue pathology in infected humans. It can be extremely difficult or impossible to ascribe subtle cell tropism differences or cellular pathology to the consensus sequence or to any "clonal" sequences recovered from a patient's cells and tissues. It has recently been observed that even the relative fitness of RNA virus clones can change rapidly, and that even clonal populations adapt rapidly to new host cell types (HOLLAND et al. 1991; MARTINEZ et al. 1991). It is important (if disturbing) to remember that clonal sequences of viruses recovered from patients can be distorted by the methods employed for recovery and amplification, whether these are growth of virus plaques, reverse transcription followed by polymerase chain reaction (PCR), or whatever. Thus RNA virology and a certain level of uncertainty go hand in hand. Finally, the recent identification of superantigens encoded by proviruses of retroviruses (MARRACK et al. 1991; DYSON et al. 1991; FRANKEL et al. 1991; WOODLAND et al. 1991) extends these concepts to T cell stimulation or deletion and immunosuppression. Any replicating RNA virus, whether retrovirus or ribovirus, might sometimes produce protein sequences with superantigen properties. When these are encoded by selected, stable, integrated proviruses they can be clearly identified (as has been done) but when such superantigens are hidden within quasispecies swarms, their presence, and their role in disease, may generally go undetected.

7 What Can Be Predicted Regarding the Future Evolution of RNA Viruses?

Very little can be predicted, except that rapid virus evolution will continue. Some "new" human RNA virus diseases will inevitably emerge, and some older diseases will disappear or become less significant. Although some RNA viruses can achieve a rather stable equilibrium in certain environments, most will generally evolve at rates exceeding by a millionfold Those of their eukaryotic hosts. Because mutation is probabilistic and produces immense and largely indeterminate quasispecies RNA virus population, the directions of RNA genome evolution must remain unpredictable.

Although new RNA virus diseases of humans will continue to emerge at indeterminate intervals, the viruses themselves will not really be new, but rather mutated and rearranged to allow infection of new hosts, or to cause new disease patterns. It is important to remember that every quasispecies genome swarm in an infected individual is unique and "new" in the sense that no identical population of RNA genomes has ever existed before and none such will ever exist again. Because a large fraction of sites on RNA virus genomes can eventually be substituted and because genomes can also be expanded, contracted, recombined and rearranged, the number of potential genome permutations which must be tried to find all viable alternatives is essentially infinite in the space time of our universe. As human populations continue to grow exponentially, the number of ecological niches for human RNA virus evolution grows apace and "new" human virus outbreaks will likely increase apace. Most "new" human viruses will be unremarkable—that is they will generally resemble "old" ones. Inevitably, some will be quite remarkable, and quite undesirable. When discussing RNA virus evolution, to call an outbreak (such as AIDS) "remarkable" is merely to state that it is of lower probability than an "unremarkable" outbreak.

8 Summary

RNA virus mutation frequencies generally approach maximum tolerable levels, and create complex indeterminate quasispecies populations in infected hosts. This usually favors extreme rates of evolution, although periods of relative stasis or equilibrium, punctuated by rapid change may also occur (as for other life forms). Because complex quasispecies populations of RNA viruses arise probabilistically and differentially in every host, their compositions and exact roles in disease pathogenesis are indeterminate and their directions of evolution, and the nature and timing of "new" virus outbreaks are unpredictable.

References

Ahmed R, Salmi A, Butler LD, Chiller JM, Oldstone MBA (1984) Selection of genetic variants of LCMV in spleens of persistently infected mice: role in suppression of cytotoxic T lymphocyte response and viral persistence. J Exp Med 160: 521–540

Balfe P, Simmonds P, Ludlam CA, Bishop JO, Leigh Brown AJ (1990) Concurrent evolution of human immunodeficiency virus type 1 in patients infected from the same source: rate of sequence change and low frequency of inactivating mutations. J Virol 64: 6221–6233

Bass BL, Weintraub H, Cattaneo R, Billeter MA (1989) Biased hypermutation of viral genomes could be due to unwinding/modification of double stranded RNA. Cell 56: 331

Batschelet E, Domingo E, Weissman C (1976) The proportion of revertant and mutant phage in a growing population as a function of mutation and growth rate. Gene 1: 27–32

Bebenek K, Kunkel TA (1990) Frameshift errors initiated by nucleotide misincorporation. Proc Natl Acad Sci USA 87: 4946–4950

Bilsel PA, Nichol ST (1990) Polymerase errors accumulating during natural evolution of the glycoprotein gene of vesicular stomatitis virus Indiana serotype isolates. J Virol 64: 4873–4883

Blank A, Gallant JA, Burgess RR, Loeb LA (1986) A RNA polymerase mutant with reduced accuracy of chain elongation. Biochemistry 25: 5920–5928

Boege U, Kobasa D, Onodera S, Parks GD, Palmenberg AC, Scraba DG (1991) Characterization of mengo virus neutralization epitopes. Virology 181: 1–13

Burns DPW, Desrosiers RC (1991) Selection of genetic variants of simian immunodeficiency virus in persistently infected rhesus monkeys. J Virol 65: 1843–1854

Cattaneo R, Schmid A, Eschle D, Baczko K, ter Meulen V, Billeter MA (1988) Biased hypermutation and other genetic changes in defective measles viruses in human brain infections. Cell 55: 255–265

Chao L (1990) Fitness of RNA virus decreased by Muller's ratchet. Nature 348: 454–455

Coffin JM (1986) Genetic variation in AIDS viruses. Cell 46: 1–4

Coffin JM (1990) Genetic variation in retroviruses. In: Kurstak E, Marusyk RG, Murphy FA, van Regenmortel MHV (eds) Applied virology research, vol 2. Plenum, New York, pp 11–33

Cullis PM, Wolfenden R (1981) Affinities of nucleic acid bases for solvent water. Biochemistry 20: 3024–3028

Daniels M (1972) Tautomerism of uracil and thymine in aqueous solution; spectroscopic evidence. Proc Natl Acad Sci USA 69: 2488–2491

De La Torre JC, Wimmer E, Holland JJ (1990) Very high frequency of reversion to guanidine resistance in clonal pools of guanidine-dependent type I poliovirus. J Virol 64: 664–671

Domingo E (1989) RNA virus evolution and the control of viral disease. Prog Drug Res 33: 93–133

Domingo E, Holland JJ (1988) High error rates, population equilibrium and evolution of RNA replication systems. In: Domingo E, Holland JJ, Ahlquist P (eds) RNA genetics, vol 3. CRC, Boca Raton, pp 3–36

Domingo E, Martinez-Salas E, Sobrino F, De la Torre JC, Portela A, Ortin J, Lopéz-Galindez C, Péres-Brena P, Villanueva N, Nájera R, VandePol S, Steinhauer D, DePolo N, Holland JJ (1985) The quasispecies (extremely heterogeneous) nature of viral RNA genome populations: biological relevance—a review. Gene 40: 1–8

Dougherty JP, Temin HM (1988) Determination of the rate of base-pair substitution and insertion mutations in retrovirus replication. J Virol 62: 2817–2822

Drake JW (1969) Comparative rates of spontaneous mutation. Nature 221: 1132

Drake JW, Allen EF, Forsberg SA, Preparata RM, Greening EO (1969) Spontaneous mutation. Nature 221: 1128–1132

Dreyfus M, Bensaude O, Dodin G, Dubois JE (1975) Tautomerism in cytosine and 3-methylcytosine. A thermodynamic and kinetic study. J Am Chem Soc 98: 6338–6349

Durbin RK, Stollar V (1986) Sequence analysis of the E1 gene of a hyperglycosylated, host restricted mutant of Sindbis virus and estimation of mutation rate from frequency of revertants. Virology 154: 135–143

Dyson PJ, Knight AM, Fairchild S, Simpson E, Tomonari K (1991) Genes encoding ligands for deletion of Vβ11 T cells cosegregate with mammary tumour virus genomes. Nature 349: 531–532

Echols H, Lu C, Burgers PMJ (1983) Mutator strains of *Escherichia coli, mutD* and *dnaQ*, with defective xonucleolytic editing by DNA polymerase III holoenzyme. Proc Natl Acad Sci USA 80: 2189–2192

Edelman P, Gallant J (1977) Mistranslation in *E coli*. Cell 10: 131–137

Eggers HJ, Tamm I (1965) Coxsackie A9 virus: mutation from drug dependence to drug resistance. Science 148: 97–98

Eigen M, Biebricher CK (1988) Sequence space and quasispecies distribution. In: Domingo E, Holland JJ, Ahlquist P (eds) RNA genetics, vol 3. CRC, Boca Raton, pp 211–245

Eigen M, Schuster P (1979) The hypercycle. A principle of natural self-organization. Springer, Berlin Heidelberg New York

Eigen M, Gardiner W, Schuster P, Winkler-Oswatitsch R (1981) The origin of genetic information. Sci Am 244: 88–188

Ellis N, Gallant J (1982) An estimate of the global error frequency in translation. Mol Gen Genet 188: 169–172

Enders J, Katz SL, Milovanovic MJ, Holloway A (1960) Studies on an attenuated measles virus vaccine. I. Development and preparation of vaccine: techniques for assay of effects of vaccination. N Engl J Med 263: 153–159

Fersht AR, Knill-Jones JW, Tsui W-C (1982) Kinetic basis of spontaneous mutation. J Mol Biol 156: 37–51

Fersht AR, Shi J-P, Tsui W-C (1983) Kinetics of base misinsertion by DNA polymerase I of *Escherichia coli*. J Mol Biol 165: 655–667

Fields BN, Joklik WK (1969) Isolation and preliminary characterization of temperature sensitive mutants of retrovirus. Virology 37: 335–342

Frankel WN, Rudy C, Coffin JM, Huber BT (1991) Linkage of *Mls* genes to endogenous mammary tumour viruses of inbred mice. Nature 349: 526–528

Fujinami RS, Oldstone MBA (1989) Molecular mimicry as a mechanism for virus-induced autoimmunity. Immunol Res 8: 3–15

Gebauer F, De La Torre JC, Gomes I, Mateu MG, Barahoma H, Tiraboschi B, Bergmann I, Augé De Mello P, Domingo E (1988) Rapid selection of genetic and antigenic variants of foot- and-mouth disease virus during persistence in cattle. J Virol 62: 2041–2049

Gorman OT, Bean WJ, Kawaoka Y, Webster RG (1990) Evolution of the nucleoprotein gene of influenza A virus. J Virol 64: 1487–1497
Gould SJ, Eldridge N (1977) Punctuated equilibria: the tempo and mode of evolution reconsidered. Paleontology 3: 115–151
Granoff A (1961) Induction of Newcastle disease virus mutants with nitrous acid. Virology 13: 402–408
Granoff A (1964) Nature of the Newcastle disease virus population. In: Hanson RP (ed) Newcastle disease virus, an evolving pathogen. University of Wisconsin Press, Madison, pp 107–108
Groenink M, Fouchier RAM, de Goede REY, de Wolf F, Gruters RA, Cuypers HTM, Huisman HG, Tersmette M (1991) Phenotypic heterogeneity in a panel of infectious molecular human immunodeficiency virus type 1 clones derived from a single individual. J Virol 65: 1968–1975
Hahn YS, Strauss EG, Strauss JH (1989a) Mapping of RNA^- temperature sensitive mutants of sindbis virus: assignment of complementation groups A, B, and G to nonstructural proteins. J Virol 63: 3142–3150
Hahn CS, Rice CM, Strauss EG, Lenches EM, Strauss JH (1989b) Sindbis virus ts103 has a mutation in glycoprotein E2 that leads to defective assembly of virions. J Virol 63: 3459–3465
Hall JD, Coen DM, Fisher BL, Weisslitz M, Randall S, Almy RE, Gelep TP, Schaffer PA (1984) Generation of genetic diversity in herpes simplex virus: an antimutator phenotype maps to the DNA polymerase locus. Virology 132: 26–37
Heinz BA, Rueckert RR, Shepard DA, Dutko FJ, McKinlay MA, Fancher M, Rossmann MG, Badger J, Smith TJ (1989) Genetic and molecular analyses of spontaneous mutants of human rhinovirus 14 that are resistant to an antiviral compounds. J Virol 63: 2476–2485
Holland JJ, Spindler K, Horodyski F, Grabau E, Nichol S, VandePol S (1982) Rapid evolution of RNA genomes. Science 215: 1577–1585
Holland JJ, De La Torre JC, Steinhauer DA, Clarke D, Duarte E, Domingo E (1989) Virus mutation frequencies can be greatly underestimated by monoclonal antibody neutralization of virions. J Virol 63: 5030–5036
Holland JJ, Domingo E, De La Torre JC, Steinhauer DA (1990) Mutation frequencies at defined single condon sites in vesicular stomatitis virus can be increased only slightly by chemical mutagenesis. J Virol 64: 3960–3962
Holland JJ, De La Torre JC, Clarke DK, Duarte E (1991) Quantitation of relative fitness and great adaptability of clonal populations of RNA viruses. J Virol (in press)
Hopfield JJ (1974) Kinetic proofreading: a new mechanism for reducing errors in biosynthetic processes requiring high specificity. Proc Natl Acad Sci USA 71: 4135–4139
Imazeki F, Omata M, Ohto M (1990) Heterogeneity and evolution rates of delta virus RNA sequences. J Virol 64: 5594–5599
Ina Y, Gojobori T (1990) Molecular evolution of human T-cell leukemia virus. J Mol Evol 31: 493–499
Ishihama A, Mizumoto K, Kawakami K, Kato A, Honda A (1986) Proofreading function associated with the RNA-dependent RNA polymerase from influenza virus. J Biol Chem 261: 10417–10421
Jakubowski H (1990) Proofreading in vivo: editing of homocysteine by methionyl-tRNA synthetase in *Escherichia coli.* Proc Natl Acad Sci USA 87: 4504–4508
Kassavetis GA, Zentner PG, Geiduschek EP (1986) Transcription at bacteriophage T4 variant late promoters: an application of a newly devised promoter-mapping method. J Biol Chem 261: 14256–14265
Kenner GW, Reese CB, Sir Todd AR (1955) The acylation of 3-methylcytosine. J Chem Soc 50C: 855–859
Kwe OM, Nottay BK, Rico-Hess R, Pollansch MA (1990) Molecular epidemiology of wild poliovirus transmission. In: Kurstak E (ed) Applied virology research, vol 2. Plenum, New York, pp 199–220
Kinnunen L, Huovilainen A, Pöyry T, Hovi T (1990) Rapid molecular evolution of wild type 3 poliovirus during infection in individual hosts. J Gen Virol 71: 317–324
Kornberg A (1974) DNA synthesis. Freeman, San Francisco, pp 67–121
Kunkel LO (1947) Variation in phytopathogenic viruses. Annu Rev Microbiol 1: 85–100
Kunkel TA (1986) Frameshift mutagenesis by eucaryotic DNA polymerases in vitro. J Biol Chem 261: 13581–13587
Kunkel TA, Alexander PS (1986) The base substitution fidelity of eucaryotic DNA polymerases. J Biol Chem 261: 160–166
Kunkel TA, Meyer RR, Loeb LA (1979) Single-strand binding protein enhances fidelity of DNA synthesis in vitro. Proc Natl Acad Sci USA 76: 6331–6335
Kurath G, Palukaitis P (1990) Serial passage of infectious transcripts of a cucumber mosaic virus satellite RNA clone results in sequence heterogeneity. Virology 176: 8–15

Kwiatkowski JS, Pullman B (1975) Tautomerism and electronic structure of biological pyrimidines. Adv Heterocycl Chem 18: 199–335
Kyuwa S, Yamaguchi K, Toyoda Y, Fujiwara K (1991) Induction of self-reactive T cells after murine coronavirus infection. J Virol 65: 1789–1795
Lahue RS, Au KG, Modrich P (1989) DNA mismatch correction in a defined system. Science 245: 160–164
Lamb RA, Dreyfuss G (1989) RNA structure. Unwinding with a vengeance [news]. Nature 337: 19–20
Lande R (1985) Expected time for random genetic drift of a population between stable phenotypic states. Proc Natl Acad Sci USA 82: 7641–7645
Loeb LA, Kunkel TA (1982) Fidelity of DNA synthesis. Annu Rev Biochem 52: 429–457
Lotfield RB, Vanderjagt D (1972) The frequency of errors in protein biosynthesis. Biochem J 128: 1353–1356
Lohrmann R, Orgel LE (1980) Efficient catalysis of polycytidylic acid-directed oligoguanylate formation by Pb^{2+}. J Mol Biol 142: 555–567
Marrack P, Kushnir E, Kappler J (1991) A maternally inherited superantigen encoded by a mammary tumour virus. Nature 349: 524–526
Martinez MA, Carillo C, Gonzalez-Candelaz F, Moya A, Domingo E, Sobrino F (1991) Fitness alteration of foot- and-mouth disease virus mutants; measurement of adaptability of viral quasispecies. J Virol 65: 3954–3957
Moses RE, Summers WC (eds) (1988) DNA replication and mutagenesis. American Society for Microbiology, Washington, p 515
Myerhans A, Cheynier R, Albert J, Seth M, Kwok S, Sninsky J, Morfeldt-Manson L, Åsjö B, Wain-Hobson S (1989) Temporal fluctuations in HIV quasispecies in vivo are not reflected by sequential HIV isolations. Cell 58: 901–910
Newman CM, Cohen JE, Kipnis C (1985) New-darwinian evolution implies punctuated equilibria. Nature 315: 400–401
O'Hara PJ, Nichol ST, Horodyski FM, Holland JJ (1984) Vesicular stomatitis virus defective interfering particles can contain extensive genomic sequence rearrangements and base substitutions. Cell 36: 915–924
Pathak VK, Temin HM (1990) Broad spectrum of in vivo forward mutations, hypermutations, and mutational hotspots in a retroviral shuttle vector after a single replication cycle: substitutions, frameshifts, and hypermutations. Proc Natl Acad Sci USA 87: 6019–6023
Petruska J, Sowers LC, Goodman MF (1986) Comparison of nucleotide interactions in water, proteins, and vacuum: model for DNA polymerase fidelity. Proc Natl Acad Sci USA 83: 1559–1562
Petruska J, Goodman MF, Boosalis MS, Sowers LC, Cheong C, Tinoco I Jr (1988) Comparison between DNA melting thermodynamics and DNA polymerase fidelity. Proc Natl Acad Sci USA 85: 6252–6256
Piccirilli JA, Krauch T, Moroney SE, Benner SA (1990) Enzymatic incorporation of a new base pair into DNA and RNA extends the genetic alphabet. Nature 343: 33–37
Preston BD, Zakour RA, Singer B, Loeb LA (1988) Fidelity of base selection by DNA polymerases. Site-specific incorporation of base analogs. In: Moses RE, Summers WC (eds) DNA replication and mutagenesis. American Society for Microbiology, Washington, pp 196–207
Pringle CR (1970) Genetic characteristics of conditional lethal mutants of vesicular stomatitis virus induced by 5-fluorouracil, 5-azacytidine, and ethyl methanesulfonate. J Virol 5: 559–567
Pringle CR, Devine V, Wilkie M, Preston CM, Dohn A, McGeoch DJ (1981)Enhanced mutability associated with a temperature-sensitive mutant of vesicular stomatitis virus. J Virol 39: 377–389
Radman M, Wagner R (1986) Mismatch repair in *Escherichia coli*. Annu Rev Genet 20: 523–538
Rodríguez-Cerezo E, Moya A, García-Arenal F (1989) Variability and evolution of the plant RNA virus pepper mild mottle virus. J Virol 63: 2198–2203
Rosenberger RF, Hilton J (1983) The frequency of transcriptional and translational errors at nonsense codons in the *lacZ* gene of *Escherichia coli*. Mol Gen Genet 191: 207–212
Sabin AB, Boulger LR (1973) History of Sabin attenuated poliovirus oral live vaccine strains. J Biol Stand 1: 115–118
Sedivy JM, Capone JP, Raj Bhandary UL, Sharp PA (1987) An inducible mammalian amber suppressor: propagation of a poliovirus mutant. Cell 50: 379–389
Simpson L (1990) RNA editing—a novel genetic phenomenon? Science 250: 512–513
Skehel JJ, Wiley DC (1988) Antigenic variation in influenza virus hemagglutinin. In: Domingo E, Holland JJ, Ahlquist P (eds) RNA genetics, vol 3. CRC, Boca Raton, pp 139–146
Smith BD, Inglis SC (1987) The mutation rate and variability of eukaryotic viruses: an analytical review. J Gen Virol 68: 2729–2740

Smith FI, Palese P (1988) Infl·ienza virus: high rates of mutation and evolution. In: Domingo E, Holland JJ, Ahlquist P (eds) RNA genetics, vol 3. CRC, Boca Raton, pp 123–135
Stec DS, Waddell A, Schmaljohn CS, Cole GA, Schmaljohn AL (1986) Antibody-selected variation and reversion in Sindbis virus neutralization epitopes. J Virol 57: 715–720
Steinhauer DA, Holland JJ (1987) Rapid evolution of RNA viruses. Annu Rev Microbiol 41: 409–433
Steinhauer DA, de la Torre JC, Holland JJ (1989a) High nucleotide substitution error frequencies in clonal pools of vesicular stomatitis virus. J Virol 63: 2063–2071
Steinhauer DA, de la Torre JC, Meier E, Holland JJ (1989b) Extreme heterogeneity in populations of vesicular stomatitis virus. J Virol 63: 2072–2080
Strauss JH, Strauss EG (1988) Evolution of RNA viruses. Annu Rev Microbiol 42: 657–683
Temin HM (1989) Is HIV unique or merely different? AIDS 2: 1–9
Ter Meulen V (1989) Virus-induced, cell mediated immunity. In: Notkins AL, Oldstone MBA (eds) Concepts in viral pathogenesis, vol 3. Springer, Berlin Heidelberg, New York, pp 297–310
Theiler M, Smith HH (1937) Use of yellow fever virus modified by in vitro cultivation for human immunization. J Exp Med 65: 787–800
Theiler M, Smith HH (1939) The effect of prolonged cultivation in vitro upon the pathogenicity of yellow fever virus. J Exp Med 65: 767–787
Topal MD, Fresco JR (1976) Complementary base pairing and the origin of substituion mutations. Nature 263: 285–289
Vartanian J-P, Meyerhans A, Åsjö B, Wain-Hobson S (1991) Selection, recombination, and G→A hypermutation of human immunodeficiency virus type 1 genomes. J Virol 65: 1779–1788
Villaverde A, Martinez MA, Sobrino F, Dopazo J, Moya A, Domingo E (1991) Fixation of mutations at the VP1 gene of foot- and-mouth disease virus. Can quasispecies define a transient molecular clock? Gene (in press)
Ward CD, Stokes MAM, Flanegan JB (1988) Direct measurement of the poliovirus RNA polymerase error frequency in vitro. J Virol 62: 558–562
Watson JD, Crick FHC (1953) The structure of DNA. Cold Spring Harbour Symp Quant Biol 48: 123–133
Wolfenden RV (1969) Tauteromeric equilibria in inosine and adenosine. J Mol Biol 40: 307–310
Woodland DL, Happ MP, Gollob KJ, Palmer E (1991) An endogenous retrovirus mediating deletion of $\alpha\beta$ T cells? Nature 349: 529–530
Wright S (1977) Experimental results and evolutionary deductions. In: Wright S (ed) Evolution and the genetics of populations, vol 3. Chicago, Chicago, pp 443–473
Wright S (1982) Character change, speciation, and the higher taxa. Evolution 36: 427–443
Yamane T, Hopfield JJ (1977) Experimental evidence for kinetic proofreading in the aminoacylation of tRNA by synthetase. Proc Natl Acad Sci USA 74: 2246–2250
Zimmern D (1988) Evolution of RNA viruses. In: Domingo E, Holland JJ, Ahlquist P (eds) RNA genetics, vol 3. CRC, Boca Raton, pp 211–240

Genetic Recombination in RNA Viruses

M. M. C. Lai

1 Introduction

Recombination in RNA viruses involves the exchange of genetic information between two nonsegmented RNA genomes, as distinct from the reassortment of RNA seen in viruses containing segmented genomes. The mechanism of RNA recombination appears to be similar to the generation of defective interfering (DI) RNA, since they both involve polymerase jumping during RNA synthesis. However, unlike the production of DI RNA, which is a relatively common phenomenon among RNA viruses, RNA recombination has so far only been demonstrated in a few RNA viruses. Homologous RNA recombination, which is defined

Howard Hughes Medical Institute and Department of Microbiology, University of Southern California School of Medicine, Los Angeles, CA 90033, USA

as the exchange of two comparable RNA regions at precise locations, was first detected in poliovirus by HIRST (1962) and LEDINKO (1963) in the early 1960s. Soon after, another member of the picornavirus family, foot-and-mouth disease virus (FMDV), an aphthovirus, also was shown to undergo recombination (PRINGLE 1965). Subsequently, a series of temperature-sensitive (ts) mutants was used to determine recombination frequencies and do obtain a linear genetic recombination map (COOPER 1968, 1977). The definitive evidence for the occurrence of RNA recombination eventually came from the biochemical analysis of protein and RNA structure of the recombinant viruses (KING et al. 1982). The second virus family to be shown to undergo RNA recombination is coronavirus (LAI et al. 1985). And more recently, several plant viruses, including brome mosaic virus and cowpea chlorotic mottle virus, also have been shown to undergo RNA recombination in rare situations (BUJARSKI and KAESBERG 1986; ALLISON et al. 1990). Thus, RNA recombination is being recognized increasingly as a general biological phenomenon among RNA viruses and probably plays an important role in viral biology and virus evolution. This chapter will deal mainly with homologous RNA recombination and will not discuss DI RNA, which is one form of nonhomologous RNA recombination.

2 RNA Recombination in Tissue Culture

2.1 Picornavirus Recombination

In poliovirus and FMDV infections, RNA recombination readily occurs between closely related strains (intratypic recombination). With more distantly related virus strains (intertypic recombination), the recombination frequency drops proportionately. A linear genetic map has been obtained, in which recombination frequencies are additive (COOPER 1968, 1977; LAKE et al. 1975). Recombination appears to occur primarily in the 3′-half of the genome, within which recombination has been demonstrated at many different sites (KING et al. 1985). However, for reasons that are not clear, recombination events have not been demonstrated in the capsid protein genes of FMDV (KING et al. 1985; KING 1988). Recombination events involve faithful and accurate crossovers, without insertions, deletions, or mismatches. Occasionally, multiple crossover events can be detected in a recombinant virus during a single growth cycle (KING et al. 1985), suggesting that the recombination frequency is quite high.

2.2 Coronavirus Recombination

Several selection markers have been used in the isolation of coronavirus recombinants, including temperature-sensitive phenotypes, monoclonal antibody neutralization-resistance phenotypes and differences in cytopathicity. Similar to picornaviruses, RNA recombination can occur almost anywhere on the genome. Furthermore, many recombinants contain multiple crossover events, some of which occur at sites outside the selection markers, and are therefore not enriched by selection. These findings suggest an extremely high frequency of RNA recombination in coronaviruses. In certain situations, recombinant viruses can become the predominant population among the viruses. For example, in a recombination study between a *ts A59* strain and a wild-type JHM strain of mouse hepatitis virus (MHV), the recombinant viruses accounted for more than 95% of the virus progeny, after only two passages in tissue culture (MAKINO et al. 1986). Thus, RNA recombination may provide a powerful evolutionary tool for coronaviruses. A linear genetic map based on recombination frequencies also has been obtained for murine coronaviruses, using a panel of ts mutants (BARIC et al. 1990). Similar to picornaviruses, the recombination frequencies are additive.

3 Recombination In Vivo

3.1 Recombination in Experimental Animals, Plants and Humans

Viral RNA recombination has been demonstrated experimentally in animals and plants, and in natural viral infections of humans. RNA recombination in animals is best illustrated in the coronavirus system. When MHV was inoculated intracerebrally into mice, progeny virus harvested from the brain contained a large percentage of recombinants (KECK et al. 1988a). The types of recombinants obtained in vivo are similar to those obtained from mixed infections in tissue culture. Although similar studies have not been performed with picornaviruses, recombinants have been detected between vaccine strains in poliovirus vaccinees (KEW and NOTTAY 1984; MINOR et al. 1986). The recombinants have been isolated from both vaccine-associated poliomyelitis patients and healthy vaccinees. Certain types of recombinants, particularly those between type 3 and type 2 poliovirus vaccine strains, are frequently isolated. One study suggests that this recombinant could become the predominant virus population in vaccinees (MINOR et al. 1986).

Several plant viruses also have been shown to undergo RNA recombination in plants or protoplasts. In general, these studies did not involve homologous recombination between two wild-type virus strains, but rather, between a defective viral RNA and a helper wild-type virus RNA. Brome mosaic virus, cowpea chlorotic mottle virus, and turnip crinkle virus underwent this type of recombination when a defective RNA was introduced to plants together with the helper viruses. RNA recombination restored the replicating ability of the defective RNA (BUJARSKI and KAESBERG 1986; ALLISON et al. 1990; RAO and HALL

1990; CASCONE et al. 1990). The ability of bromovirus RNAs to undergo homologous recombination is variable and probably depends on the conditions of infection. Recently nonhomologous recombination involving these RNAs also has been reported (RAO and HALL 1990).

3.2 RNA Recombination in Natural Viral Evolution

The sequence analysis of RNA viruses has suggested that, in some cases, these RNA viruses might have been derived by RNA recombination with other viruses during natural viral infections. For example, western equine encephalitis virus may be a recombinant derived from Sindbis virus and eastern equine encephalitis virus as the result of a crossover event (HAHN et al. 1988). Also, based on the degree of divergence of different parts of the viral genome, it has been argued that some of the natural isolates of the avian coronavirus, infectious bronchitis virus (IBV), may have undergone recombination with each other, resulting in the exchange of portions of their genomes (KUSTERS et al. 1989). An even more dramatic example of recombination may have occurred in MHV. This virus contains a hemagglutinin-esterase (HE) gene, which closely resembles the analogous gene of influenza C virus (LUYTJES et al. 1988). This gene potential could have been acquired by MHV recombination with influenza C virus. It is not clear whether the local sequence homology between MHV and influenza C virus is sufficient to allow homologous recombination, nor is there experimental proof that these two viruses have indeed undergone recombination; however, sequence information provides a strong argument for the occurrence of RNA recombination in nature. Several plant viruses, including cowpea chlorotic mottle virus (ALLISON et al. 1989) and tobacco rattle virus (ANGENENT et al. 1990), also have sequence arrangements which suggest that recombination events have occurred during the evolution of these viruses. Furthermore, several positive-strand RNA animal and plant viruses, which have dissimilar genomic organizations, possess conserved functional domains in their genomes (HASELOFF et al. 1984). RNA recombination involving these functional modules best explains the mechanism of evolution of these viruses.

4 Recombination Frequency

Although RNA recombination generally is a rare event among RNA viruses, picornaviruses and coronaviruses show a surprisingly high frequency of recombination. Genetic mapping studies have suggested that the recombination frequency is approximately 2.2% for the entire poliovirus RNA genome (COOPER 1968, 1977; LAKE et al. 1975). Using a series of temperature-sensitive mutants of FMDV, MCCAHON et al. (1977) found a recombination frequency of 0.9% for a region of approximately 3 kb. Considering the possibility that recombination probably occurs in both directions, and occurs not only between different parents, but also between different molecules of the same virus, the authors argued that the recombination frequency for the entire picornavirus RNA could be extrapolated to between 10% and 20% (KING 1988). KIRKEGAARD and BALTIMORE (1986) reported a recombination frequency of 0.1% between two selection markers separated by only 190 nucleotides. Based on a similar argument, it was suggested that the recombination frequency for the entire poliovirus genome would be roughly 15% (KING 1988). This frequency is extraordinarily high, but has never been experimentally shown. The recombination frequency estimates should be viewed with caution, since different regions of the RNA recombine with different efficiencies and the selection methods used often favor certain types of recombinants. An example of this bias is the observation that the cross over sites in picornavirus RNA are clustered in the 3′-half of the genome (MCCAHON et al. 1977). Rarely has recombination been detected in the 5′-half of the genome. Recombination frequency was significantly lower when more distantly related picornaviruses was studied.

The recombination frequency of coronavirus has been measured directly and proved to be even higher than the figure estimated for picornaviruses. That recombinants could be detected even in the absence of any selection pressure was an indication of the extraordinarily high recombination frequency of coronaviruses (MAKINO et al. 1986). In a study in which recombinants were detected randomly without selection pressure, recombinants accounted for 10% of the progeny released from a mixed infection (MAKINO et al. 1986). Also, in several recombination studies using two selection markers, many recombinants not only had the expected crossover sites between the two selection markers, but also had crossover sites outside the selection markers (MAKINO et al. 1981; KECK et al. 1988b). The presence of the latter type of crossover sites strongly suggests that recombination occurred at such a high frequency that no selection pressure was needed for the detection of crossovers. Furthermore, many recombinants demonstrate multiple crossovers in the viral genome after only a single growth cycle (KECK et al. 1987, 1988b). Each of these findings suggests that coronavirus recombination can be detected readily. The recombination frequency for the entire coronavirus genome (31 kb) has been determined from a series of recombination studies using a large panel of temperature-sensitive mutants. These studies estimated the recombination frequency of MHV to be nearly 25% (BARIC et al. 1990). Since the recombinant viruses analyzed covered more than two-thirds of the genome, the estimated recombination frequency should be very close to the actual recombination frequency of coronavirus. These recombination frequencies are translated into roughly 1% recombination per 1300 nucleotides for coronavirus RNA and 1700 nucleotides for poliovirus RNA (BARIC et al. 1990). These frequencies compare favorably with the figures (1% per 200 bp for T4 phage, and per 1750 bp for *Escherichia coli*) for DNA recombination (HAYES 1968). Thus, the studies with picornavirus and coronavirus indicated a recombination frequency much higher than expected. No figure is available for the recombination frequency of plant RNA viruses; however, it appears to be lower.

5 Nonhomologous Recombination Between Viral RNA and Unrelated Viral or Cellular RNAs

Besides homologous recombination, some RNA viruses can incorporate either unrelated viral genes or cellular genes into the viral genome, possibly by a nonhomologous recombination mechanism. A characteristic of this type of recombination is that the cellular RNAs or individual viral RNAs involved either do not replicate by themselves or replicate by a mechanism different from that of the RNA virus in question. Therefore, the recombination cannot be explained simply by polymerase jumping from one viral RNA to a different RNA during the course of RNA synthesis. There are several examples of this kind of recombination:

1. Coronavirus MHV contains a HE gene, which was probably derived from influenza C virus by recombination (LUYTJES et al. 1988). These two viruses are unrelated, and the mechanisms of their RNA synthesis are quite different.
2. The pestivirus bovine viral diarrhea virus occasionally incorporates a cellular gene into its viral genome. One of the cellular genes frequently incorporated is the ubiquitin gene (MEYERS et al. 1991). The incorporation of cellular genes, particularly ubiquitin, appears to correlate well with the cytopathogenic potential of the virus. The acquisition of this cellular gene by the virus via a nonhomologous recombination mechanism seems most likely.
3. A mechanism of nonhomologous recombination could also account for the gene rearrangements observed in some RNA viruses. For instance, between the coronaviruses MHV and IBV, the gene order for the matrix protein and a nonstructural protein, i.e., genes 5 and 6 of MHV, respectively, is reversed (LAI 1990). This reversion of gene order could be explained by the recombination of viral RNA with a postulated RNA cassette containing an individual viral gene. Since each coronavirus gene is flanked by similar intergenic sequences (LAI 1990), each viral gene could be considered a gene cassette which can recombine and rearrange within the viral genome. RNA recombination also could explain the conservation of certain functional elements among the RNA genomes of many animal and plant viruses, which have dissimilar genomic organization (HASELOFF et al. 1984).

6 The Mechanism of RNA Recombination

6.1 The Copy-Choice Mechanism

There are two possible mechanisms of RNA recombination. In one case, the recombination would occur on the double-stranded RNA replicative intermediates, possibly by a breakage and reunion mechanism similar to that described for DNA recombination. The second case would be a copy-choice mechanism involving polymerase jumping from one template to a different template during RNA replication. Thus, RNA recombination would be concomitant with RNA replication in this model. The majority of evidence currently available favors the latter mechanism. The most definitive evidence came from studies by KIRKEGAARD and BALTIMORE (1986), who examined poliovirus RNA recombination under conditions in which the replication of one parental virus was selectively blocked before superinfecting with a second virus. The results showed that recombination was dependent on RNA replication, and thus involved polymerase jumping from one template to another during RNA synthesis. The detailed mechanism of copy-choice recombination is still not known. Presumably, RNA synthesis proceeds by a discontinuous process, pausing at various sites of strong secondary structure. This transcriptional pausing would allow RNA polymerase, together with the incomplete RNA products, to be dissociated from the original RNA template and subsequently bind to the same or a different RNA template and continue transcription. When this polymerase complex binds to a different template, the transcriptional product would be a recombinant RNA. This RNA recombination model is consistent with the following observations:

1. Transcriptional pausing has been demonstrated in many experimental systems, including RNA-dependent RNA synthesis in RNA phages and DNA-dependent RNA transcription in bacteria (KASSAVETIS and CHAMBERLIN 1981; MILLS et al. 1978). It appears that both DNA-dependent and RNA-dependent RNA synthesis is inherently discontinuous. Conceivably, some viral RNA-dependent RNA polymerases may be nonprocessive, thus allowing for pausing RNA products to be dissociated from templates.
2. In coronavirus MHV-infected cells, pausing RNA transcripts of various sizes, all of which initiated from the 5′-end of the genome, have been detected (BARIC et al. 1987). The sizes of these RNA intermediates suggest that they result from polymerase pausing at sites of strong secondary structure. In addition, some of these RNA species were separated from the template RNA (BARIC et al. 1987), and potentially could be the precursor RNAs for recombination. Direct biochemical evidence that these RNA intermediates actually participate in the reinitiation of RNA synthesis and RNA recombination has not yet been obtained.

6.2 Does RNA Recombination Occur During Negative- or Positive-Strand RNA Synthesis?

The study by KIRKEGAARD and BALTIMORE (1986), using conditions where the RNA replication of one of the parental viruses was blocked suggested that RNA recombination occurs primarily during the negative-strand RNA synthesis of poliovirus. However, it is possible that RNA recombination also could occur during positive-strand RNA synthesis, since more positive-strand RNA is synthesized, allowing more ample opportunities for RNA recombination. In a study of coronavirus RNA recombination involving transfected RNA fragments, it was shown that only the positive-strand RNA fragment could recombine with the viral genome (C.L. LIAO and M.M.C. LAI, unpublished observation). It is likely that RNA recombination can take place during both positive- and negative-strand RNA synthesis; this issue remains to be investigated.

6.3 Are There Specific Sequence Requirements for RNA Recombination and Are There Recombination "Hot Spots"?

If RNA recombination proceeds by a copy-choice mechanism whereby pausing RNA products dissociate and rebind to a different RNA template, one would predict that RNA recombination should occur at sites of strong sequence homology between the two parental viruses and also occur more readily between closely related viral RNAs (MCCAHON et al. 1977, 1985; KING 1988). In picornaviruses, recombination frequency is indeed higher between the more closely related strains than distantly related ones. Furthermore, sequence analysis of some recombinants suggested that recombination occurred more frequently at sites of strong secondary structure (TOLSKAYA et al. 1987). In addition, there is evidence for recombinational hot spots in MHV (BANNER et al. 1990). One of the putative recombinational hot spots corresponds to a hypervariable region in which frequent deletions occur after virus passage in tissue culture or animals. Thus, it appears that the same secondary structure of RNA is responsible for deletions and recombination. All of these studies suggest that RNA recombination occurs at sites corresponding to the presence of RNA secondary structure or similar nucleotide sequences between the two parental RNAs. However, the study by KIRKEGAARD and BALTIMORE (1986) suggested that recombination could occur practically anywhere within a 190-nucleotide stretch of poliovirus RNA, and there was no requirement for sequence homology between the parental viruses, suggesting that there were no preferred recombination sites. Nevertheless, this study did not rule out the possibility that, when the entire RNA genome is concerned, there may be preferred recombination sites. In the case of MHV, no common sequences are observed among the individual recombination sites, although there is clustering of recombination sites (BANNER et al. 1990).

All the recombination studies reported so far involved the selection of viable recombinant viruses. Thus, the types of recombinants obtained may not reflect the actual mechanism of RNA recombination, but result from selection pressures. A recent study examining MHV RNA recombination in the absence of artificial selection pressure (BANNER and LAI, 1991) supported this possibility. In this study, two MHVs were coinfected into a susceptible cell line, and the intracellular RNA and viruses released were screened for recombinants using the polymerase chain reaction (PCR) without selection pressure. It was found that recombination sites were distributed almost evenly throughout the region encompassed by the two primers used for PCR. However, when these viruses were passaged further in tissue culture, the crossover sites of most surviving recombinants were clustered in a particular region of the genome (BANNER and LAI, 1991). These data suggest that while recombination events are random, certain types of recombinants confer selective advantages. Thus, the types of recombinants isolated in any recombination study are likely to represent only those which have selective advantages under the conditions used. Nevertheless, it cannot be ruled out that certain RNA structures may indeed favor RNA recombination. In particular, the clustering of recombination sites in the noncoding regions of viral RNA may reflect actual recombinational hot spots in mechanistic terms.

Many questions remain unanswered concerning the mechanism of RNA recombination. For instance, what are the enzymatic requirements for RNA recombination? And are there any particular properties associated with enzymes which allow RNA recombination, in contrast to enzymes which do not, e.g., vesicular stomatitis virus (VSV) RNA polymerase?

7 The Biological Significance of RNA Recombination

Why have picornaviruses and coronaviruses acquired the ability to undergo a high frequency of homologous RNA recombination, in contrast to other RNA viruses? The answers may lie in the properties of their RNA polymerases. The RNA polymerases of these viruses may have nonprocessive properties, thus allowing the pausing RNA transcription products to be dissociated from the RNA template during RNA replication. The dissociated, incomplete RNA products may then participate in RNA recombination. Obviously, RNA recombination provides evolutionary advantages for these viruses, which may have special needs because of the properties of their RNA genomes:

1. Recombination may be a mechanism to eliminate errors in RNA synthesis. In the VSV system, it has been shown that RNA polymerase has an enormously high error frequency, in the order of 10^{-4} (STEINHAUER and HOLLAND 1986). For most RNA viruses, deleterious mutations can be partially overcome by genetic complementation. Since picornaviruses synthesize a polyprotein, most of their gene products function *in cis* and cannot be complemented easily. Thus, RNA recombination provides an escape mechanism in lieu of genetic complementation. In the case of coronaviruses, the need for RNA recombination is dictated by the extremely large size of its RNA genome, which ranges from 27 to 31 kb (LEE et al. 1991). In the absence of a proofreading mechanism, many RNA molecules would likely be nonfunctional due to the accumulation of multiple errors during RNA synthesis. RNA recombination may allow the virus to eliminate the defective segments and thereby retain the biological activities of its RNA. It is not clear whether picornavirus and coronavirus polymerases differ from the polymerases of other RNA viruses. It is known that coronavirus RNA transcription involves a discontinuous process (LAI 1990); thus, coronavirus RNA polymerase is quite adept at

jumping or switching templates during RNA synthesis. This inherent polymerase property may account for the extremely high frequency of RNA recombination observed in coronaviruses.

2. RNA recombination may be a mechanism for virus evolution. RNA recombination may allow viruses to adapt quickly to a change in environment. For example, in children receiving poliovirus vaccines, recombination of the virus populations in the gastrointestinal tract occurs very quickly. The recombinants, which commonly involve type 2 and type 3 vaccine strains (MINOR et al. 1986), apparently have a selective advantage under these conditions and become the predominant population in a few days after vaccination. Even in tissue culture cells, recombinants may outgrow parental viruses under certain conditions, as demonstrated by coronavirus recombination.
3. Although recombination may lead to the divergence and heterogeneity of RNA viruses, it potentially may result in the convergence of viral sequences, particularly in viruses such as coronavirus which undergo a high frequency of recombination. Frequent recombination among poliovirus serotypes could have resulted in the disappearance of serotype barriers. Therefore, the maintenance of such serotype differences must require some selective pressure.
4. Nonhomologous recombination generates DI RNA, gene rearrangement, or insertion of cellular genes, all of which have significant biological consequences on viral biology.

RNA recombination also can have deleterious effects. Recombination between viruses of low virulence may yield recombinant viruses of unexpected virulence. This has been demonstrated by the emergence of neurotropic poliovirus as a result of recombination between poliovirus vaccine strains (KEW and NOTTAY 1984). Similar results have been shown with several DNA virus recombinants. For example, two avirulent herpes simplex virus strains can recombine in vivo to yield a highly virulent virus (JAVIER et al. 1986). Similar observations also have been made with pseudorabies virus (KATZ et al. 1990). Thus, RNA recombination could pose a potentially serious problem in the administration of live, attenuated vaccines.

8 Epilogue

Although RNA recombination so far has been demonstrated only in a few viruses, the list of RNA viruses able to generate recombinants is growing. Many can undergo either homologous or nonhomologous recombination. Thus, RNA recombination plays an important role in the biology and evolution of RNA viruses. From certain points of view, RNA recombination is similar to the recombination seen in retroviruses, which also have a very high frequency of recombination and a nonprocessive polymerase (reverse transcriptase) (HU and

Temin 1990). Although the enzymes involved in retrovirus and RNA virus recombination are different, they are similar from the mechanistic point of view. It seems likely that most RNA viruses have an ability to recombine, as implied from their ability to undergo RNA rearrangement and to generate DI RNA. The failure to detect homologous recombination in them may be due simply to inappropriate selection pressures. It will be a challenge to demonstrate the possible occurrence of genetic recombination in other RNA viruses.

Acknowledgments. I thank Drs. John Polo, Tom MacNaughton, Lisa Welter and Lisa Banner for critical comments on the manuscript. The research conducted in my laboratory were supported by US Public Health Services Research Grant AI-19244 and National Multiple Sclerosis Society Grant RG 1449.

References

Allison RF, Janda M, Ahlquist P (1989) Sequence of cowpea chlorotic mottle virus RNAs 2 and 3 and evidence of a recombination event during bromovirus evolution. Virology 172: 321–330

Allison RF, Thompson C, Ahlquist P (1990) Regeneration of a functional RNA virus genome by recombination between deletion mutants and requirement for cowpea chlorotic mottle virus 3a and coat genes for systemic infection. Proc Natl Acad Sci USA 87: 1820–1824

Angenent GC, Posthumus E, Brederode FT, Bol JF (1990) Genome structure of tobacco rattle virus strain PLB: further evidence on the occurrence of RNA recombination among tobraviruses. Virology 171: 271–274

Banner LR, Keck JG, Lai MMC (1990) A clustering of RNA recombination sites adjacent to a hypervariable region of the peplomer gene of murine coronavirus. Virology 175: 548–555

Banner LR, LAI MMC (1991) Random nature of coronavirus RNA recombination in the absence of selection pressure. Virology 185: 441–445

Baric RS, Shieh C-K, Stohlman SA, Lai MMC (1987) Analysis of intracellular small RNAs of mouse hepatitis virus: evidence for discontinuous transcription. Virology 156: 342–354

Baric RS, Fu K, Schaad MC, Stohlman SA (1990) Establishing a genetic recombination map for murine coronavirus strain A59 complementation groups. Virology 177: 646–656

Bujarski JJ, Kaesberg P (1986) Genetic recombination between RNA components of a multipartite plant virus. Nature 321: 528–531

Cascone PJ, Carpenter CD, Li XH, Simon AE (1990) Recombination between satellite RNAs of turnip crinkle virus. EMBO J. 9: 1709–1715

Cooper PD (1968) A genetic map of poliovirus temperature-sensitive mutants. Virology 35: 584–596

Cooper PD (1977) Genetics of picornaviruses. In: Fraenkel-Conrat H, Wagner RR (eds) Comprehensive virology, vol 9. Plenum, New York, pp 133–208

Hahn CS, Lustin S, Strauss EG, Strauss JH (1988) Western equine encephalitis virus is a recombinant virus. Proc Natl Acad Sci USA 85: 5997–6001

Haseloff J, Goelet P, Zimmern D, Ahlquist P, Dasgupta R, Kaesberg P (1984) Striking similarities in amino acid sequence among nonstructural proteins encoded by RNA viruses that have dissimilar genomic organization. Proc Natl Acad Sci USA 81: 4358–4362

Hayes W (1968) In: The genetics of bacteria and their viruses, 2nd edn. Blackwell, Oxford

Hirst GK (1962) Genetic recombination with Newcastle disease virus, polioviruses and influenza virus. Cold Spring Harbor Symp Quant Biol 27: 303–309

Hu W-S, Temin HM (1990) Genetic consequences of packaging two RNA genomes in one retroviral particle: pseudodiploidy and high rate of genetic recombination. Proc Natl Acad Sci USA 87: 1556–1560

Javier RT, Sedarati F, Stevens JG (1986) Two avirulent herpes simplex viruses generate lethal recombinants in vivo. Science 234: 746–749

Kassavetis GA, Chamberlin MJ (1981) Pausing and termination of transcription within the early region of bacteriophage T7 DNA in vitro. J Biol Chem 256: 2777–2786

Katz JB, Henderson LM, Erickson GA (1990) Recombination in vivo of pseudorabies vaccine strains to produce new virus strains. Vaccine 8: 286–288

Keck JG, Stohlman SA, Soe LH, Makino S, Lai MMC (1987) Multiple recombination sites at the 5'-end of murine coronavirus RNA. Virology 156: 331–341
Keck JG, Matsushima GK, Makino S, Fleming JO, Vannier DM, Stohlman SA, Lai MMC (1988a) In vivo RNA–RNA recombination of coronavirus in mouse brain. J Virol 62: 1810–1813
Keck JG, Soe LH, Makino S, Stohlman SA, Lai MMC (1988b) RNA recombination of murine coronaviruses: recombination between fusion-positive MHV-A59 and fusion-negative MHV-2. J Virol 62: 1989–1998
Kew OM, Nottay BK (1984) Evolution of the oral polio vaccine strains in humans occurs by both mutation and intramolecular recombination. In: Chanock RM, Lerner RA (eds) Modern approaches to vaccines: molecular and chemical basis of virus virulence and immunogenicity. Cold Spring Harbor Laboratory, Cold Spring Harbor, pp 357–362
King AMQ (1988) Recombination in positive strand RNA viruses. In: Domingo E, Holland JJ, Ahlquist P (eds) RNA genetics, vol 2. CRC, Boca Raton, FL, pp 149–165
King AMQ, McCahon D, Slade WR, Newman JWI (1982) Recombination in RNA. Cell 29: 921–928
King AMQ, McCahon D, Saunders K, Newman JWI, Slade WR (1985) Multiple sites of recombination within the RNA genome of foot-and-mouth disease virus. Virus Res 3: 373–384
Kirkegaard K, Baltimore D (1986) The mechanism of RNA recombination in poliovirus. Cell 47: 433–443
Kusters JG, Niesters HGM, Lenstra JA, Horzinek MC, van der Zeijst BAM (1989) Phylogeny of antigenic variants of avian coronavirus IBV. Virology 169: 217–221
Lai MMC (1990) Coronavirus: organization, replication and expression of genome. Annu Rev Microbiol 44: 303–333
Lai MMC, Baric RS, Makino S, Keck JG, Egbert J, Leibowitz JL, Stohlman SA (1985) Recombination between nonsegmented RNA genomes of murine coronaviruses. J Virol 56: 449–456
Lake JR, Priston RAJ, Slade WR (1975) A genetic recombination map of foot- and-mouth disease virus. J Gen Virol 27: 355–367
Ledinko N (1963) Genetic recombination with poliovirus type 1: studies of crosses between a normal horse serum-resistant mutant and several guanidine-resistant mutants of the same strain. Virology 20: 107–119
Lee HJ, Shieh C-K, Gorbalenya AE, Koonin EV, La Monica N, Tuler J, Bagdzhadzhyan A, Lai MMC (1991) The complete sequence (22 kilobases) of murine coronavirus gene 1 encoding the putative proteases and RNA polymerases. Virology 180: 567–582
Luytjes W, Bredenbeek PJ, Noten AFH, Horzinek MC, Spaan WJM (1988) Sequence of mouse hepatitis virus A59 mRNA 2: indications for RNA-recombination between coronavirus and influenza C virus. Virology 166: 415–422
Makino S, Keck JG, Stohlman SA, Lai MMC (1986) High-frequency RNA recombination of murine coronaviruses. J Virol 57: 729–737
Makino S, Fleming JO, Keck JG, Stohlman SA, Lai MMC (1987) RNA recombination of coronaviruses: localization of neutralizing epitopes and neuropathogenic determinants on the carboxyl terminus of peplomers. Proc Natl Acad Sci USA 84: 6567–6571
McCahon D, King AMQ, Roe DS, Slade WR, Newman JWI, Cleary AM (1985) Isolation and biochemical characterization of intertypic recombinants of foot- and-mouth disease virus. Virus Res 3: 87–100
McCahon D, Slade WR, Priston RA, Lake JR (1971) An extended genetic recombination map of foot-and-mouth disease virus. J Gen Virol 35: 555–565
Meyers G, Tautz N, Dubovi EJ, Thiel H-J (1991) Viral cytopathogenicity correlated with integration of ubiquitin-coding sequences. Virology 180: 602–616
Mills DR, Dobkin C, Kramer FR (1978) Template-determined, variable rate of RNA chain elongation. Cell 15: 541–550
Minor PD, John A, Ferguson M, Icenogle JP (1986) Antigenic and molecular evolution of the vaccine strain of type 3 poliovirus during the period of excretion by a primary vaccine. J Gen Virol 67: 693–706
Pringle CR (1965) Evidence of genetic recombination in foot- and-mouth disease virus. Virology 25: 48–54
Rao ALN, Hall TC (1990) Requirement for a viral trans-acting factor encoded by brome mosaic virus RNA-2 provides strong selection in vivo for functional recombinants. J Virol 64: 2437–2441
Steinhauer DA, Holland JJ (1986) Direct method for quantitation of extreme polymerase error frequencies at selected single base sites in viral RNA. J Virol 57: 219–228
Tolskaya EA, Romanova LI, Blinov VM, Victorova EG, Sinyakov AN, Kolesnikova MS, Agol VI (1987) Studies on the recombination between RNA genomes of poliovirus: the primary structure and nonrandom distribution of crossover regions in the genomes of intertypic poliovirus recombinants. Virology 161: 54–61

Foot-and-Mouth Disease Virus Populations Are Quasispecies

E. DOMINGO, C. ESCARMIS, M. A. MARTINEZ, E. MARTINEZ-SALAS, and M. G. MATEU

1 Introduction

The term "quasispecies" describes complex distributions of replicating molecules subject to mutation and competitive selection (EIGEN 1971; EIGEN and SCHUSTER 1979; EIGEN and BIEBRICHER 1988). The original theoretical concept of EIGEN and colleagues concerned populations of infinite numbers of individual molecules and ideal, steady-state equilibrium conditions (recent review on the theoretical concept in EIGEN et al. 1989). It is clear that in spite of their large population size, RNA viruses deviate from such idealized behaviour. However, several key features of RNA viruses such as nucleotide sequence heterogeneity, generally high mutation rates, and potential for very rapid evolution are best understood in the framework of the quasispecies concept (see the chapter by HOLLAND et al.). Viral isolates, either in their natural niche or disturbed by adaptation to growing in cell culture, consist of a multitude of viable and defective mutants termed the "mutant spectrum" of the population. During replication, each genomic distribution is dominated by one (or several) "master sequence (s)," that generally coincides with the average or consensus sequence

Centro de Biologia Molecular, Universidad Autónoma de Madrid, Canto Blanco, 28049 Madrid, Spain

Current Topics in Microbiology and Immunology, Vol. 176

of the population. With the levels of genetic heterogeneity for foot- and-mouth disease virus (FMDV) documented in the following paragraphs, the master sequence often represents as little as 1% or less of the population of molecules, and it may have a brief life span. Here we review the evidence for the quasispecies structure of FMDV and its biological implications, notably the antigenic diversity of this widespread pathogen.

2 The Process of Infection by FMDV

The basic features of this picornavirus are summarized in Table 1. FMDV displays a surprising ability to spread among a wide range of host animals, including cattle, swine, sheep, goats, and several wild species. The ease of contagion stems from a requirement for a few infectious units to initiate infection at several portals of entry (respiratory tract, skin lesions). Transmission often constitutes a population bottleneck in which one or a few of the many infectious particles from an infected animal (estimated at 10^9–10^{12}) are sampled and amplified in the new host (BACHRACH 1968; PEREIRA 1981; DOMINGO et al. 1990, and references therein). This founder event is relevant to the interpretation of FMDV variation in the field (Sect. 6). FMDV generally causes a systemic, acute infection, characterized by fever, vesicular lesions (mainly in the mouth and feet), and myocarditis among young animals. In ruminants, the acute phase may be followed by an inapparent persistent infection involving limited viral replication in the esophageal-

Table 1. General features of FMDV

Virus particle

Icosahedral symmetry, 300 Å in diameter
Sedimentation 146 S
Buoyant density in CsCl 1.43–1.50 g/cm^3
Unstable at pH < 7 and physiological temperatures
Proteins per particle: 60 copies of each VP1, VP2, VP3 (M.W. 23 000–25 000), and VP4 (M.W. 8500); 1–2 copies of VP0 (uncleaved VP2, VP4 precursor); VPg covalently linked to 5' end of RNA
Antigenic diversity: seven serotypes (A, O, C, SAT1, SAT2, SAT3, Asia1) and multiple variants

Genome

Single-stranded infectious RNA (~8500 nucleotides)
Genetic map, where VPg is the protein covalently linked to the 5′ end, and $(A)_n$ is the poly A tail at the 3′ end of the RNA:

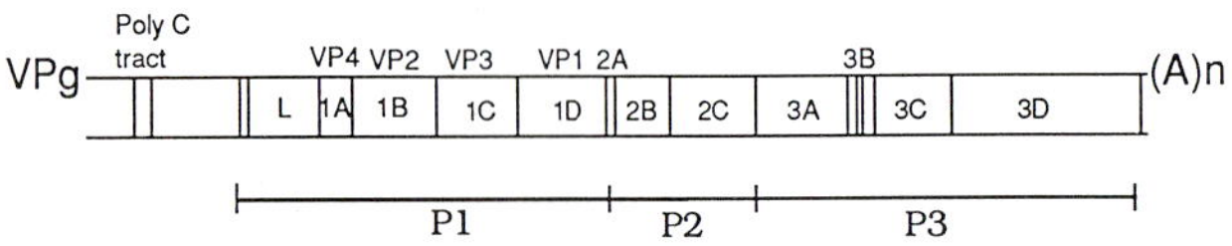

pharyngeal region. Persistent infections constitute an important reservoir of FMDV in nature. (Review on FMDV pathogenesis in TIMONEY et al. 1988.)

In spite of considerable progress in the knowledge of FMDV at the molecular level (Table 1) the mechanisms by which those various disease patterns are initiated, maintained, and terminated are not understood. During acute and persistent infections FMDV displays continuous genetic heterogeneity. Probably, this is the adaptive strategy that has contributed most to the prevalence of the virus, in spite of vast efforts to control its spread.

3 Genetic Heterogeneity of FMDV Populations

Genomic RNA from viruses isolated during a single outbreak of disease differed in an estimated 0.7%–2.2% of nucleotides, as quantitated by T_1 oligonucleotide fingerprinting (DOMINGO et al. 1980; KING et al. 1981; ANDERSON et al. 1985). Subsequent work on nucleotide sequencing of RNA or complementary DNA (cDNA) has confirmed that FMDVs from a single disease episode are heterogeneous (Table 2). Analysis of RNA from individual viral plaques, derived from one isolate, revealed two FMDV subpopulations whose genomes differed in at least one residue. These observations led to the proposal that FMDV in nature is a quasispecies (DOMINGO et al. 1980).

Table 2. Variability of FMDV

Genetic heterogeneity[a]
During a disease outbreak
Among consensus sequences of different isolates: 60–100 substitutions per genome
Among consensus sequences of contemporary isolates: 2–20 substitutions per genome
Among individual genomes of one isolate: 0.6–2 substitutions per genome
Of clonal populations in cell culture
Among consensus sequences of independently passaged plaque-purified viruses: 14–57 substitutions per genome
Among individual genomes of clonal, passaged population: 2–8 substitutions per genome
Frequency of MAb-resistant mutants
In virus from lesions of infected animals; 2.9×10^{-6}–2.6×10^{-5}
In virus from cell culture fluid: 4×10^{-5}
Evolution[b]
Rate of fixation of mutations
Acute disease: $< 0.04 \times 10^{-2}$–4.5×10^{-2} substitutions per nucleotide per year
Persistent infection in cattle (VP1 gene): 0.9×10^{-2}–7.4×10^{-2} substitutions per nucleotide per year

[a] Based on data from DOMINGO et al. (1980), SOBRINO et al. (1986), DE LA TORRE et al. (1988), VILLAVERDE et al. (1988, 1991), CARRILLO et al. (1990a), and MARTINEZ et al. (1991a)

[b] It varies for different genomic segments. Rates are not always proportional to the time intervals between isolations. Based on data from SOBRINO et al. (1986) and GEBAUER et al. (1988)

4 Mutations Are Continuously Arising at Many Sites of the FMDV Genome

It could be argued that coinfections with preexisting variant FMDVs were responsible for the observed heterogeneities in the field. Analysis of viruses rescued from animals or cell cultures acutely or persistently infected with plaque-purified FMDV strongly suggests that FMDV variants are generated de novo at high rates.

4.1 Evolution of FMDV During Experimental Infection of Animals with Cloned Virus

Persistent infections of cattle were established with clones of FMDV C_3 Resende Br/55 characterized by either a short or a long genomic poly (C) tract (Table 1) (Costa Giomi et al. 1984, 1988; Gebauer et al. 1988). Viruses were rescued from the esophageal/pharyngeal region of the animals during 539 days of inapparent infection and analyzed. The length of the poly (C) tract fluctuated from about 145–280 residues. Two genomic subpopulations with poly (C) of different size indicated genetic heterogeneity of FMDV replicating in one animal at a given time. The function of the poly (C) tract and the biological significance of its size variations are unknown. Transfection with infectious RNA transcripts from cloned cDNA have shown that at least 32 C residues are required for a productive infection (Zibert et al. 1990). However, progeny virus included a poly (C) tract of 60 or 80 nucleotides, and this size did not vary after 30 serial passages in BHK-21 cells. Thus, both in cell culture and in persistently infected cattle there appears to be a range in the number of C residues compatible with active FMDV multiplication.

In the viruses persisting in carrier cattle, charge shifts in capsid proteins VP1, VP2, and VP3 were detected by electrofocusing (Gebauer et al. 1988). Double bands at the positions of VP1 and VP3 revealed heterogeneity in the isolates. Nucleotide sequencing of the VP1 gene of sequential isolates indicated a rate of nucleotide replacement that ranged from 0.9×10^{-2} to 7.4×10^{-2} substitutions per nucleotide per year (Table 2). Some of the viruses did not react with monoclonal antibodies (MAbs) that recognize the main antigenic determinant on protein VP1 (Gebauer et al. 1988; see also Sect. 5). Thus, during persistent infections of cattle, FMDV became genetically heterogeneous and there was a rapid emergence and dominance of antigenic variants.

In another line of research, swine were infected with plaque-purified FMDV C_1 Santa Pau Spain 70 (clone C-S8c1) and in the course of the acute infection viruses were rescued from organs and vesicular lesions (Carrillo et al. 1990a). The proportion of variant viruses resistant to neutralizing MAbs was measured directly on vesicular fluids, avoiding viral replication in cell culture. The frequency of MAb-resistant (MAR) genotypes was about 3×10^{-5}, a value very similar to that found for the parental FMDV C-S8c1 in cell culture (Table 2). In addition to MAR mutants, a variant was isolated from blood during the viremic phase that induced, upon reinoculation into swine, an early emergence of disease symptoms (CARRILLO et al. 1990a and manuscript in preparation). Thus, as in persistent infections, genetic and phenotypic variants of FMDV arise during acute infections in vivo.

4.2 Rapid Generation of FMDV Mutants During Acute and Persistent Infections in Cell Culture

The genetic diversity attained upon limited replication of FMDV was evaluated by serial passage in cell culture of multiple FMDV populations, all derived from plaque-purified FMDV (SOBRINO et al. 1983). After 28–30 virus passages, the average nucleotide sequence of the RNA of each of the populations differed from the others in an estimated 14–57 nucleotides. Analysis of individual clones indicated that each infectious RNA molecule differed from the parental sequence by an average of two to eight mutations. The serial passage led to an increase in the yield of infectious FMDV particles per cell.

Application of a new in situ enzyme-linked immunosorbent assay (ELISA) that allows visualization of the reactivity of individual viral plaques with antibodies (DÍEZ et al. 1989), revealed that passaged FMDV (clone C-S8c1) rapidly became antigenically heterogeneous. Since no anti-FMDV antibodies were present during the propagation of virus, antigenic variation of FMDV was independent of immune selection. These and other observations suggest that the antigenic variation of FMDV may follow from fluctuations in the quasispecies distribution of genomes, driven by mutations unrelated to immune selection (this point is further discussed in Sects. 5 and 7).

FMDV C-S8c1 was also used to establish persistent infections in cloned BHK-21 cells (DE LA TORRE et al. 1985). Analysis of the virus shed from such cultures demonstrated that there was a gradual modification of its genome and of several phenotypic properties (acquisition of a *ts* character, small plaque morphology, virion instability) of FMDV. At cell passage 58, the consensus RNA coding for the VP1 protein differed in about 0.3% of residues from the initial FMDV C-S8c1 RNA. Sequencing of VP1 RNA from nine viral clones from this population showed a genetic heterogeneity of 5×10^{-4} substitutions per nucleotide. Gradually, the resident FMDV became more virulent for the parental BHK-21 cells and the latter, in turn, became progressively more resistant to FMDV C-S8c1. Since both the virus and the cells used to initiate persistence had been cloned, variant FMDVs and variant cells were generated during the persistent infection (DE LA TORRE et al. 1988, 1989a, b; review in DOMINGO et al. 1990). In spite of their increased virulence for BHK-21 cells, the viruses were highly attenuated for mice and cattle (DÍEZ et al. 1990a). Thus, attenuation was not an inherent property of the mutant FMDVs, but was a host-dependent trait. The hypervirulence for BHK-21 cells was probably selected by the increased resistance of the cells to FMDV infection. Cell fusion studies suggested that such a resistance was mediated by trans-acting cellular products (De La Torre et al. 1989a). Such products have not been identified.

Nucleotide sequencing of the RNA from virus after 100 passages of the persistently infected cells showed multiple mutations at several genomic sites Diez et al., unpublished results). Thus, the molecular basis of the phenotypic alterations observed is unknown. Nine amino acid substitutions were fixed in the viral capsid during the 100 cell passages. Three of the variant amino acids are not represented in the corresponding position of any picornavirus sequenced to date (Palmenberg 1989; Díez et al. 1990b). Cysteine at position 7 of VP3, that provides disulfide bridges at the virion fivefold axis (Acharya et al. 1989) (and which is conserved in all other FMDVs that have been sequenced) was substituted by valine. This shows that even structurally critical amino acids may be replaced when viral replication occurs in a modified environment (in this case provided by the prolonged residence of FMDV in BHK-21 cells). It is not known whether the substitution of cysteine by valine represents a positive selective advantage for the modified virus, or if it simply reflects a relaxation of the cysteine requirement. This, and other substitutions that appear to cluster around the fivefold axis of the capsid, probably underlie the particle instability observed during virus purification. Stability was partially restored in high ionic strength media. Molecular modeling studies suggested that hydrophobic interactions between the methyl side chain of valines contributed to keep the modified virions assembled (Díez et al. 1990b).

The main conclusion from the above paragraphs is the evolution of FMDV was driven to produce a variety of distinct phenotypes selected in response to different infection conditions. In all cases tested, evolution occurred via complex, heterogeneous distributions of genomes, in agreement with the quasispecies nature of the virus.

FMDV undergoes high frequency recombination in cell culture (King 1988). The extent of FMDV recombination in nature is not known. It may provide a mechanism for more drastic evolutionary jumps than those mediated by point mutations. Recombination may also rescue high-fitness genomes from highly mutated (low-fitness) parental viruses (see the chapter by Lai).

5 Antigenic Diversity and the Dynamics of Antigenic Variation

Among all phenotypic changes of FMDV, antigenic diversification is highly significant for disease control, since it is a major obstacle to the design of effective vaccines (Domingo 1989; Brown 1990). Use of MAbs in both neutralization and binding assays has revealed that contemporary isolates of the same geographical origin, or even viral clones derived from one isolate, may be antigenically distinct (Rowlands et al. 1983; Mateu et al. 1987, 1988, 1989).

In most cases, antigenic variation has been traced to amino acid replacements at hypervariable, exposed sites on the viral capsid. The first such site recognized as important for virus neutralization (site A) (STROHMAIER et al. 1982) is now known to involve a protruding, disordered loop on protein VP1 (the GH loop, at residues 130–160; ACHARYA et al. 1989). At least for serotype C this site contains many (at least 11) distinguishable, partly overlapping continuous epitopes (MATEU et al. 1988, 1989, 1990). For serotype O, some epitopes at this site appear to be more complex, involving residues from the carboxy terminal segment of VP1 (PARRY et al. 1989) or other capsid regions (PARRY et al. 1990). KITSON et al. (1990) have located four distinct sites on FMDV O_1 involved in neutralization of infectivity, and several sites are also found in other serotypes (THOMAS et al. 1988; BAXT et al. 1989). In all cases these antigenic sites were located on exposed loops on VP1, VP2, and VP3 (KITSON et al. 1990).

Several lines of evidence suggest that site A of FMDV is highly immunodominant (reviewed by BROWN 1990), perhaps due to its accessibility and structural flexibility. Peptides representing this VP1 segment were necessary to afford protection by synthetic vaccine formulations (reviewed by BROWN 1990; DOMINGO et al. 1990). Serological variants of one type A strain differed in two amino acids of this loop, and the serological specificity of the variants was adequately mimicked by synthetic peptides representing only such sequences (ROWLANDS et al. 1983; CLARKE et al. 1983).

Two mechanisms of antigenic diversification of site A have been distinguished by relating VP1 sequences of field isolates of FMDV type C with the reactivity of the viruses with MAbs. One is a gradual increase in antigenic distance brought about by accumulation of amino acid replacements at the two most variable sequence stretches within site A (Figs. 1 and 2). The other is an abrupt antigenic change entailing loss of many epitopes, caused by single, critical amino acid substitutions at the same site (MATEU et al. 1990; MARTINEZ et al. 1991). In particular, replacement of Asp or His by Gln, Arg, or Leu at VP1 position 146 caused a remarkable antigenic difference. The use of substituted synthetic peptides proved that even chemically conservative substitutions (such as Leu → Ile or Leu → Val) affected reactivity of FMDV with neutralizing antibodies (MATEU et al. 1989 and unpublished results). These substitutions occur frequently in the quasispecies distribution of FMDV genomes. The above observations again implicate quasispecies as an important element of viral pathogenesis. (For a more extensive review on the antigenic structure of FMDV see DOMINGO et al. 1990.)

Antigenic variants of FMDV have been selected under a number of conditions: in partially immune animals (FAGG and HYSLOP 1966), in persistently infected cattle (GEBAUER et al. 1988) (Sect. 4.1), and in cell culture. In the latter case, they emerged both in the presence (CARRILLO et al. 1989) and absence of anti-FMDV antibodies (BOLWELL et al. 1989; DÍEZ et al. 1989, 1990b). These findings suggest that the antigenic variants result from the generally high mutation rates during picornaviral replication (EGGERS and TAMM 1965; HEINZ et al. 1989; DE LA TORRE et al. 1990; see also the chapter by HOLLAND et al.) and

VIRUS	FMDV LOOP
	`133                    158`
O Consensus	`ECRYSRNAVPNLRGDLQVLAQKVART`
O_1 BFS 1860, 7 others[1]	
O_1 BFS 67	`G`
O_1 Kaufbeuren, O Zusmarhausen	`    N`
O_1 Campos	`           V`
O Wien	`           V       D  A`
O_2 Normandie	` S         V     A G  A`
O Wuppertal, O Thalheim	`S K  DAR S V          AE A`
O Israel	`N   GNV  T V          A`
O ISA 7/83 2	`N   GAHT T V          A`
O ISA 7/83 1	`    GTYTTT V          A`
O_6 V1	`V K  KT    V   T   D   S A`
O Hong Kong	`S K  DTHMS V       T  AS A`
A Consensus	`TNKYSTGGS..RRGDMGSLAARVAKQ`
A_5 Allier, 2 others[2]	`      D P             A`
A_5 Spain 83, 3 others[3]	`      D P          T  A`
A_5 Morocco	`      D P    D        A`
A_5 France	`      D P    D    P   A`
A_5 Westerwald	`        P         A   A`
A Modena	`               T  T   A`
A Parma, A Salerno	`               T  TT  A`
A_{12} 119	`     AS  G V   F    P   R`
A_{10} 61	`     ASD    S  L  I     T`
A Ostdeutschland	` S   AS L  GP  L  P     T`
A_{27}	`     N  Q   A`
A Venceslau	` S  TVS  G`
A Argentina 79	` S  TV   G`
A_{24}	` S  AV   G       T     V`
A_{32}	`VS  AV   G     L P`
A_{22} Iraq	` S   A  TG     L P      A`
A_{22} USSR	` S   A  MG     LEP      A`
C Consensus	`TTTYTTSA....RGDLAHLTATHARH`
C-S8, 3 others[4]	`     A              T`
C-S20	`     A T`
C-S15, 5 others[5]	`       T          I`
C-S30	`       T          V`
C-S35	`       T          IA`
C-S9	`    AA              T    Y`
C_1 Oberbayern	`     A T              R G`
C_3 Resende, C_3 Argentina 84	`           R       ATA`
C_3 Resende c12, c3B	`           R     D ATA`
C_3 Argentina 85	`  A  AG    R       A A`
C_3 Indaial 78	`  A  A     R       A A`
C_3 Indaial 71	`  A   GV   R       A A`

Fig. 1. Sequence alignment of the main antigenic site (site A) of FMDVs of serotypes O, A, C. Amino acid sequence (single letter code) given corresponds to the central, disordered region of the VP1 GH loop (residues 133–158 of FMDV O_1 BFS, ACHARYA et al. 1989). Only amino acids that differ from the consensus sequence defined for each serotype are indicated. A *dot* is a deletion. [1]Isolates O_1 BFS 1848, O_1 Lausanne, O_1 Aulendorf, O_1 Austrian vaccine, O Murchin, O Funen I and II; [2]A Lérida, A Bernbeuren; [3]A_5 Portugal, A_5 Spain 86, A Valladolid; [4]C-S10, C-S14, C-S18; [5]C-S16, C-S17, C-S21, C-S22, C-S33. The consensus amino acid was assigned to undefined positions in viruses A_5 Allier, A Bernbeuren, A Lérida, A_5 Spain 86, A Valladolid, C-S18, C-S30, and C-S33. Data from KURZ et al. (1981), KLEID et al. (1981), BOOTHROYD et al. (1982), MAKOFF et al. (1982), VILLANUEVA et al. (1983), BECK et al. (1983), CHEUNG et al. (1983), WEDDELL et al. (1985), SOBRINO et al. (1986), OULDRIDGE et al. (1986), BECK and STROHMAIER (1987), MARTINEZ et al. (1988), PICCONE et al. (1988), GEBAUER et al. (1988), MATEU et al. (1989), BOLWELL et al. (1989), CARRILLO et al. (1990b)

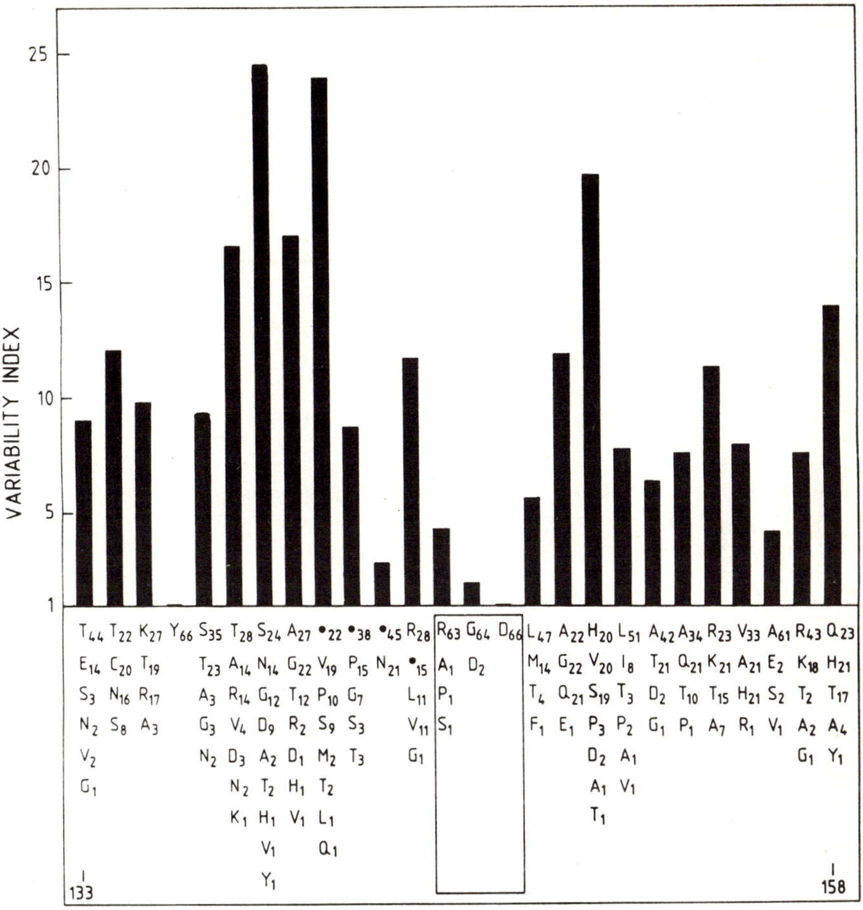

Fig. 2. Amino acid variability at antigenic site A of FMDV serotypes O, A, C. The number of times that an amino acid is found at any given position (counted from the alignment of Fig. 2) is indicated. Undefined amino acids because of sequence ambiguities were not taken into account. The variability index is the ratio between the number of different amino acids found at the considered position and the frequency of the most common amino acid at the same position (WU and KABAT 1970); the range of possible values is 1–330. The highly conserved tripeptide Arg-Gly-Asp (proposed to be involved in receptor recognition, FOX et al. 1989) is boxed

from the negative selection imposed on most mutant genomes (DOMINGO et al. 1978; DOMINGO and HOLLAND 1988; DOMINGO et al. 1990; COFFIN 1990). In this model (DÍEZ et al. 1989, 1990b), substitutions at antigenic sites are regarded as likely to be tolerated, due to the loose structural constraints of exposed, flexible loops. That is, variant FMDVs with replacements at those sites may not be subject to intense negative selection. Genomic fluctuations (driven by selective mutations at other loci, or by random sampling events) will be often accompanied by a mutation at those permissive sites (see also Sect. 7).

An alternative model of high-frequency replacements at antigenic domains is that the FMDV RNA polymerase depicts decreased fidelity when copying RNA which encodes those domains (WEDDELL et al. 1985). There is little solid evidence in favour of substantial variations in mutation rates among different RNA viruses or different sites within one RNA virus (reviewed by EIGEN and BIEBRICHER 1988, see also the chapter by HOLLAND et al.). However, the possibility cannot be excluded that due to secondary structure of the RNA template (or other sequence effects), RNA polymerases could be driven to be more or less error prone than when copying unstructured RNA.

6 Evolution of FMDV in the Field

Sequence alignments and phylogenetic relationships among picornaviruses were first established by PALMENBERG (1989). For FMDV, the most parsimonious tree relating the VP1 gene of type A, O, and C isolates depicted several clusters that reflected the groupings of classical serology (DOPAZO et al. 1988). The tree was extremely ramified, as expected due to the fact that each isolate sequenced to date has proven genetically unique. The analysis documented that mutations accumulate preferentially (but not exclusively) at a limited number of VP1 residues. A corresponding bias for certain amino acid substitutions at the antigenic sites of VP1 presumably has limited the extent of antigenic diversification undergone by FMDV in the field (MARTINEZ et al. 1991).

The rate of fixation of mutations in the FMDV genome may be modulated either by differential mutability at various genomic loci, or by selective forces, or both. Results with FMDV and other viral systems suggest that selection is the main contributor to differential diversification of gene segments (DOMINGO and HOLLAND 1988; COFFIN 1990). VILLAVERDE et al. (1988, 1991) have compared the rates of fixation of mutations at the VP1 and 3D (polymerase) genes among epidemiologically closely related FMDV isolates. The rates were significantly different for the two genes. Interestingly, however, no difference was found in the genetic heterogeneity of VP1 and 3D RNA segments among cocirculating FMDVs. This suggests that the conservation of the polymerase gene is not caused by low mutability but by a limitation in the fixation of substitutions.

For brief, acute episodes of disease, a relatively steady accumulation of mutations was observed (VILLAVERDE et al. 1991). It was proposed that such a transient "molecular clock" was the result of random sampling and amplification in a new host of mutants from the FMDV quasispecies mutant spectrum. The clock was rapidly lost, warning against conclusions about the time of origin of viral strains, based on nucleotide or amino acid sequence comparisons (PICCONE et al. 1988; DOMINGO 1989; COFFIN 1990).

It has not been possible to define any trend in the evolution of FMDV in the field. Extreme genetic and antigenic heterogeneities are observed along with surprising long-term conservations of sequences (PICCONE et al. 1988; MATEU et al. 1988; DOMINGO et al. 1990; MARTINEZ et al. 1991). Such complex molecular epidemiology may partly be due to the behavior of quasispecies, endowed with a double potential for either relative population stability or rapid evolution (DOMINGO et al. 1978, 1985; HOLLAND et al. 1982; STEINHAUER and HOLLAND 1987; DOMINGO and HOLLAND 1988). A disturbing problem in foot- and-mouth disease (FMD) epidemiology is the accidental reintroduction of vaccine strains in the field (BECK and STROHMAIER 1987). Unless traced to a vaccine origin by other evidence, such reintroductions are difficult to distinguish from long-term conservation (in natural reservoirs) solely on the basis of nucleotide sequence analysis.

Thus, evolution of FMDV in the field appears to be a complex and unpredictable process. This may be due, at least in part, to the multiple variants present in any infected animal (Sect. 4), and to the unknown nature of the selective constraints and random sampling events during virus multiplication and spread.

7 Conclusions and Prospects

Acute and persistent FMDV infections proceed via genetically heterogeneous virus populations termed quasispecies. This designation emphasizes that viral populations do not consist of one defined molecular species, but of distributions of nonidentical, related species. This feature is not unique to FMDV but extends to most (if not all) RNA viruses and other RNA genetic elements (HOLLAND et al. 1982; DOMINGO et al. 1985; STEINHAUER and HOLLAND 1987; DOMINGO and HOLLAND 1988: TEMIN 1989; KURSTAK et al. 1990; other chapters of this volume).

The fleeting dominance of FMDV variants (Sect. 4) is best explained by the population equilibrium model of RNA genomes (DOMINGO and HOLLAND 1988), implicit in the quasispecies concept. Each variant is continuously rated in competition with all other mutants present and arising in the population. Positive selection is exerted on the best-adapted members that arise in the mutant spectra. Negative selection is imposed on variants bearing deleterious mutations. As a result of such rating, the most neutral mutants in a given environment will predominate in the quasispecies. This has been invoked as a possible explanation of the ease of antigenic variation of FMDV in the absence of immune selection (Sect. 5).

Population complexity in the field (Sect. 6) is a drawback for disease control, in particular for the design of synthetic vaccines. To diminish the likelihood of selecting FMDVs able to overcome an immune response, synthetic vaccines should be formulated with multiple, independent B- and T-cell epitopes (DOMINGO 1989). This is an important challenge, since whole-virus, inactivated vaccines are effective in controlling FMD, but it would be desirable to avoid the handling of infectious virus.

The error prone replication of RNA viruses opens interesting prospects. HOLLAND et al. (1990) have observed that the mutation frequency at defined genomic loci during poliovirus and vesicular stomatitis virus replication was near the maximum compatible with maintaining viral infectivity. Thus, if drugs could be designed to decrease even further the viral replication fidelity, their use could divert viral multiplication from a productive into an abortive infection. This could provide the immune system with an enhanced opportunity to clear the infection. In addition to such practical possibilities, quasispecies pose the challenge of elucidating the biological role that variant viruses play in disease processes.

Acknowledgements. We are indebted to D. Andreu, C. Carrillo, M. Dávila, J.C. de la Torre, J. Diez, J. Dopazo, E. Giralt, M. Medina, A. Moya, F. Sobrino, N. Villanueva, and A. Villaverde for important contributions to the FMDV project at the C.B.M., Madrid (Spain). Work supported by CICYT (Spain), European Community (programs Science and Bridge) and Fundación Ramón Areces (Spain).

References

Acharya R, Fry E, Stuart D, Fox G, Rowlands D, Brown F (1989) The three-dimensional structure of foot-and-mouth disease virus at 2.9 Å resolution. Nature 337: 709–716

Anderson EC, Underwood BO, Brown F, Ngichabe CK (1985) Variation in foot- and-mouth disease virus isolates in Kenya: an examination of field isolates by T_1 oligonucleotide fingerprinting. Vet Microbiol 10: 409–423

Bachrach HL (1968) Foot-and-mouth disease virus. Annu Rev Microbiol 22: 201–244

Baxt B, Vakharia V, Moore DM, Franke AJ, Morgan DO (1989) Analysis of neutralizing antigenic sites on the surface of type A_{12} foot- and-mouth disease virus. J Virol 63: 2143–2151

Beck E, Strohmaier K (1987) Subtyping of european FMDV outbreak strains by nucleotide sequence determination. J Virol 61: 1621–1629

Beck E, Feil G, Strohmaier K (1983) The molecular basis of the antigenic variation of foot- and-mouth disease virus. EMBO J 2: 555–559

Bolwell C, Brown AL, Barnett PV, Campbell RO, Clarke BE, Parry NR, Ouldridge EJ, Brown F, Rowlands D (1989) Host cell selection of antigenic variants of foot- and-mouth disease virus. J Gen Virol 70: 45–57

Boothroyd JC, Harris TJR, Rowlands DJ, Lowe PA (1982) The nucleotide sequence of cDNA coding for the structural proteins of foot- and-mouth disease virus. Gene 17: 153–161

Brown F (1990) Picornaviruses. In: van Regenmortel MHV, Neurath AR (eds) Immunochemistry of viruses II. The basis for serodiagnosis and vaccines. Elsevier, Amsterdam, pp 153–169

Carrillo EC, Rieder Rojas E, Cavallaro L, Schiappacassi M, Campos R (1989) Modification of foot- and-mouth disease virus after serial passages in the presence of antiviral polyclonal sera. Virology 171: 599–601

Carrillo C, Plana J, Mascarella R, Bergadá J, Sobrino F (1990a) Genetic and phenotypic variability during replication of foot- and-mouth disease virus in swine. Virology 179: 890–892

Carrillo C, Dopazo J, Moya A, González M, Martínez MA, Saiz JC, Sobrino F (1990b) Comparison of vaccine strains and the virus causing the 1986 foot- and-mouth disease outbreak in Spain: epizootiological analysis. Virus Res 15: 45–56

Cheung A, DeLamarter J, Weiss S, Küpper H (1983) Comparison of the major antigenic determinants of different serotypes of foot- and-mouth disease virus. J Virol 48: 451–459

Clarke BE, Carroll AR, Rowlands DJ, Nicholson BH, Houghten RA, Lerner RA, Brown F (1983) Synthetic peptides mimic subtype specificity of foot- and-mouth disease virus. FEBS Lett 157: 261–264

Coffin JM (1990) Genetic variation in retroviruses. In: Kurstak E, Marusyk RG, Murphy FA, van Regenmortel MHV (eds) Applied virology research, vol 2. Plenum, New York, pp 11–33

Costa Giomi MP, Bergmann IE, Scodeller EA, Augé de Mello P, Gomes I, La Torre JL (1984) Heterogeneity of the polyribocytidylic acid tract in aphtovirus: biochemical and biological studies of viruses carrying polyribocytidylic acid tracts of different lengths. J Virol. 51: 799–805

Costa Giomi MP, Gomes I, Tiraboschi B, Augé de Mello P, Bergmann IE, Scodeller EA, La Torre JL (1988) Heterogeneity of the polyribocytidylic acid tract in aphtovirus: changes in the size of the poly (C) of viruses recovered from persistently infected cattle. Virology 162: 58–64

De la Torre JC, Dávila M, Sobrino F, Ortín J, Domingo E (1985) Establishment of cell lines persistently infected with foot-and-mouth disease virus. Virology 145: 24–35

De la Torre JC, Martínez-Salas E, Díez J, Villaverde A, Gebauer F, Rocha E, Dávila M, Domingo E (1988) Coevolution of cells and viruses in a persistent infection of foot- and-mouth disease virus in cell culture. J Virol 62: 2050–2058

De la Torre JC, De la Luna S, Díez J, Domingo E (1989a) Resistance to foot- and-mouth disease virus mediated by trans-acting cellular products. J Virol 63: 2385–2387

De la Torre JC, Martínez-Salas E, Díez J, Domingo E (1989b) Extensive cell heterogeneity during a persistent infection with foot- and-mouth disease virus. J Virol 63: 59–63

De la Torre JC, Wimmer E, Holland JJ (1990) Very high frequency of reversion to guanidine resistance in clonal pools of guanidine-dependent type I poliovirus. J Virol 64: 664–671

Díez J, Mateu MG, Domingo E (1989) Selection of antigenic variants of foot- and-mouth disease virus in the absence of antibodies, as revealed by an in situ assay. J Gen Virol 70: 3281–3289

Díez J, Hofner M, Domingo E, Donaldson AI (1990a) Foot- and-mouth disease virus strains isolated from persistently infected cell cultures are attenuated for mice and cattle. Virus Res 18: 3–8

Díez J, Dávila M, Escarmís C, Mateu MG, Domínguez J, Pérez JJ, Giralt E, Melero JA, Domingo E (1990b) Unique amino acid substitutions in the capsid proteins of foot-and-mouth disease virus from a persistent infection in cell culture. J Virol 64: 5519–5528

Domingo E (1989) RNA virus evolution and the control of viral disease. Prog Drug Res 33: 93–133

Domingo E, Holland JJ (1988) High error rates, population equilibrium and evolution of RNA replication systems. In: Domingo E, Holland JJ, Ahlquist P (eds) RNA genetic vol 3. CRC, Boca Raton, pp 3–36

Domingo E, Sabo D, Taniguchi T, Weissmann C (1978) Nucleotide sequence heterogeneity of an RNA phage population. Cell 13: 735–744

Domingo E, Dávila M, Ortín J (1980) Nucleotide sequence heterogeneity of the RNA from a natural population of foot-and-mouth disease virus. Gene 11: 333–346

Domingo E, Martínez-Salas E, Sobrino F, de la Torre JC, Portela A, Ortín J, López-Galíndez C, Pérez Breña P, Villanueva N, Nájera R, VandePol S, Steinhauer D, de Polo N, Holland J (1985) The quasispecies (extremely heterogeneous) nature of viral RNA genome population: biological relevance—a review. Gene 40: 1–8

Domingo E, Mateu MG, Martinez MA, Dopazo J, Moya A, Sobrino F (1990) Genetic variability and antigenic diversity of foot- and-mouth disease virus. In: Kurstak E, Marusyk RG, Murphy FA, van Regenmortel MHV (eds) Applied virology research, vol 2. Plenum, New York, pp 233–266

Dopazo J, Sobrino F, Palma EL, Domingo E, Moya A (1988) Gene encoding capsid protein VP1 of foot- and-mouth disease virus: a quasispecies model of molecular evolution. Proc Natl Acad Sci USA 85: 6811–6815

Eggers HJ, Tamm I (1965) Coxsackie A9 virus: mutation from drug dependence to drug independence. Science 148: 97–98

Eigen M (1971) Self-organization of matter and the evolution of biological macromolecules. Naturwissenschaften 58: 465–523

Eigen M, Biebricher CK (1988) Sequence space and quasispecies distribution. In: Domingo E, Holland JJ, Ahlquist P (eds) RNA genetics, vol 3. CRC, Boca Raton, pp 211–245

Eigen M, Schuster P (1979) The hypercycle—a principle of natural self-organization. Springer, Berlin Heidelberg New York

Eigen M, Mc Caskill J, Schuster P (1989) The molecular quasispecies. In: Prigogine I, Rice SA (eds) Advances in chemical physics, vol 75. Wiley, New York, pp 149–263

Fagg RH, Hyslop NSG (1966) Isolation of a variant strain of foot- and-mouth disease virus (type O) during passage in partly immunized cattle. Hyg 64: 397–404

Fox G, Parry NR, Barnett PV, McGinn B, Rowlands DJ, Brown F (1989) The cell attachment site of foot-and-mouth disease virus includes the amino acid sequences RGD (arginine-glycine-aspartic acid). J Gen Virol 70: 625–637

Gebauer F, de la Torre JC, Gomes I, Mateu MG, Barahona H, Tiraboschi B, Bergmann I, Augé de Mello P, Domingo E (1988) Rapid selection of genetic and antigenic variants of foot- and-mouth disease virus during persistence in cattle. J Virol 62: 2041–2049

Heinz BV, Rueckert RR, Shepard DA, Dutko FJ, McKinlay MA, Fancher M, Rossmann MG, Berger J Smith TJ (1989) Genetic and molecular analyses of spontaneous mutants of human rhinovirus 14 that are resistant to an antiviral compound. J Virol 63: 2476–2485

Holland JJ, Spindler K, Horodyski F, Grabau E, Nichol S, VandePol S (1982) Rapid evolution of RNA genomes. Science 215: 1577–1585

Holland JJ, Domingo E, de la Torre JC, Steinhauer DA (1990) Mutation frequencies at defined single codon sites in vesicular stomatitis virus and poliovirus can be increased only slightly by chemical mutagenesis. J Virol 64: 3960–3962

King AMQ (1988) Genetic recombination in positive strand RNA viruses. In: Domingo E, Holland JJ, Ahlquist P (eds) RNA genetics, vol 2. CRC, Boca Raton, pp 149–165

King AMQ, Underwood BO, McCahon D, Newman JWI, Brown F (1981) Biochemical identification of viruses causing the 1981 outbreak of foot-and-mouth disease in UK. Nature 293: 497–480

Kitson JD, McCahon D, Belsham GJ (1990) Sequence analysis of monoclonal antibody resistant mutants of type O foot-and-mouth disease virus: evidence for the involvement of the three surface exposed capsid proteins in four antigenic sites. Virology 179: 26–34

Kleid DG, Yansura D, Small B, Dowbenko D, Moore DM, Grubman MJ, McKercher PD, Morgan DO, Robertson BH, Bachrach HL (1981) Cloned viral protein vaccine for foot-and-mouth disease: responses in cattle and swine. Science 214: 1125–1129

Kurstak E, Marusyk RG, Murphy FA, van Regenmortel MHV (eds) (1990) Applied virology research, vol 2. Plenum, New York

Kurz C, Forss S, Küpper H, Strohmaier K, Schaller H (1981) Nucleotide sequence and corresponding amino acid sequence of the gene for the major antigen of foot-and-mouth disease virus. Nucleic Acids Res 9: 1919–1931

Makoff AJ, Paynter CA, Rowlands DJ, Boothroyd JC (1982) Comparison of the amino acid sequence of the major immunogen from three serotypes of foot-and-mouth disease virus. Nucleic Acids Res 10: 8285–8295

Martínez MA, Carrillo C, Plana J, Mascarella R, Bergadá J, Palma EL, Domingo E, Sobrino F (1988) Genetic and immunogenic variations among closely related isolates of foot-and-mouth disease virus. Gene 62: 75–84

Martinez MA, Carrillo C, Gonzalez-Candelas F, Moya A, Domingo E, Sobrino F (1991a) Fitness alteration of foot-and-mouth disease virus mutants: measurement of adaptability of viral quasispecies J Virol 65: 3954–3957

Martnez MA, Hernandez J, Piccone ME, Palma EL, Domingo E, Knowles NJ, Mateu MG (1991b) Two mechanism of antigenic diversification of foot-and-mouth disease virus. Virology 184: 695–706

Mateu MG, Rocha E, Vicente O, Vayredà F, Navalpotro C, Andreu D, Pedroso E, Giralt E, Enjuanes L, Domingo E (1987) Reactivity with monoclonal antibodies of viruses from an episode of foot- and-mouth disease. Virus Res. 8: 261–274

Mateu MG, da Silva JL, Rocha E, de Brum DL, Alonso A, Enjuanes L, Domingo E, Barahona H (1988) Extensive antigenic heterogeneity of foot-and-mouth disease virus of serotype C. Virology 167: 113–124

Mateu MG, Martínez MA, Rocha E, Andreu D, Parejo J, Giralt E, Sobrino F, Domingo E (1989) Implications of a quasispecies genome structure: effects of frequent, naturally occurring amino acid substitutions on the antigenicity of foot-and-mouth disease virus. Proc Natl Acad Sci USA 86: 5883–5887

Mateu MG, Martínez MA, Capucci L, Andreu D, Giralt E, Sobrino F, Brocchi E, Domingo E (1990) A single amino acid substitution affects multiple overlapping epitopes in the major antigenic site of foot-and-mouth disease virus of serotype C. J Gen Virol 71: 629–637

Ouldridge EJ, Parry NR, Barnett PV, Bolwell C, Rowlands DJ, Brown F, Bittle JL, Houghten RA, Lerner RA (1986) Comparison of the structures of the major antigenic sites of foot-and-mouth disease viruses of two different serotypes. In: Brown F, Chanock RM, Lerner RA (eds) Vaccines'86. Cold Spring Harbor Laboratory, New York, pp 45–49

Palmenberg A (1989) Sequence alignments of picornavirus capsid proteins. In: Semler BL, Ehrenfeld E (eds) Molecular aspects of picornavirus infection and detection. American Society for Microbiology, Washington, pp 211–241

Parry NR, Barnett PV, Ouldridge EJ, Rowlands DJ, Brown F (1989) Neutralizing epitopes of type O foot-and-mouth disease virus. II. Mapping three conformational sites with synthetic peptide reagents. J Gen Virol 70: 1493–1503

Parry NR, Fox G, Rowlands D, Brown F, Fry E, Acharya R, Logan D, Stuart D (1990) Structural and serological evidence for a novel mechanism of antigenic variation in foot-and-mouth disease virus. Nature 347: 569–572

Pereira HG (1981) Foot-and-mouth disease. In: Gibbs EPJ (ed) Virus diseases of food animals, Vol 2. Academic, New York, pp 333–363

Piccone ME, Kaplan G, Giavedoni L, Domingo E, Palma EL (1988) VP1 of serotype C foot-and-mouth disease virus: long-term conservation of sequences. J Virol 62: 1469–1473

Rowlands DJ, Clarke BE, Carroll AR, Brown F, Nicholson BH, Bittle JL, Houghten RA, Lerner RA (1983) Chemical basis of antigenic variation in foot-and-mouth disease virus. Nature 306: 694–697

Sobrino F, Dávila M, Ortín J, Domingo E (1983) Multiple genetic variants arise in the course of replication of foot-and-mouth disease viruse in cell cultures. Virology 128: 310–318

Sobrino F, Palma EL, Beck E, Dávila M, de la Torre JC, Negro P, Villanueva N, Ortin J, Domingo E (1986) Fixation of mutants in the viral genome during an outbreak of foot-and-mouth disease: heterogeneity and rate variations. Gene 50: 149–159

Steinhauer D, Holland JJ (1987) Rapid evolution of RNA viruses. Annu Rev Microbiol 41: 409–433

Strohmaier K, Franze R, Adam KH (1982) Location and characterization of the antigenic portion of the FMDV immunizing protein. J Gen Virol 59: 295–306

Temin HM (1989) Is HIV unique or merely different? J AIDS 2: 1–9

Thomas AAM, Woortmeijer RJ, Puijk W, Barteling SJ (1988) Antigenic sites of foot-and-mouth disease virus type A10. J Virol 62: 2782–2789

Timoney JF, Gillespie JH, Scott FW, Barlough JE (1988) Hagan and Bruner's microbiology and infectious diseases of domestic animals. Cornell University Press, Ithaca, pp 647–667

Villanueva N, Dávila M, Ortín J, Domingo E (1983) Molecular cloning of cDNA from foot- and-mouth disease virus C_1-Santa Pau (C-S8). Sequence of protein VP1 coding segment. Gene 23: 185–194

Villaverde A, Martínez-Salas E, Domingo E (1988) 3D gene of foot- and-mouth disease virus. Conservation by convergence of average sequences. J Mol Biol 204: 771–776

Villaverde A, Martínez MA, Sobrino F, Dopazo J, Moya A, Domingo E (1991) Fixation of mutations at the VP1 gene of foot-and-mouth disease virus: can quasispecies define a transient molecular clock? Gene 103: 147–153

Weddell GN, Yansura DG, Dowbenko DJ, Hoatlin ME, Grubman MJ, Moore DM, Kleid DG (1985) Sequence variation in the gene of the immunogenic capsid protein VP1 of foot-and-mouth disease virus type A. Proc Natl Acad Sci USA 82: 2618–2622

Wu TT, Kabat EA (1970) An analysis of the sequences of the variable regions of Bence-Jones proteins and myeloma light chains and their implications for antibody complementarity. J Exp Med 132: 211–250

Zibert A, Maass G, Strebel K, Falk MM, Beck E (1990) Infectious foot-and-mouth disease virus derived from a cloned full-length cDNA. J Virol 64: 2467–2473

Genetic Diversity and Rapid Evolution of Poliovirus in Human Hosts

L. KINNUNEN, T. PÖYRY, and T. HOVI

1 Introduction

Rapid changes in phenotypic markers of polioviruses during replication in man were already reported in the 1950s but studies examining the mode and rate of genetic variation of the viruses only started in the 1980s. Recent studies have revealed that like other RNA viruses, polioviruses show typical features of a quasispecies with a multitude of variants present in a host at a given time and drifts in the composition of the mixture in relation to time. In this review we discuss the pattern of genetic variation of polioviruses and its relation to virus-host relationships.

2 Polioviruses and Poliovirus Infections in Man

Polioviruses are members of the enterovirus subgroup in the *Picornaviridae* family. Polioviruses have a single-stranded messenger-sense RNA genome of about 7440 nucleotides and an icosahedral capsid consisting of 60 copies of

---

Enterovirus Laboratory, Department of Virology and Molecular Biology Unit, National Public Health Institute, Mannerheimintie 166, 00300 Helsinki, Finland

Current Topics in Microbiology and Immunology, Vol. 176

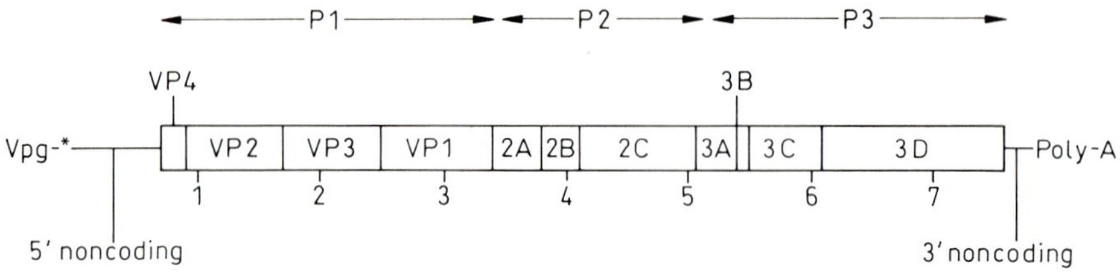

Fig. 1. Genome organization of poliovirus. The *top line* shows the genomic regions P1, P2, and P3. Untranslated regions are shown as a *single line* and translated products as *open boxes*

four structural proteins. A small protein VPg is covalently linked to the 5′-end of the RNA followed by a unique 750-nucleotide noncoding region (5′NCR), one long reading frame about 6600 nucleotides, a short 70-nucleotide 3′NCR, and a genomic poly A tail. The coding region can be divided into three functionally distinct domains P1, P2, and P3 (Fig. 1). The coding region of the genome is translated as a large polyprotein and cleaved by virus-coded proteases to eleven proteins: VP1, VP2, VP3, and VP4 are capsid proteins; nonstructural proteins 2A and 3C are proteases; 3D is a polymerase; 2C and the genome-linked protein VPg (3B) are involved in replication events; the function of proteins 2B and 3A is so far unknown (Fig. 1). Replication of the RNA takes place in the cytoplasm and involves at least two virus-coded proteins. Poliovirus infection is typically lytic and relatively efficient: 10^4–10^5 daughter viruses are produced per infected cell.

Man is the only natural host of polioviruses and transmission takes place mainly through the fecal-oral route. There are some differences in the epidemiological characteristics of the three serotypes of poliovirus, e.g., poliovirus type 1 is more often associated with paralytic poliomyelitis than serotypes 2 or 3. The principal site of virus replication in the body is the gastrointestinal mucosa and the adjacent lymphoid tissues. Paralytic poliomyelitis, the "typical" disease caused by the polioviruses is actually a relatively rare (less than 1%) consequence of infection. Neutralizing antibodies appear in the circulation 1–2 weeks after onset of infection but viral replication in the intestines usually continues for several weeks thereafter. Immunity following natural infection is considered to be lifelong as regards protection from the disease, but asymptomatic reinfections have been described. Systematic use of vaccines, developed more than three decades ago, has practically eliminated poliomyelitis from the Americas, Europe, and several other countries; however, in many developing countries poliomyelitis continues to be a serious public health problem.

3 Variation Within a Serotype

3.1 General Aspects

All three serotypes of poliovirus, showing about 70% of nucleotide identity (TOYODA et al. 1984), have a common phylogenetic origin. While extensive amino acid variation within a serotype can be seen in most of the known antigenic sites, all strains of poliovirus can be easily classified into one of the three serotypes by using hyperimmune animal antisera and the neutralization test. Information concerning serotype-specific antigenic sites and the corresponding genomic regions is incomplete as the entire sequence of the capsid coding region of the genome is known only for a couple of strains in each serotype.

Partial RNA sequence is known at selected genomic regions for a number of strains, and our discussion is based mainly on this information. The oldest strains in this collection go back to the late 1930s or early 1940s when they were inoculated into monkeys. We thus have in principle a time span of about five decades of poliovirus evolution in man to follow. Unfortunately, the sequenced strains are not evenly distributed within this range of time and are not representative of different geographic regions either. The picture we can construct today is therefore rather fragmentary. However, several trends are already obvious from this information.

The methods used to demonstrate variation and evolution of poliovirus are numerous. T1 oligonucleotide mapping and monoclonal antibodies have been used to show heterogeneity between strains belonging to the same serotype (NOTTAY et al. 1981; MINOR 1982; CRAINIC et al. 1983). The rapid evolution rate of polioviruses (CRAINIC et al. 1983; MINOR et al. 1986; HUOVILAINEN et al. 1988; KINNUNEN et al. 1990), however, limits the use of these methods in epidemiological studies and in systematic "population genetics" of polioviruses. In this respect, oligonucleotide mapping can be used only to study closely related strains (KEW et al. 1981; TAKEDA et al. 1984; TRENT et al. 1989); the fact that one amino acid replacement is sufficient to modify or abolish neutralization by a given monoclonal antibody also limits the usefulness of these reagents. Partial RNA sequencing is the most direct method to assess variation, allowing the detection of even remote epidemiological linkeages (RICO-HESSE et al. 1987; PÖYRY et al. 1990).

Within a serotype, polioviruses form a population of extremely heterogenous genomes, a so-called quasispecies (HOLLAND et al. 1982). Virus strains isolated from one individual or even a single specimen are genetically and antigenically different (KEW et al. 1981; MINOR et al. 1986; HUOVILAINEN et al. 1987, 1988; KINNUNEN et al. 1990). The degree of variation increases when isolates from different host individuals within an epidemic, or from geographically more distinct areas are compared. As an example a dendrogram based on nucleotide differences in the whole 5′ noncoding region (749 nucleotides) was constructed. Four strains from one individual (C), isolates collected from other individuals during the outbreak in Finland in 1984, nearest known relatives to these strains

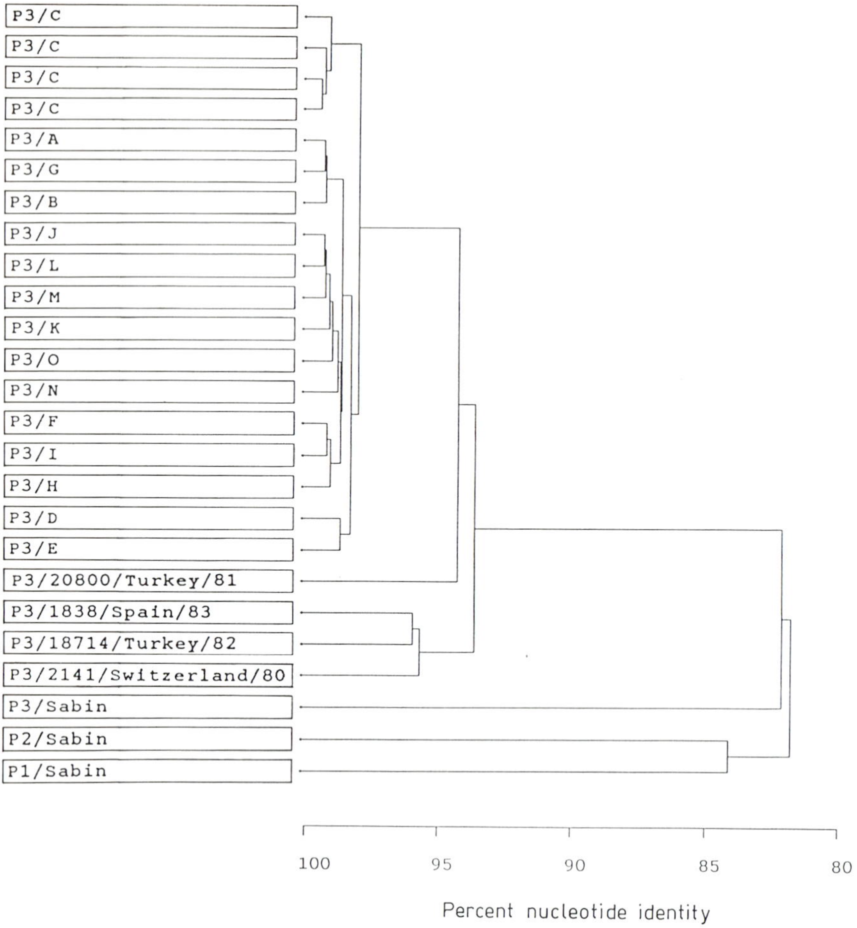

Fig. 2. Genetic relationships among type 3 polioviruses and type 1 and type 2 Sabin strain shown as a dendrogram based on nucleotide identity in the entire 5′ noncoding region. A–O represent strains collected during one epidemic. From one individual four strains were isolated and they are marked by the same symbol (C). Other wild-type 3 strains shown are the nearest known relatives of the epidemic virus. Sabin strains illustrate the distance to epidemiologically unrelated strains

isolated outside Finland, and the vaccine strains (Sabin) are compared and show different ranges of relative nucleotide substitutions (Fig. 2).

3.2 Variation of the Noncoding Regions

As a whole, the noncoding regions of poliovirus RNA are the most conserved parts of the genome between serotypes, e.g., as regards the three Sabin vaccine strains the first 650 nucleotides are $>85\%$ identical and the last 70 nucleotides before the poly A tail are >95% identical (TOYODA et al. 1984). The last 100 nucleotides or so before the polyprotein initiation codon form a striking exception to the general conservation of the noncoding regions. This so-called "hypervariable region" is, in fact, the most variable region of the genome and shows as much as or more than 50% interstrain difference between and within serotypes (TOYODA et al. 1984; PÖYRY et al. 1990). Interestingly, neither the relatively conserved 650 nucleotides of the 5′NCR nor the 100-nucleotide hypervariable region shows any signs of serotype specificity. A dendrogram comparing the first 650 nucleotides of the 5′NCR from several representatives of all three serotypes shows no grouping according to serotype (Fig. 3).

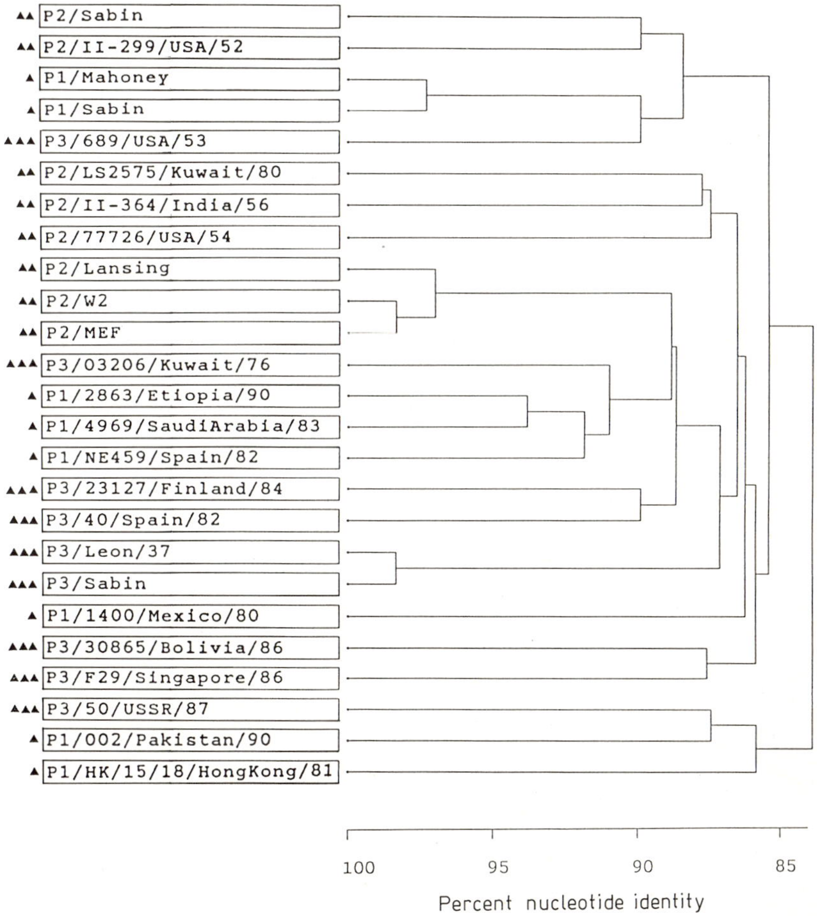

Fig. 3. Genetic relatinships among type 1, 2, and 3 polioviruses shown as a dendrogram based on nucleotide identity of the first 650 nucleotides in the 5′ noncoding region. ▲, serotype 1; ▲▲, serotype 2; ▲▲▲, serotype 3

Secondary structure models that share several identical features have been constructed for the conserved part of the 5′NCR of poliovirus RNA (PILIPENKO et al. 1989; SKINNER et al. 1989; RIVERA et al. 1988). Sequence variation seen in this region does not interfere with the proposed hairpin-loop structures (PÖYRY et al., manuscript). Conserved secondary structure may be relevant to the biological functions assigned to this genomic region e.g., internal initiation of translation, neurovirulence and replication (TRONO et al. 1988; BIENKOWSKA-SZEWCZYK and EHRENFELD 1988; PELLETIER et al. 1988; DEL ANGEL et al. 1989; ANDINO et al. 1990).

3.3 Variation of the Coding Region

The structural proteins and especially the antigenic sites are variable between and within serotypes whereas the nonstructural proteins are more conserved (Table 1). Variation can be envisaged to be advantageous for the virus in the regions of the capsid proteins which are targets of immunological surveillance, while it could be dangerous to the function of the nonstructural proteins which are mostly enzymes.

In the noncoding regulatory regions of RNA the need to maintain the secondary structure is one important factor limiting sequence variation. In the coding region the variation is mainly limited because of the requirement for a functional polypeptide structure. Most of the genetic variation seen in the coding region is silent, i.e., it does not lead to amino acid replacements, and in the capsid protein genes mutations resulting in amino acid replacements are concentrated at the known antigenic sites and the amino terminal 35 amino acids of VP1.

Table 1. Amino acid difference of poliovirus proteins between five strains[a]

Genomic region	Protein	Amino acid difference (%)
P1	VP4	≦7
P1	VP2	≦22
P1	VP3	≦19
P1	VP1	≦33
P2	2A	≦13
P2	2B	≦16
P2	2C	≦7
P3	3A	≦3
P3	3B	≦9
P3	3C	≦7
P3	3D	≦6

[a] P1/Sabin (NOMOTO et al. 1982), P2/Sabin (TOYODA et al. 1984) P2/Lansing (LA MONICA et al. 1986), P3/Sabin (TOYODA et al. 1984) P3/Finland/23127/84 (HUGHES et al. 1986)

The sequences of an interval of 150 nucleotides encoding parts of the capsid protein VP1 and the protease 2A has been used to determine variation among poliovirus type 1 and 3 strains in nature (RICO-HESSE et al. 1987; PÖYRY et al. 1990). The maximum divergence both between 60 wild poliovirus type 1 and 18 poliovirus type 3 strains tested independently was about 22%. The difference between Sabin 1 and wild type 1 strains varied between 15% and 22% and the difference between Sabin 3 and all studied wild type 3 strains was about 27%. This is remarkable, as the three Sabin vaccine strains diverge from each other only by 29% at this region of the genome. In Fig. 4 the genetic relationships of 12

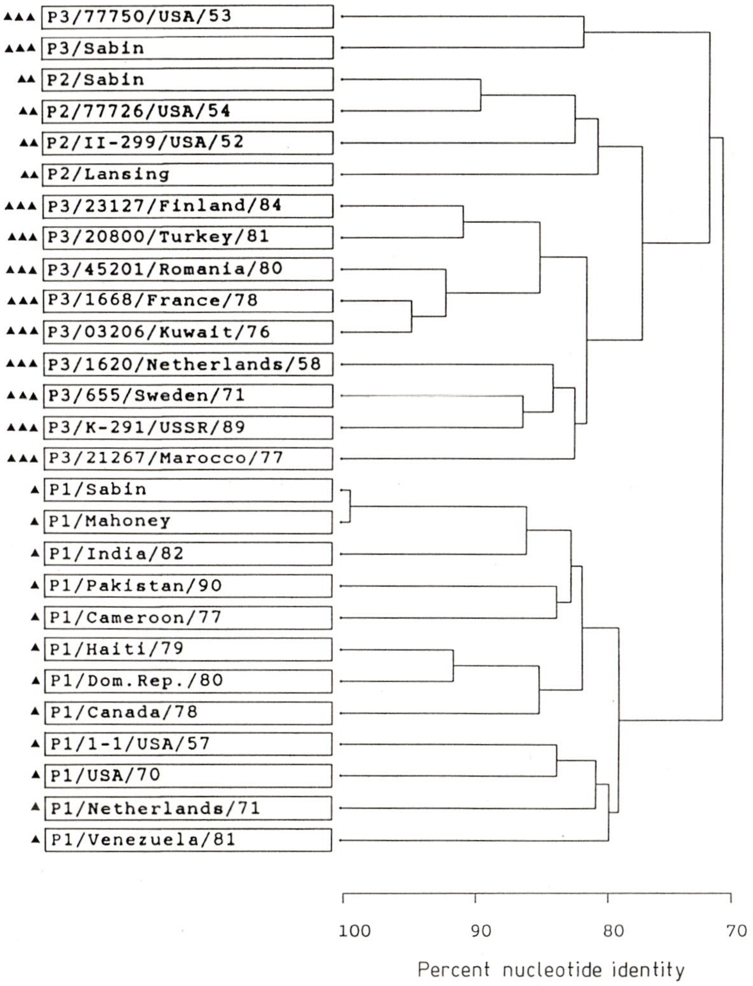

Fig. 4. Genetic relationships among type 1, 2, and 3 poliovirus shown as a dendrogram based on nucleotide identity in the region of 150 nucleotides covering the VP1-2A junction. ▲, serotype 1; ▲▲, serotype 2; ▲▲▲, serotype 3

type 1 strains, 4 type 2 strains, and 11 type 3 strains are compared. Poliovirus strains belonging to serotype 1 are clustered together, but serotypes 2 and 3 can not be separated in this analysis.

It is typical of polioviruses that several genotypes within a serotype cocirculate at a given time. Epidemiologically related strains usually form a cluster more or less clearly separated from the other strains. RICO-HESSE et al. (1987) defined a 15% difference in the nucleotide sequence of the VP1-2A region, a likely limit for a reliable epidemiological linkage. The remarkable difference between Sabin 3 vaccine strain and the present European strains could be due to geographic or temporal reasons, or both. The parental type 3-Leon strain was isolated in the USA in 1937.

4 Evolution

4.1 Generation of Variation

Mutation and recombination are the mechanistic alternatives on which the genetic variation observed in poliovirus populations is based. The probability of one nucleotide mutating during a single replication cycle through, for example, substitution or recombination is defined as the mutation rate. The estimates of poliovirus mutation rate vary between 10^{-3} and $> 10^{-5}$ (PINCUS et al. 1986; EMINI et al. 1983; DIAMOND et al. 1985; BLONDEL et al. 1986; PARVIN et al. 1986) for poliovirus structural genes. Recombination between poliovirus strains has been demonstrated (ROMANOVA et al. 1980; KING et al. 1982) and it is considered to take place by a copy choice mechanism (KIRKEGAARD and BALTIMORE 1986). Interserotypic recombinants are readily isolated from vaccinees who have received the oral trivalent live virus Sabin vaccine (OPV) (KEW and NOTTAY 1984; MINOR et al. 1986). This suggests that recombination is possible and apparently advantageous under these conditions. One can envisage that, as the vaccinee gets simultaneously an attenuated representative of all three poliovirus serotypes (each of which has a low fitness, i.e., a low relative capacity for progeny production in a natural host as compared to a wild-type virus), recombination makes it possible to quickly create a new genotype without some of the attenuating mutations and thus with a higher fitness. In a natural infection in which the host is usually infected by one serotype only, it is difficult to detect or study recombination but this is likely to happen between closely related genomes even more frequently than that between the three serotypes in OPV vaccines.

A virus population lies between two fires; it must maintain enough variation to optimize its adaptability to changing environments, but on the other hand, it should not risk its immediate fitness in the present environment by overproduction of mutations. A high mutation rate leads to accumulation of deleterious mutations (genetic load) into the genome (MULLER 1950) and thus to a lowered immediate fitness (CHAO 1990). Recombination is probably the most rapid means to generate the genotype that is best adapted to a given environment. One could assume that capability to use recombination allows higher mutation rates with both immediate fitness and adaptability being kept as high as possible.

4.2 The Role of Selection and Chance in Virus Evolution

The reason why viruses are readily adapted to their environment is most likely natural selection: those which in the existing variation are most fit for the present environment will be enriched. Selection can operate because the variants have different fitness in a particular environment.

Environments vary in time and space, and selective forces change in respect to both. When the environment of a virus population changes (e.g., antibodies are formed by the host individual) new antigenic variants can overgrow the old ones (HUOVILAINEN et al. 1987, 1988). In one host organism there are numerous micro-environments (habitats) with diverse selective forces affecting the virus population, e.g., invasion of different tissues and cell types may result in selection of different properties. For example, while analyzing the evolution of type 3 poliovirus we found that sensitivity of one of the major antigenic sites in the virion to the host serine protease trypsin, appeared to be a positive selecting property in some individuals (HUOVILAINEN et al. 1987; MINOR et al. 1987). Sensitivity to trypsin is a conserved property among type 2 and type 3 poliovirus strains at this otherwise variable surface loop (MINOR et al. 1987; ROIVAINEN and HOVI 1988).

Selection can operate with a varying intensity through many chemical, physical, and biological factors at any stage during the virus life cycle. Transmission from one host to another, survival outside the body, or possible competition for resources with other viruses are further situations where selection could operate.

There is no simple correlation between the mutation rate and the evolution rate of a given RNA virus. All RNA viruses have about equally high mutation rates but the rate by which mutations are fixed in the population varies. The observed evolution rate can vary in different virus species but it is also influenced by virus-host interactions during infection by a given virus. Although virus population is a pool of variants the probability for one mutation to be fixed into the population without positive selection is low and the same average sequence will be maintained (SPINDLER et al. 1982; STEINHAUER et al. 1989; DE LA TORRE and HOLLAND 1990).

The role of genetic changes caused by chance, i.e., genetic drift in virus evolution is difficult to assess. It can be assumed that when the number of replication cycles increases the number of mutations being fixed by chance increases too. Another factor that randomly directs evolution operates when a population is established by a few founders carrying only a small sample of the variation from a larger population. This so called "founder principle" or "bottleneck effect" could occur when the virus is transmitted from one host individual to an other. In this situation, different paths of evolution may be initiated depending on the original content of the sample.

4.3 Evolution of Poliovirus

During an epidemic, nucleotide substitution rates of 1%–2% per year for wild poliovirus strains have been suggested, based on oligonucleotide mapping (NOTTAY et al. 1981). By the same method similar rates of base substitutions of the Sabin vaccine strain were observed during virus passage in only one or two individuals (KEW et al. 1981). Genetic and antigenic evolution of the type 3 vaccine straln during the period of excretion by a primary vaccinee have also been reported (MINOR et al. 1986).

Antigenic and genetic properties of wild type 3 poliovirus strains isolated during the Finnish epidemic of 1984–1985 were studied. A panel of nine neutralizing monoclonal antibodies was used to analyze the antigenic properties of 188 plaque-purified strains from 17 fecal specimens, derived from eight people during a 2-month period. It was demonstrated that a human host excretes a mixture of antigenic variants and that the composition of the mixture changes rapidly during infection in one individual, indicating antigenic evolution. The apparent direction of this evolution varied, as judged by neutralization of the variants by a set of vaccine strain-specific monoclonal antibodies (KINNUNEN et al. 1990). The fact that evolution occurs so rapidly in one individual is a consequence of selection. The various paths of evolution can be a result of different composition of antibody specificities in different individuals, or a consequence of pure chance. Chance can play a role by selecting from alternative, equally good ways to escape from a similar immunological pressure, or chance can act through a "founder effect".

Silent mutation rates were used to estimate the overall evolution rate of the virus genome as silent mutation frequency between different genes is approximately similar for all genes, even when the amino acid-altering mutation frequency is different (KIMURA 1981; HAYASHIDA et al. 1985). In our study, sequential specimens collected from one individual showed maximally 0.5% of silent mutations, which corresponds to about 30–40 silent nucleotide substitutions for the whole genome during a few weeks observation period. The silent nucleotide substitution frequency between specimens from different individuals was usually between 0.8% and 2%, which corresponds to about 60–150 silent nucleotide substitutions for the whole genome.

The phylogenetic relationships of 36 strains from 15 persons collected during the epidemic were studied by the DNAPARS program (JOSEPH FELSENSTEIN 1990, University of California, Berkeley, California) and are shown as an unrooted tree (Fig. 5). The tree is based on nucleotide sequences in regions of RNA coding for the known antigenic sites. Strains derived from one person often form

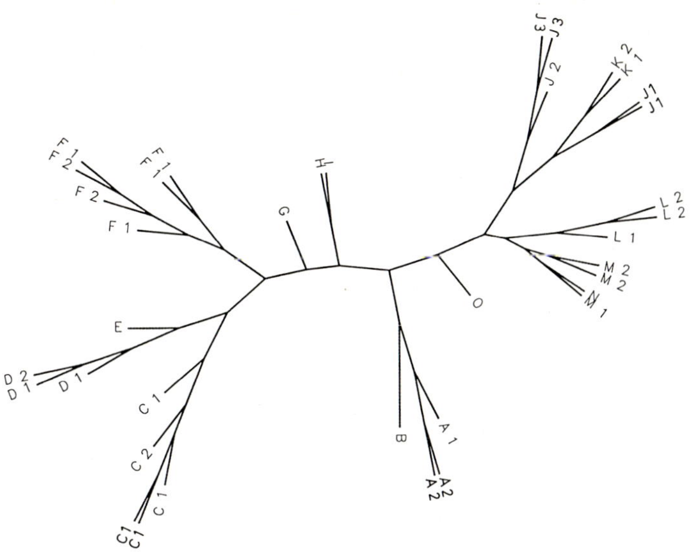

Fig. 5. An unrooted tree constructed by the maximum parsimony method showing the phylogenetic relationships between 36 strains collected during an epidemic from 15 persons. The tree is based on 637 nucleotides in a discontinuous region coding for the known major antigenic sites. Each strain (ends of the branches) isolated from a given individual is marked by the same letter. The number indicates the sequential specimen from which the strain is isolated. The number of divergence points between two strains indicates the "distance" of genetic relationship

one branch in the phylogenetic tree, i.e., A, C, D, F, and L. Strains from the individual marked K seem to be phylogenetically closest relatives to the first specimen of J. It could be assumed that J, who was a playmate of K and of her brother L, has transmitted the virus to K in the beginning of infection. Strains from individual N also seem to have the closest relative in the first specimen of M. The evolutionary relationships suggest that spreading of the outbreak in the host population took place before most of the variation was generated. A likely explanation could be that the transmission in the host population is so rapid that the original strain will reach most susceptible hosts before they are exposed to the variants generated during the following weeks.

5 Conclusions

The genetic variation of poliovirus demonstrates typical features of quasi-species which are shared by all studied RNA viruses. Relatively long infection episodes in a given host individual enables the poliovirus to search for new potentially successful genomic constellations, as reflected by the branched structure of phylogenetic trees constructed from strains isolated from a single host. On the other hand, rapid spreading of the virus between hosts sharing close contacts limits the spreading of the later variants. Hence, only very few of the new branches seen in a host individual represent a founder of new genetic lineages, but once generated, several of them may cocirculate simultaneously during an epidemic.

Mutations due to "errors" of the RNA polymerase are complemented by recombination as fuel for genetic variation. Immunological pressure and other selection forces during the several weeks or months infection episode in a given host, as well as chance in the transmission of the infection from one host to another, are responsible for enrichment of the variants that we isolate from clinical specimens.

References

Andino R, Rieckhof GE, Trono D, Baltimore D (1990) Substitutions in the protease ($3C^{pro}$) gene of poliovirus can suppress a mutation in the 5′ noncoding region. J Virol 64: 607–612

Bienkowska-Szewczyk K, Ehrenfeld E (1988) An internal 5′ noncoding region required for translation of poliovirus RNA in vitro. J Virol 62: 3068–3072

Blondel B, Crainic R, Fichot O, Dufraisse G, Candrea A, Diamond D, Girard M, Horaud F (1986) Mutations conferring resistance to neutralization with monoclonal antibodies in type 1 poliovirus can be located outside or inside the antibody binding site. J Virol 57: 81–90

Chao L (1990) Fitness of RNA virus decreased by Muller's ratchet. Nature 348: 454–455

Crainic R, Couillin P, Blondel B, Cabau N, Boue A, Horodniceanu F (1983) Natural variation of poliovirus neutralization epitopes. Infect Immun 41: 1217–1225

Del Angel RM, Papavassiliou AG, Fernandez-Tomas C, Silverstein SJ, Racaniello VR (1989) Cell proteins bind to multiple sites within the 5′ untranslated region of poliovirus RNA. Proc Natl Acad Sci USA 86: 8299–8303

De la Torre JC, Holland JJ (1990) RNA virus quasispecies populations can suppress vastly superior mutant progeny. J Virol 64: 6278–6281

Diamond DC, Jameson BA, Bonin J, Kohara M, Abe M, Itoh H, Komatsu T, Arita M, Kuge S, Nomoto A, Osterhaus ADME, Crainic R, Wimmer E (1985) Antigenic variation and resistance to neutralization in poliovirus type 1. Science 229: 1090–1093

Emini EA, Kao S, Lewis AJ, Crainic R, Wimmer E (1983) Functional basis of poliovirus neutralization determined with monospecific neutralizing antibodies. J Virol 46: 466–474

Hayashida H, Toh H, Kikuno R, Miyata T (1985) Evolution of influenza virus genes. Mol Biol Evol 2: 289–303

Holland J, Spindler K, Horodyski F, Grabau E, Nichol S, VandePol S (1982) Rapid evolution of RNA genomes. Science 215: 1577–1585

Hughes PJ, Evans DMA, Minor PD, Schild GC, Almond JW, Stanway G (1986) The nucleotide sequence of a type 3 poliovirus isolated during a recent outbreak of poliomyelitis in Finland. J Gen Virol 67: 2093–2102

Huovilainen A, Hovi T, Kinnunen L, Takkinen K, Ferguson M, Minor PD (1987) Evolution of poliovirus during an outbreak: sequential type 3 poliovirus isolates from several persons show shifts of neutralization determinants. J Gen Virol 68: 1373–1378

Huovilainen A, Kinnunen L, Ferguson M, Hovi T (1988) Antigenic variation among 173 strains of type 3 poliovirus isolated in Finland during the 1984 to 1985 outbreak. J Gen Virol 69: 1941–1948

Kew OM, Nottay BK (1984) Evolution of oral poliovirus vaccine strain in humans occurs by both mutation and intermolecular recombination. In: Chanock R, Lerner R (eds) Modern approaches to vaccines. Cold Spring Harbor, New York

Kew OM, Nottay BK, Hatch MH, Nakano JH, Obijeski JF (1981) Multiple genetic changes can occur in the oral poliovaccines upon replication in humans. J Gen Virol 56: 337–347

Kimura M (1981) Estimation of evolutionary distances between homologous nucleotide sequences. Proc Natl Acad Sci USA 78: 454–458

King AMQ, McCahon D, Slade WR, Newman JWI (1982) Recombination in RNA. Cell 29: 921–928

Kinnunen L, Huovilainen A, Pöyry T, Hovi T (1990) Rapid molecular evolution of wild type 3 poliovirus during infection in individual hosts. J Gen Virol 71: 317–324

Kirkegaard K, Baltimore D (1986) The mechanism of RNA recombination in poliovirus. Cell 47: 433–443

La Monica N, Meriam c, Racaniello VR (1986) Mapping of sequences required for mouse neurovirulence of poliovirus type 2 Lansing. J Virol 57: 515–525

Minor PD (1982) Characterization of strains of type 3 poliovirus by oligonucleotide mapping. J Gen Virol 59: 307–317

Minor PD, John A, Ferguson M, Icenogle JP (1986) Antigenic and molecular evolution of the vaccine strain of type 3 poliovirus during the period of excretion by a primary vaccine. J Gen Virol 67: 693–706

Minor PD, Ferguson M, Phillips A, Magrath DI, Huovilainen A, Hovi T (1987) Conservation in vivo of protease cleavage sites in antigenic sites of poliovirus. J Gen Virol 68: 1857–1865

Muller HJ (1950) Our load of mutations. Am J Hum Genet 2: 111–176

Nomoto A, Omata T, Toyoda H, Kuge S, Horie S, Kataoka Y, Genba Y, Nakano Y, Imura N (1982) Complete nucleotide sequence of the attenuated poliovirus Sabin 1 strain genome. Proc Natl Acad Sci USA 79: 5793–5797

Nottay BK, Kew OM, Hatch MH, Heyward JT, Obijeski JF (1981) Molecular variation of type 1 vaccine-related and wild poliovirus during replication in humans. Virology 108: 405–423

Parvin JD, Moscona A, Pan A, Leider JM, Palese P (1986) Measurement of the mutation rates of animal viruses: influenza A virus and poliovirus type 1. J Virol 59: 377–383

Pelletier J, Kaplan G, Racaniello VR, Sonenberg N (1988) Cap-independent translation of poliovirus mRNA is conferred by sequence elements within the 5′ non-coding region. Mol Cell Biol 8: 1103–1112

Pilipenko EV, Blinov VM, Romanova LI, Sinyakov AN, Maslova SV, Agol VI (1989) Conserved structural domains in the 5′ untranslated region of picornaviral genomes. An analysis of the segment controlling translation and neurovirulence. Virology 168: 201–209

Pincus SE, Diamond DC, Emini EA, Wimmer E (1986) Guanidine-selected mutants of poliovirus: mapping of point mutations to polypeptide 2C. J Virol 57: 638–646

Pöyry T, Kinnunen L, Kapsenberg J, Kew O, Hovi T (1990) Type 3 poliovirus/Finland/1984 is genetically related to common Mediterranean strains. J Gen Virol 71: 2535–2541

Rico-Hesse R, Pallansch MA, Nottay BK, Kew OM (1987) Geographic distribution of wild poliovirus type 1 genotypes. Virology 160: 311–322

Rivera VM, Welsh JD, Maizel JV (1988) Comparative sequence analysis of the 5′ noncoding region of the enteroviruses and rhinoviruses. Virology 165: 42–50

Roivainen M, Hovi T (1988) Cleavage of VP1 and modification of antigenic site 1 of type 2 polioviruses by intestinal trypsin. J Virol 62: 3536–3539

Romanova LI, Tolskaya EA, Kolesnokova MS, Agol VI (1980) Biochemical evidence for intertypic genetic recombination of polioviruses. FEBS Lett 118: 109–112

Skinner MA, Racaniello VR, Dunn G, Cooper J, Minor PD, Almond JW (1989) New model for the secondary structure of the 5′ noncoding RNA of poliovirus is supported by biochemical and genetic data that also show that RNA secondary structure is important in neurovirulence. J Mol Biol 207: 379–392

Spindler KR, Horodyski FM, Holland JJ (1982) High multiplicities of infection favor rapid and random evolution of vesicular stomatitis virus. Virology 119: 96–108

Stanway G, Cann AJ, Hauptmann R, Hughes P, Clarke LD, Mountford RC, Minor PD, Schild GC, Almond JW (1983) The nucleotide sequence of poliovirus type 3 Leon $12a_1b$: comparison with poliovirus type 1. Nucleic Acids Res 11: 5629–5643

Steinhauer DA, de la Torre JC, Meier E, Holland JJ (1989) Extreme heterogeneity in populations of vesicular stomatitis virus. J Virol 63: 2072–2080

Takeda N, Miyamura K, Ogino T, Natori K, Yamazaki S, Sakurai N, Nakazono N, Ishii K, Kono R (1984) Evolution of enterovirus type 70: oligonucleotide mapping analysis of RNA genome. Virology 134: 375–388

Toyoda H, Kohara M, Kataoka Y, Suganuma T, Omata T, Imura N, Nomoto A (1984) Complete nucleotide sequence of all three poliovirus genomes. J Mol Biol 174: 561–585

Trent DW, Grant JA, Monath TP, Manske CL, Corins M, Fox GE (1989) Genetic variation and microevolution of Dengue 2 virus in Southeast Asia. Virology 172: 523–535

Trono D, Andino R, Baltimore D (1988) An RNA sequence of hundreds of nucleotides at the 5′ end of poliovirus RNA is involved in allowing viral protein synthesis. J Virol 62: 2291–2299

Mutations and A/I Hypermutations in Measles Virus Persistent Infections

R. CATTANEO and M. A. BILLETER

1 Persistent Measles Virus Infections

The molecular biology of measles virus (MV) and of other nonsegmented negative strand RNA viruses is currently subject to intense scrutiny for several reasons. First, acute MV infection is among the primary causes of infant death in third world countries (BLOOM 1989). Second, on rare occasions, MV persistence induces lethal syndromes of the central nervous system known as subacute sclerosing panencephalitis (SSPE) and measles inclusion body encephalitis (MIBE) (reviewed in TER MEULEN et al. 1983). Third, unexpected phenomena such as biased hypermutation and RNA editing recently have been described for these viruses (reviewed in BILLETER and CATTANEO 1991; CATTANEO 1990).

SSPE is one of the most thoroughly studied persistent viral infections of the human central nervous system and serves as a model for the study of persistent infections by RNA viruses suspected to cause· other human syndromes (KRISTENSSON and NORRBY 1986). The clinical manifestations of SSPE and MIBE are similar, but SSPE, developing in immunologically noncompromised children 5–10 years after acute MV infection, is accompanied by a hyperimmune response, whereas MIBE occurs in immunosuppressed patients after a shorter incubation period (TER MEULEN et al. 1983).

Infectious virus is not detectable in the brain of SSPE or MIBE victims, but occasionally cell-associated defective viruses can be isolated by cocultivation of

Institut für Molekularbiologie I, Universität Zürich, Hönggerberg, 8093 Zürich, Switzerland

Current Topics in Microbiology and Immunology, Vol. 176

brain cells with fibroblasts (for review see WECHSLER and MEISSNER 1982). Most of these cell-associated MVs are characterized by defects in expression of the matrix protein (M; WECHSLER and FIELDS 1978; HALL et al. 1979). The M protein as well as the other viral envelope proteins, mediating fusion (F), and hemagglutination (H), often cannot be detected in brain autopsy material (NORRBY et al. 1985; BACZKO et al. 1986). A generally reduced production of the viral envelope proteins in human brain infections is due to a steep gradient of transcription leading to low-level expression of the distally located genes M, F, and H (CATTANEO et al. 1987b). SSPE-derived cell lines harboring cell-associated MVs show transcript ratios which are similar to those of lytically infected cells (CATTANEO et al. 1987a), standing in contrast to infected rat brains which exhibit steep transcription gradients (SCHNEIDER-SCHAULIES et al. 1989). Thus, down-regulation of transcription of the genes coding for the viral envelope proteins appears to be a specific property of brain tissue. Low expression of viral envelope proteins would tend to hide brain cells from immune attack, thereby facilitating viral latency.

A typical phenomenon associated with SSPE and MIBE are the numerous mutational alterations of MV genomes (CATTANEO et al. 1989b). Some of these mutations are likely to be crucial for the transition from innocuous latency to the destructive spread of the infection. The envelope protein genes appear to be particularly affected, whereas the genes for the replication-associated nucleocapsid protein (N) and phosphoprotein (P) did not accumulate mutations leading to striking alterations of their reading frames. Here we discuss the effects of single point mutations and of clusters of U to C or A to G transitions (biased hypermutation; CATTANEO et al. 1988) on measles virus gene expression and replication in persistent infections of human brains. Moreover, cases of biased hypermutation monitored in other viral and cellular systems are reviewed.

2 Mutations in Measles Virus Genomes: Types and Distribution

In the SSPE and MIBE cases discussed here, as in most viral infections of humans, it is impossible to unambiguously define the mutations fixed during persistence, since the genomic sequences of the individual lytic viruses initiating the diseases are not known. To somehow circumvent this problem, a "consensus" sequence consisting of the nucleotides found most frequently in MV sequences derived from all lytic and persistent viruses analyzed was constructed (CATTANEO et al. 1989b). This consensus covers the first five MV genes, that is, more than 9000 nucleotides (Fig. 1, top). In the following, nucleotides deviating from the consensus will be referred to as "mutations", although this term is correct only for an unknown number of these deviations.

Most mutations are presumably due to the relatively error prone viral RNA replicase (for review see STEINHAUER and HOLLAND 1987); in the MV genes

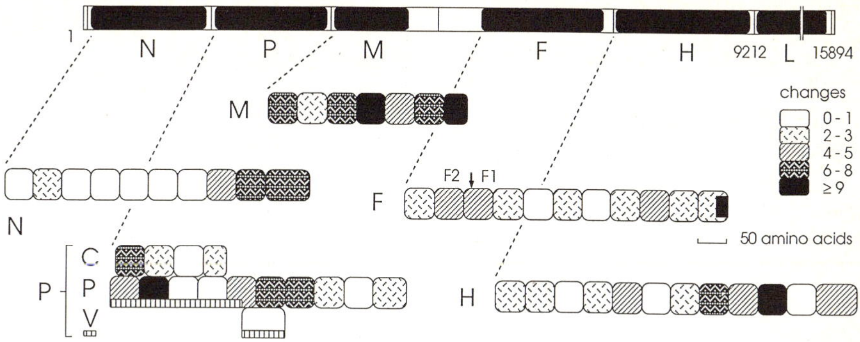

Fig. 1. *TOP*, MV genome coding regions are represented by *black areas*, untranslated regions by *white areas*, and gene boundaries by *vertical lines*. *Bottom*, Variability of MV proteins. For segments of 50 consecutive amino acids, represented as *boxes*, the sum of all differences of the sequences of SSPE cases A and B, MIBE case C, and SSPE cell line IP-3-Ca (CATTANEO et al. 1989b) is indicated by different shading as specified on the right. In the carboxyl terminal parts of proteins, segments of variable length were considered, but the darkness of shading was normalized to a segment length of 50 amino acids. In the M gene, the sequence of case C has been substituted by that of case K (CATTANEO et al. 1986; Fig. 2) to exclude the extreme biased hypermutation event of case C. The part of the F gene which is often altered has been indicated by a small *black rectangle*. The site of endoproteolytic cleavage of the F_0 precursor protein is indicated with an *arrow*. (Modified from CATTANEO et al. 1989b)

considered here, substitutions prevail by a factor of at least 100 over deletions or insertions. Among the substitution mutations, transitions prevail by a factor of about ten over transversions, as in other viral and cellular genes (BILLETER and CATTANEO 1991). Interestingly, a major bias is apparent for replacement of U residues by Cs, which are at least twice as frequent as the other three types of transitions. This bias results from more or less extensive "biased hypermutation" events, characterized as clusters of U to C (or, less frequently, A to G) transitions. We discuss in Sects. 3 and 4 the consequences of point mutations on MV gene expression, whereas in Sect. 5, the characteristics and the mechanism of biased hypermutation events is presented.

In the only four SSPE or MIBE cases for which a complete sequence of the N, P, M, F, and H genes is available, silent mutations accumulated at remarkably uniform levels around 0.8%–0.9% in almost all reading frames (CATTANEO et al. 1989b). The region containing the two overlapping P and C reading frames of the P gene (Fig. 1, bottom left), with silent mutation levels of only ~0.6% is not a true exception, since the number of possible sites for silent mutations is reduced by the reading frame overlap. The untranslated regions (white areas in the top bar of Fig. 1) accumulated three to four times more mutations than the expressed reading frames, a value close to the statistical expectation, assuming generally no negative selection value for either silent mutations in reading frames or total mutations in untranslated regions. In this respect, the M–F untranslated region (about 1000 nucleotides long) did not differ from the other untranslated regions, which are five to ten times shorter.

The mutations leading to amino acid changes (replacement site mutations) are distributed in a less random fashion. They show a frequency of $\sim 0.5\%$ over the N and F coding regions, of $\sim 0.8\%$ over the P, C, and H coding regions, and of $\sim 1.2\%$ over the M coding region (CATTANEO et al. 1989b). It should be noted that a comparison of the different members of the *Paramyxoviridae* shows a different pattern of protein variability: the most variable protein is P, followed by H and N, whereas F and M are the most conserved (RIMA 1989); for L, probably even more conserved, the data do not allow valid statistics as yet. It is striking that in the persistent MVs studied here, M is the most variable protein, an observation which indicates that this protein is subject to low or even no selective constraints in persistent infections.

3 Conservation of the Reading Frames for the Replication-Associated Proteins

The distribution of replacement site mutations in the single reading frames of genes N, M, F, and H and in the three reading frames of gene P is illustrated in the lower part of Fig. 1. From this representation, showing by darker shadings increasing levels of mutations, it is clear that the N reading frame (left) is modified by mutations almost exclusively in the carboxyl terminal region. It is interesting to note that the major antigenic sites of the N protein have been localized in this region which protrudes from the viral nucleocapsid structure (BUCKLAND et al. 1989). The variable region of the N gene of many different MV isolates has been analyzed, and the comparison of these sequences has allowed identification of several different MV lineages (TAYLOR et al. 1991).

The MV P protein accumulated mutations in its amino terminal region (Fig. 1, bottom left), a domain which is thought to interact electrostatically with the polymerase during transcription, as described for the related rhabdovirus vesicular stomatitis virus (VSV) (CHATTOPADHYAY and BANERJEE 1988). This domain is poorly conserved in paramyxo- and rhabdoviruses (MASTERS and BANERJEE 1987; RIMA 1989), and its variability is not surprising. The carboxyl terminal region of the P protein, which apparently interacts directly with the template, is more highly conserved both in lytic as well as in persistent infections.

The V protein (indicated by a ribbon marked with vertical dashes in Fig. 1, bottom left) consists of the amino terminal half of the P protein joined to a cysteine-rich carboxyl terminal region. This protein is expressed from edited messenger RNAs (mRNAs) containing an additional G residue, thus accessing a different reading frame (CATTANEO et al. 1989a). The carboxyl terminal region of V is highly conserved, not only in the persistent viruses studied here but also in general in lytic *Paramyxoviridae* (THOMAS et al. 1988). Its function has not been defined yet, and the same is true for the poorly conserved C protein.

Not much is known about the polymerase (or L) genes of persistent MV strains; only partial L gene sequences of SSPE case K, comprising about 2000 nucleotides, have been determined, and they can be compared only with the Edmonston strain sequence (BLUMBERG et al., unpublished observations). This comparison suggests that in persistent MVs, the replacement site mutations in L accumulate at the lowest level of all genes.

4 Alterations of the Envelope Proteins

The reading frames of the three envelope proteins are differentially conserved. The M protein coding region is characterized by the highest number of mutation of all reading frames (Fig. 1, center). Note that this representation is an underestimation of the mutations accumulated in M, because data from a gene in which an extreme case of biased hypermutation had occurred were not considered (case C, legend to Fig. 1). This observation reinforces the suggestion that M protein is dispensable, or its absence possibly constitutes even an advantage in MV persistent infections (WECHSLER and FIELDS 1978; HALL et al. 1979).

On the other hand, the F protein coding region is remarkably well conserved over most of its length (Fig. 1, center right), but in many cases striking mutations appear very close to the carboxyl terminus (CATTANEO et al. 1989b). In all ten SSPE F genes examined, at least a significant fraction of cloned complementary DNAs (cDNAs) contained point mutations or, less frequently, nucleotide deletions resulting in truncation or alteration of part of the 33 amino acid long F protein intracellular domain (indicated as a small black box in Fig. 1); in seven of these ten cases, exclusively cDNAs encoding truncated forms of the F protein were monitored (SCHMID et al., unpublished).

The conservation of the H gene coding region is intermediate (Fig. 1, bottom right). However, it must be noted that in the H gene of case A, two of the five potential glycosylation sites were eliminated, and in a different case, an additional potential glycosylation site was added by point mutations. The high levels of mutations appearing in a segment of the second half of gene H are largely due to a cluster of 20 A to G mutations in the cell line IP-3-Ca, resulting in 16 amino acid changes. These 20 As (as read in the plus, or antigenome, strand) are concentrated in a region spanning only 333 nucleotides, containing a total of 97 As (Fig. 2, left, IP-3-Ca).

Proteins of RNA viruses not directly involved in replication or transcription are expected to accumulate some alterations during persistence (ROWLANDS et al. 1980; HOLLAND et al. 1982). In the case of the MV M protein, there is indirect evidence that some of the alterations induced by mutations do favor persistence (reviewed in BILLETER and CATTANEO 1991). Another mutational event which might favor viral persistence is the truncation of the F protein intracellular

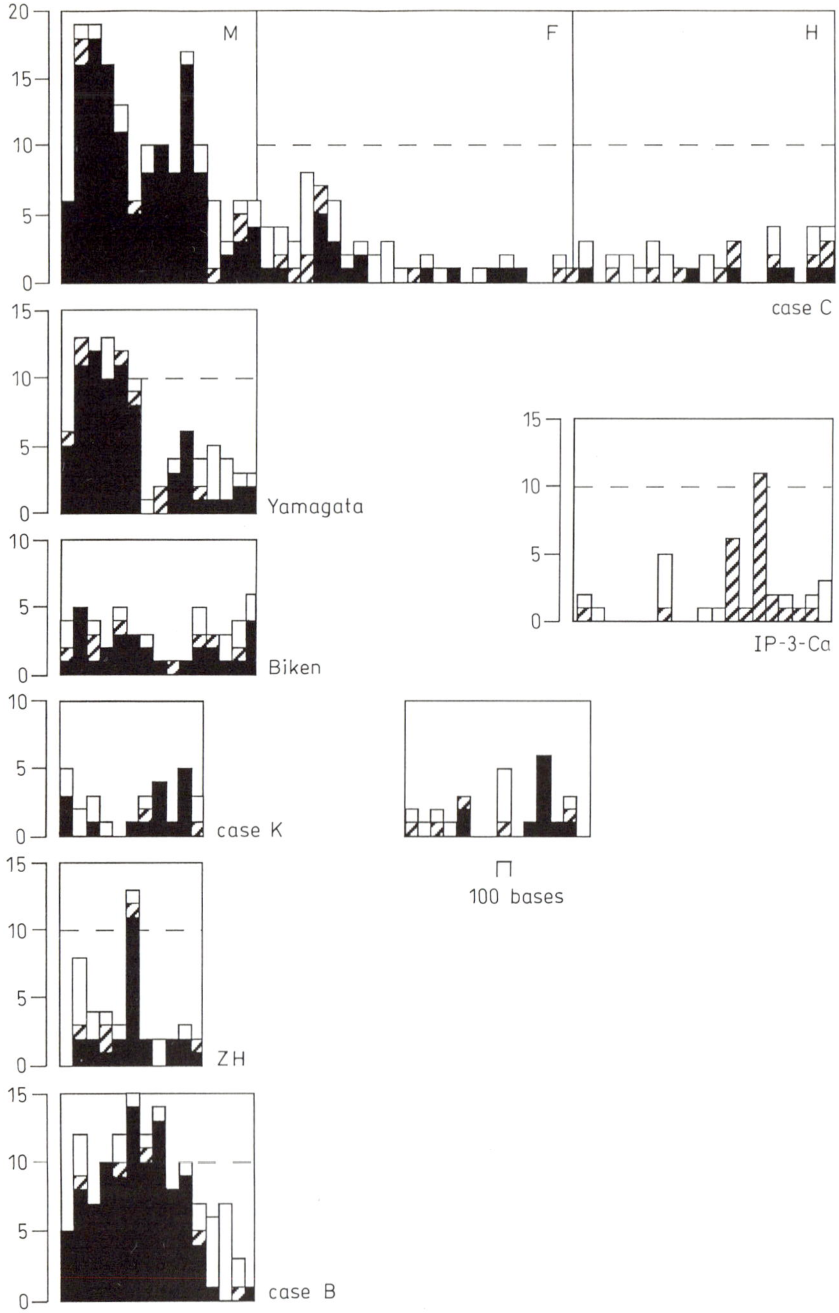

Fig. 2. Mutations and hypermutations in persistent MV genomes. For segments of 100 nucleotides, represented as columns, the number of accumulated mutations is proportional to the height of the columns (see *scale* on the *left*). The M, F, and H genes of case C; part of the M, F, and H genes of case K; the M genes of cell lines Yamagata, Biken, and ZH, and of case B; and the H gene of cell line IP-3-

domain. The fusion function probably permits local transit of MV genomes from cell to cell, and, therefore, must be retained, as suggested also by the conservation of the sequence of the F_1 protein fusogenic peptide (CATTANEO et al. 1988). In a more subtle fashion, however, alteration of the F protein intracellular domain might negatively influence the stability of this protein, contributing to its diminished exposure to the cell surface, and thus "hiding" the infection from immune attack. From studies with the single envelope protein of VSV, it appears that small alterations of its intracellular domain affect intracellular transport, and strongly compromise viral budding (WHITT et al. 1989). H protein expression is probably also not dispensable in persistent infections, because both F and H proteins must be present simultaneously at the cell surface to provide efficient fusion to a neighboring uninfected cell (WILD et al. 1991).

5 A/I Hypermutation of RNA Viruses and mRNA Targeting for Degradation: The Mechanism

In addition to single point mutations which most likely were introduced by the viral polymerase, clusters of U to C or A to G transitions were identified in some MV genes. In the most extreme case, 132 of 266 U residues of the M gene of one MIBE case (case C, Fig. 2, top left) were mutated to C. This event was named "biased hypermutation" (CATTANEO et al. 1988), and soon evidence accumulated that other, less extreme, biased hypermutation events occurred in SSPE cases. In Fig. 2, U to C substitutions are represented by black boxes. These transitions are particularly frequent in the M genes of the MIBE case C, of the SSPE cell lines Yamagata (WONG et al. 1989), Biken (AYATA et al. 1989) and ZH (ENAMI et al. 1989), of the SSPE cases K and B (CATTANEO et al. 1986; BACZKO et al., unpublished), and in a short region of the F gene of case K (SCHMID et al., unpublished). A to G substitutions, represented by stippled boxes in Fig. 2, are particularly frequent in a limited area of the H gene of the SSPE cell line IP-3-Ca (CATTANEO et al. 1989b). For comparison, the less frequent other two types of transitions and eight types of transversions are represented cumulatively as white boxes.

A model for the mechanism of introduction of clustered U to C transitions in MV genomes was proposed after the discovery by BASS and WEINTRAUB (1988) that an enzymatic activity called "double-stranded RNA unwindase" converts up

Fig. 2. (*Continued*)
Ca are shown. *Black shading* represents U to C mutations, *stippled shading* A to G mutations, and *no shading* the other ten different types of mutation. When more than one cDNA clone for each gene was studied, only the mutations present in a relevant fraction of the cDNAs were considered. In cell line Yamagata and in case B, different hypermutation events were defined (WONG et al. 1989; BACZKO et al., unpublished), which are represented cumulatively here. Note that in case B, the first three M cDNAs analyzed did not reveal numerous U to C transitions (CATTANEO et al. 1988). When many more clones from the same and from four additional brain areas were examined, however, U to C transitions were found in a large majority of the cDNAs (BACZKO et al., unpublished)

to 50% of the A residues in duplex RNA to inosine (I). In brief, the aberrant formation of a double-stranded RNA structure involving the MV genome and an M mRNA was suggested (BASS et al. 1989). After unwinding/modification, many biased mutations would have arisen concomitantly with the first replication round by introduction of C residues opposite to I residues. The hypermutated MV genomes, defective in M protein function, presumably had a selective advantage in persistently infected brains. That clonal selection of a virus bearing a hypermutated M gene has indeed occurred is suggested by the nature of the cDNAs obtained from the brain of case C: all five M gene cDNAs analyzed showed the same 132 U to C transitions (CATTANEO et al. 1988).

The cluster of A to G mutations in the H gene of cell line IP-3-Ca is reminiscent of the biased hypermutation event detected in M genes; however, it involves A to G rather than U to C mutations, and only a gene segment rather than the whole gene (Fig. 2, right, IP-3-Ca). We suggested that the IP-3-Ca hypermutation event involved replicative copying of an antigenome which had hybridized over a short stretch with newly synthesized genomic RNA and thus had been modified (CATTANEO et al. 1989b). For this reason, A to G (as read in the plus strand orientation) rather than the corresponding U to C mutations are monitored.

It must be stressed that the relatively high frequency of biased hypermutation events detected in persistent infections, and there particularly in the M gene, is probably a reflection of the lower selective pressures operating in these infections. In our view, biased hypermutation events are probably as frequent in lytic as in persistent infections, but are usually propagated only in cases where selective pressure is released, e.g., in the genome of persistent viruses or in defective interfering particles. Indeed, biased hypermutation events have been detected in defective interfering particles of VSV (O'HARA et al. 1984), and in the 3′ termini of the genomic RNA in persistent infections of human parainfluenza virus 3 (MURPHY et al. 1991). A very limited hypermutation event might have occurred, however, in a substrain of Edmonston virus: In the P gene of this strain, six U to C changes distributed over 600 nucleotides are the only differences from another Edmonston sequence (KAELIN 1989). The frequency and the extent of biased hypermutation events might be influenced by the levels of double-stranded RNA unwinding/modifying activity present in different cell types (WAGNER et al. 1990).

Clusters of A to G transitions have also been detected in the *Xenopus* basic fibroblast growth factor (bFGF) mRNAs (KIMELMAN and KIRSCHNER 1989). From this cellular gene, an "antisense" transcript can be produced in addition to the "sense" mRNA, exclusively at a certain stage of embryonic development and at levels about 20 times higher than the sense mRNA. Over the region of transcript overlap, 50% of the A residues were altered to G (Fig. 3B). From Fig. 3A and 3B, it is also evident that biased hypermutations in MV M genes (resulting from the modification of the negative strand genome, and thus read as U to C in the plus strand orientation shown here), as well as modification of the bFGF transcripts (resulting from direct alteration of the mRNA sequence, and thus read as A to G), do not show a strong bias to involve particular residues in the sequence; the

A. **Mutations in matrix genes of persistent measles viruses**

```
           3901     .         .         .         .         .         .
consensus  UCCGUGUUGUUUAUAUGAGCAUCACCCGUCUUUCGGAUAACGGGUAUUACACCGUUCCUA
case C     ......CC....................................C........C....
Yamagata   ......C...C..C................CC.u...C........C...........C.
Biken      .....................................C......C.............C.
case K     ............................C...............................
ZH         ....C........C..............C.C......C.....a..CC......C...C.
case B     ....C.CC..CC.C................C...a..C......C.CC..........C.
```

B. **Mutations in Xenopus basic fibroblast growth factor transcripts**

```
           651      .         .         .         .         .         .
wild type  GACUGGAAGCUAAUAACUACAACACUUACCGGUCUCGGAAAUACAGCAGCUGGUAUGUGG
clone 211  .......G...G...G....GG.....G...........GG......G......G.....
clone 217  ......GG......GG..G....G...G...........GG.............G.....
clone 218  .......G....G.....G..G.G...G...........GG......G......G.....
clone 220  .......G....G.GG....GG.....G...........GG......G......G.....
clone 238  ...........G..G.....GG.....G...........GG.G....G............
```

Fig. 3 A, B. Clusters of U to C or A to G transitions in viral RNA genomes and in a cellular mRNA. **A** Sequence of a 60-nucleotide-long region of MV matrix genes of six SSPE or MIBE cases, corresponding to part of the sixth column of Fig. 2. U to C mutations are shown by *capital letters*, other mutations by *small letters*. **B** A 60-nucleotide-long region of the transcript for *Xenopus laevis* bFGF, as deducted from the sequence of five different cDNA clones (Kimelman and Kirschner 1989). Note that in the five bFGF cDNAs examined, always about 50% of the as were altered, whereas only in three of the six MV M genes examined was a similarly high level of mutations monitored over the limited region shown.

distribution of modified residues is however not completely random, and it is possible that the neighboring nucleotides influence the choice of the modification sites. In the case of bFGF, mutational modification correlates with reduced transcript stability which is needed to achieve rapid inactivation of function. The bFGF data are fully compatible with the suggestion by Bass and Weintraub (1988) that the double-stranded RNA unwinding/modifying activity could be a housekeeping enzyme implicated in the initial step for elimination of double-stranded RNA hybrids by RNases.

One should also note that G/A hypermutation, possibly due to polymerase slippage during DNA synthesis, has been recently observed in human immunodeficiency virus I genomes (Pathak and Temin 1990; Vartanian et al. 1991). In this review and in future we will use "A/I hypermutation," rather than biased hypermutation (Cattaneo et al. 1988), to define the mutational mechanism described originally in persistent measles virus genomes.

6 Role of Mutations in Disease Development

Mutations in MV genomes related to SSPE and MIBE cause important alterations of the envelope proteins, whereas the reading frames for the proteins involved in replication are generally well conserved. Could mutations introduced during persistence be only a fortuitous byproduct of viral replication? The clonal nature of the viral genomes characterized in several SSPE and MIBE brains strongly suggests that this is not the case, and that certain viral mutations have a decisive influence on the propagation of infection.

Two observations are in line with this suggestion. First, the hypermutated M gene detected in MIBE case C must have arisen in one single MV genome after the initial infection (Sect. 5), and then must have prevailed over all the competing "normal" genomes. Second, and more generally, the number of differences between cDNA clones recovered from one case is about ten times lower than the number of differences between cases (BILLETER and CATTANEO 1991). In the absence of any positive selection for the prevalence of one successful genomic clone a much broader distribution of mutations would be expected.

It should be mentioned that in brain autopsy material of four different SSPE cases, two or more populations of viral genomes have been identified, at least one of which encoding a protein product with clearly altered properties (SCHMID et al. in preparation; BACZKO et al., unpublished). It is conceivable that in these mixed populations the altered genomes prevail, showing a "dominant phenotype," while the normal genomes are carried along without being fully eliminated.

Acknowledgements. We thank Knut Baczko and other colleagues for communicating unpublished information, and Karin Kaelin for critical reading of the manuscript. This work was supported by grant 3.166–88 of the Schweizerische Nationalfonds and by the Kanton Zürich.

References

Ayata M, Hirano A, Wong TC (1989) Structural defect linked to nonrandom mutations in the matrix gene of Biken strain subacute sclerosing panencephalitis virus defined by cDNA cloning and expression of chimeric genes. J Virol 63: 1162–1173

Baczko K, Liebert UG, Billeter M, Cattaneo R, Budka H, ter Meulen V (1986) Expression of defective measles virus genes in brain tissues of patients with subacute sclerosing panencephalitis. J Virol 59: 472–478

Bass BL, Weintraub H (1988) An unwinding activity that covalently modifies its double-stranded RNA substrate. Cell 55: 1089–1098

Bass BL, Weintraub H, Cattaneo R, Billeter MA (1989) Biased hypermutation of viral RNA genomes could be due to unwinding/modification of double-stranded RNA. Cell 56: 331

Billeter MA, Cattaneo R (1991) Molecular biology of defective measles viruses persisting in the human central nervous system. In: Kingsbury DW (Ed) The paramyxoviruses. Plenum, New York, pp 323–345

Bloom BR (1989) Vaccines for the Third World. Nature 342: 115–120

Buckland R, Giraudon P, Wild F (1989) Expression of measles virus nucleoprotein in *Escherichia coli*: use of deletion mutants to locate the antigenic sites. J Gen Virol 70: 435–441

Cattaneo R (1990) Messenger RNA editing and the genetic code. Experientia 46: 1142–1148

Cattaneo R, Schmid A, Rebmann G, Baczko K, ter Meulen V, Bellini WJ, Rozenblatt S, Billeter MA (1986) Accumulated measles virus mutations in a case of subacute sclerosing panencephalitis: interrupted matrix protein reading frame and transcription alteration. Virology 154: 97–107

Cattaneo R, Rebmann G, Schmid A, Baczko K, ter Meulen V, Billeter MA (1987a) Altered transcription of a defective measles virus genome derived from a diseased human brain. EMBO J 6: 681–688

Cattaneo R, Rebmann G, Baczko K, ter Meulen V, Billeter MA (1987b) Altered ratios of measles virus transcripts in diseased human brains. Virology 160: 523–526

Cattaneo R, Schmid A, Eschle D, Baczko K, ter Meulen V, Billeter MA (1988) Biased hypermutation and other genetic changes in defective measles viruses in human brain infections. Cell 55: 255–265

Cattaneo R, Kaelin K, Baczko K, Billeter MA (1989a) Measles virus editing provides an additional cysteine-rich protein. Cell 56: 759–764

Cattaneo R, Schmid A, Spielhofer P, Kaelin K, Baczko K, ter Meulen V, Pardowitz J, Flanagan S, Rima BK, Udem SA, Billeter MA (1989b) Mutated and hypermutated genes of persistent measles viruses which caused lethal human brain diseases. Virology 173: 415–425

Chattopadhyay D, Banerjee AK (1988) NH_2-terminal acidic region of the phosphoprotein of vesicular stomatitis virus can be functionally replaced by tubulin. Proc Natl Acad Sci USA 85: 7977–7981

Enami M, Sato TA, Sugiura A (1989) Matrix protein of cell-associated subacute sclerosing panencephalitis viruses. J Gen Virol 70: 2191–2196

Hall WW, Lamb RA, Choppin PW (1979) Measles and subacute sclerosing panencephalitis virus proteins: lack of antibodies to the M protein in patients with subacute sclerosing panencephalitis. Proc Natl Acad Sci USA 76: 2047–2051

Holland J, Spindler K, Horodyski F, Grabau E, Nichol S, VandePol S (1982) Rapid evolution of RNA genomes. Science 215: 1577–1585

Kaelin K (1989) RNA editing in the measles virus phosphoprotein gene provides an additional protein. Diploma thesis, University of Zurich

Kimelman D, Kirschner MW (1989) An antisense mRNA directs the covalent modification of the transcript encoding fibroblast growth factor in Xenopus oocytes. Cell 59: 687–696

Kristensson K, Norrby E (1986) Persistence of RNA viruses in the central nervous system. Annu Rev Microbiol 40: 159–184

Masters PS, Banerjee AK (1987) Sequences of Chandipura virus N and NS genes: evidence for high mutability of the NS gene within vesiculoviruses. Virology 157: 298–306

Murphy DG, Dimock K, Kang CY (1991) Numerous transitions in human parainfluenza virus 3 RNA recovered from persistently infected cells. Virology 181: 760–763

Norrby E, Kristensson K, Brzosko WJ, Kapsenberg JG (1985) Measles virus matrix protein detected by immune fluorescence with monoclonal antibodies in the brain of patients with subacute sclerosing panencephalitis. J Virol 56: 337–340

O'Hara PJ, Nichol ST, Horodyski FM, Holland JJ (1984) Vesicular stomatitis virus defective interfering particles can contain extensive genomic sequence rearrangements and base substitutions. Cell 36: 915–924

Pathak VK, Temin HM (1990) Broad spectrum of in vivo forward mutations, hypermutations, and mutational hotspots in a retroviral shuttle vector after a single replication cycle: substitutions, frameshifts and hypermutations. Proc Natl Acad Sci USA 87: 6019–6023

Rima BK (1989) Comparison of amino acid sequences of the major structural proteins of the paramyxo and morbilliviruses. In: Mahy BWJ, Kolakofsky E (Eds.) Genetics and pathogenicity of negative strand viruses. Elsevier, Amsterdam, pp 254–263

Rowlands D, Grabau E, Spindler K, Jones C, Semler B, Holland J (1980) Virus protein changes and RNA termini alterations evolving during persistent infection. Cell 19: 871–880

Schneider-Schaulies S, Liebert UG, Baczko K, Cattaneo R, Billeter M, ter Meulen V (1989) Restriction of measles virus gene expression in acute and subacute encephalitis of Lewis rats. Virology 171: 525–534

Steinhauer DA, Holland JJ (1987) Rapid evolution of RNA viruses. Annu Rev Microbiol 41: 409–433

Taylor MJ, Godfrey E, Baczko K, ter Meulen V, Wild TF, Rima BK (1991) Identification of several different lineages of measles virus. J Gen Virol 72: 83–88

Ter Meulen V, Stephenson JR, Kreth HW (1983) Subacute sclerosing panencephalitis. Compr Virol 18: 105–159

Thomas SM, Lamb RA, Paterson RG (1988) Two mRNAs that differ by two nontemplated nucleotides encode the amino coterminal proteins P and V of the paramyxovirus SV5. Cell 54: 891–902

Vartanian J-P, Meyerhans A, Asiö B, Wain-Hobson S (1991) Selection, recombination and G/A hypermutation of human immunodeficiency virus type I genomes. J Virol 65: 1779–1788

Wagner RW, Yoo C, Wrabetz L, Kamholz J, Buchhalter J, Hassan NF, Khalili K, Kim SU, Perussia B, McMorris FA, Nishikura K (1990) Double-stranded RNA unwinding and modifying activity is detected ubiquitously in primary tissues and cell lines. Mol Cell Biol 10: 5586–5590

Wechsler SL, Fields BN (1978) Differences between the intracellular polypeptides of measles and subacute sclerosing panencephalitis virus. Nature 272: 458–460

Wechsler SL, Meissner HC (1982) Measles and SSPE viruses: similarities and differences. Prog Med Virol 28: 65–95

Whitt MA, Chong L, Rose JK (1989) Glycoprotein cytoplasmic domain sequences required for rescue of a vesicular stomatitis virus glycoprotein mutant. J Virol 63: 3569–3578
Wild TF, Malvoisin E, Buckland R (1991) Measles virus: both the haemagglutinin and fusion glycoproteins are required for fusion. J Gen Virol 72: 439–442
Wong TC, Ayata M, Hirano A, Yoshikawa Y, Tsuruoka H, Yamanouchi K (1989) Generalized and localized biased hypermutation affecting the matrix gene of a measles virus strain that causes subacute sclerosing panencephalitis. J Virol 63: 5464–5468

Evolutionary Processes in Influenza Viruses: Divergence, Rapid Evolution, and Stasis

O. T. GORMAN[1,2], W. J. BEAN[1], and R. G. WEBSTER[1]

1 Divergent Evolution of Influenza A Viruses

1.1 Separation of Influenza Virus Gene Pools

Interspecies transmissions combined with isolation of host species contribute to the evolutionary divergence of viruses because of the separation of host-specific virus gene pools. Barriers to frequent interspecies transmissions maintain the separation of progeny and parent virus gene pools and allow independent evolution of host-specific strains. These barriers may be in the form of infrequent likelihood of transmission because of different ecologies of host species, a lack of infectivity of the virus in new hosts, or interference from established viruses

[1] Department of Virology and Molecular Biology, St. Jude Children's Research Hospital, 332 North Lauderdale, P. O. Box 318, Memphis, Tennessee 38101, USA
[2] Current Address: U.S. Fish and Wildlife Service, 835 E. David Drive, Flagstaff, AZ 86001, USA

Current Topics in Microbiology and Immunology, Vol. 176

mediated by host immunity. Partitioning of avian influenza virus gene pools can result from geographic separation of waterfowl populations by separation of flyways and breeding and overwintering grounds. This mechanism has been suggested for the divergence of H4 hemagglutinin lineages in avian viruses (DONIS et al. 1989). The subdivision of host populations provides a great deal of heterogeneity to virus populations and enhances the maintainence of a large number of virus subtypes.

Interspecies transmission of viruses does not necessarily result in a net gene flow between host-specific virus gene pools; reassorted progeny virions with new genes may have lower fitness (reduced replication and virus shedding) relative to virions with host-adapted genes, and thus may not persist. In mixed infections of different virus strains in the same host cells, gene segments of the different strains behave like alleles in populations of eukaryote organisms; all possible combinations of gene subtypes are theoretically generated. However, independent reassortment of some genes may not be observed, indicating that only certain gene combinations may be viable. The reasons for a lack of independent reassortment and evolution among virus genes may vary. One possibility is that coevolution of functionally interdependent proteins results in an evolutionary linkage of the associated genes. In this situation, a mutation that arises in one protein requires complementary mutations in other proteins in order to maintain an optimal functional protein interaction and to maintain virus fitness. Reassortment of these genes from virus strains that have undergone significant host-specific evolution is likely to produce progeny virions of lower relative fitness because the accumulated mutations in the different proteins are not likely to be complementary. A possible example of this type of linkage occurs between RNA gene segments 4 and 7 (HA and M proteins, respectively) of the virulent A/Chicken/Pennsylvania/83 (H5N2) virus isolates (WEBSTER et al. 1989). Another factor contributing to a lack of independent reassortment of virus genes is host-specific adaptation of virus proteins that may or may not be functionally interdependent. In this case the loss of host-adapted genes through reassortment results in progeny virions of lower relative fitness. The third mechanism contributing to a lack of independent reassortment is chance. Reassortment may not decrease fitness, but does not occur because isolation of the different host species provides few opportunities for mixed infections of host-specific virus strains.

1.2 Selection Pressures and Evolutionary Constraints on Influenza Viruses

Each virus gene may evolve differently because of different selective pressures and evolutionary constraints. Genes that code for surface proteins, HA and NA, may be subject to strong selection pressure by neutralizing antibodies of host immune systems. Genes for internal proteins may not be subjected to strong host immune selection pressure but are thought to undergo significant host-specific adaptive evolution (e.g., NP: GAMMELIN et al. 1990; GORMAN et al. 1990a). Internal protein genes such as polymerases may have virus-specific functional constraints on evolution (e.g., PB2 gene: GORMAN et al. 1990b). Because of host immune selection pressure, surface proteins are expected to evolve more rapidly and to be replaced by reassortment more frequently. Reassortant viruses with new genes for surface proteins have a selective advantage over the parent virus to which the host has had considerable antigenic exposure; the new viruses are able to escape (at least temporarily) the host immune response. If these new viruses are sufficiently infectious they can cause pandemics and replace previous strains, resulting in "antigenic shifts" (WEBSTER and LAVER 1975). Thus, surface protein genes may not be expected to have a long evolutionary history within hosts that subject the virus to considerable immune selection pressure, e.g., humans. Internal protein genes that show a high degree of host-specific evolution and cause virus attenuation when experimentally reassorted with different host-specific viruses (e.g., NP gene: SCHOLTISSEK et al. 1985; TIAN et al. 1985; SNYDER et al. 1987) are not expected to reassort frequently. However, internal protein genes that evolve slowly and do not show a high degree of host-specific evolution may be replaced more frequently because new reassorted viruses are not likely to show any attenuation (e.g., PB1 genes in human viruses: KAWAOKA et al. 1989). In the case of PB1 genes, virus-specific constraints on the viral polymerases may prevent any significant host-specific divergent evolution. Thus, the conserved nature of these proteins does not present a barrier to reassortment, i.e., reassorted viruses do not suffer a loss of relative fitness.

1.3 Host-Specific Evolution of Influenza Viruses

The putative role of the NP protein gene as a determinant of host range (SCHOLTISSEK et al. 1985; TIAN et al. 1985; SNYDER et al. 1987) has lead to the use of the NP gene as a model for long-term host-specific evolution of influenza viruses (GORMAN et al. 1990a, 1991; GAMMELIN et al. 1990). Using RNA hybridization techniques BEAN (1984) showed that NP genes of influenza, A viruses fall into five host-specific groups. Subsequently, GORMAN et al. (1990a, 1991) showed in phylogenetic analyses that NP genes have evolved into five major host-specific lineages that correspond to five NP gene RNA hybridization groups (BEAN 1984) (Fig. 1). These lineages are: (a) EQPR56 (Equine/Prague/56) (equine 1 viruses); (b) recent equine viruses, i.e., those related to Equine/Miami/63 (equine 2 viruses); (c) human viruses joined with classical swine viruses, i.e., those related to Swine/Iowa/15/30; (d) H13 gull viruses; (e) all other avian viruses. Geographic patterns of evolution are evident in avian virus NP genes; North American, Australian, and Old World isolates form separate sublineages.

At present, phylogenies for the six internal protein influenza virus genes that include H1N1 and H3N2 human and swine viruses have been determined (PB1: KAWAOKA et al. 1989; PA: OKAZAKI et al. 1989; PB2: GORMAN et al. 1990b; NP: GAMMELIN et al. 1990; GORMAN et al. 1990a, 1991; M: ITO et al. 1991; NS: KAWAOKA

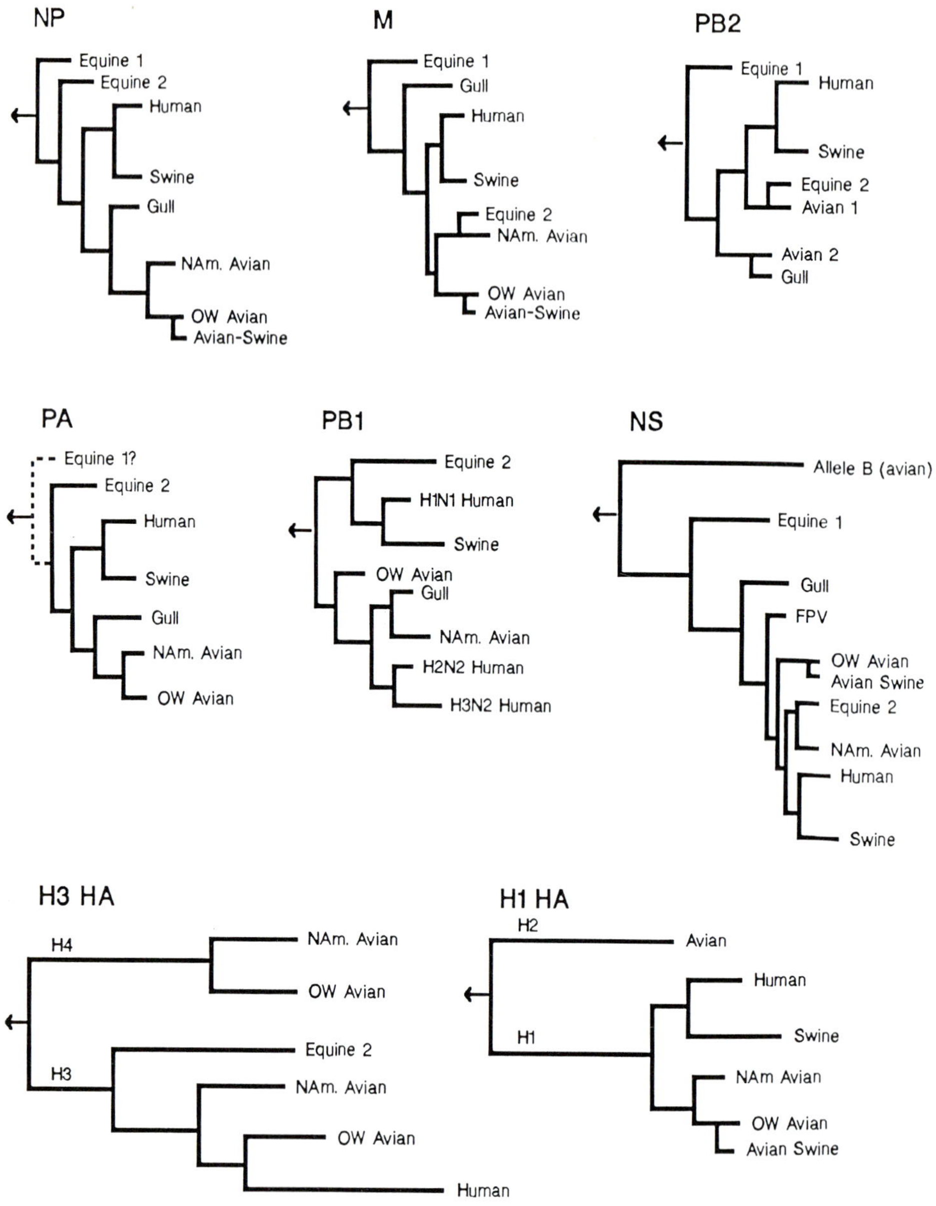

Fig. 1. Generalized phylogenies (cladograms) of influenza virus genes. Phylogenies were determined with PAUP software version 2.4 (David Swofford, Illinois Natural History Survey), which uses a maximum parsimony algorithm to find the shortest length trees. *Horizontal distance* is proportional to the minimum number of nucleotide changes needed to join the gene sequences (no scale is given). *Vertical lines* are for spacing branches and labels. The *arrow* at the left of each tree represents the node connecting the influenza B virus homologue. *Equine 1*, Eq/Prague/56 (H7N7) virus isolate; *Equine 2*, recent H3N8 equine viruses; *Human* (unless noted otherwise), human H1N1, H2N2, and H3N2 viruses; *Swine*, classical swine viruses (i.e., those related to Sw/Iowa/15/30); *Gull*, H13 gull

et al. 1991). Phylogenies for surface protein subtype genes H1, H3, and H4 HAs are available (KAWAOKA et al. 1990; BEAN et al. 1991; DONIS et al. 1989; KAWAOKA, unpubl. data). Generalized phylogenetic trees (cladograms) showing the major branching topologies for the phylogenies of these genes are shown in Fig. 1. Of the eight gene phylogenies shown in Fig. 1 none show identical topologies. This indicates that past reassortment events and differential extinction have affected patterns of evolution for each gene.

For those gene phylogenies that include EQPR56 (equine 1), this virus always shows an outgroup relationship to other virus lineages. This pattern indicates that the EQPR56 (equine 1) is the most divergent and possibly the oldest of the nonavian influenza A virus lineages. As such, its relationship to other gene lineages permits us to estimate the relative order of ages of divergence (vicariance) among the gene lineages. Cladograms for the NP and PA genes are very similar and would be identical if the EQPR56 PA gene (sequence not done) shows the same relative position (Fig. 1). The close match in the phylogenies of NP and PA genes indicates that they share a common evolutionary history in each host; they form a gene constellation and apparently have not reassorted independently.

The M gene shows significant differences compared to the NP and PA cladograms. First, the equine 2 M genes appear to have been recently derived from North American avian viruses in contrast to the much older origin of equine 2 NP and PA genes. Second, the H13 gull virus M gene is closer to EQPR56 and more distant from other virus M genes suggesting that the gull M gene may have an older origin compared to the H13 gull NP and PA genes. Like the recent equine M genes, the PB2 gene of H13 gull viruses shows a more recent origin than the NP, PA, and M gull virus genes.

In the NS gene phylogeny there is a very old b allele (TREANOR et al. 1989) avian lineage that predates the divergence of the EQPR56 (equine 1) lineage. The H13 gull NS gene shows the same relative evolutionary position as the H13 gull M gene, i.e., the origins of these genes are older than the origin of the NP, PA, PB1, and PB2 gull H13 genes. The fowl plague virus (FPV) NS genes, which are from the earliest avian virus isolates, appear to be derived from a lineage that diverged prior to the split between Old World avian, North American avian, and human and classical swine groups. The recent equine NS, like the M and PB2 genes, is derived from the North American avian group and shows a more recent origin than NP, PA, and PB1 genes.

The PB1 lineage shows less congruence with other gene lineages. Human virus PB1 genes show three different origins: H1N1 human viruses form a sister

◄

viruses; *FPV*, fowl plague viruses; *NAm. Avian*, North American avian viruses; *OW Avian*, Old World or Eurasian avian viruses; *Avian Swine*, avian-like H1N1 swine viruses. There are two distinct avian lineages in the PB2 tree, *Avian 1* and *Avian 2* which contain Eurasian and North American avian viruses. Nucleotide phylogenies represented are taken from KAWAOKA et al. (1989; PB1), GORMAN et al. (1990b; PB2), OKAZAKI et al. (1989; PA), GORMAN et al. (1990a, 1991; NP), KAWAOKA (unpubl. data, H1HA), BEAN et al. (1991; H3HA), ITO et al. (1991; M), KAWAOKA et al. (1991; NS)

group to classical swine viruses, and H2N2 and H3N2 human viruses each form separate sublineages derived from avian virus PB1 genes. The H13 gull PB1 gene, like the PB2, appears to have a more recent origin than for other genes, but the recent equine PB1 gene appears to have an older origin like the NP and PA genes.

A comparison of nucleotide and amino acid sequences of H3 hemagglutinin genes shows that the progenitor of the 1968 human pandemic (Hong Kong) strain was derived from an avian virus very similar to those currently circulating in ducks in Asia, and the transfer of the avian virus H3 gene to human viruses probably occurred in 1965 (BEAN et al. 1991). Since then, the H3 human viruses have diverged rapidly from this progenitor. This rapid accumulation of nucleotide and amino acid changes is in contrast to the much lower rates observed in avian H3 viruses and, like the avian virus NP protein, the avian virus H3 protein appears to be in evolutionary stasis. Unlike human H3 viruses the equine 2 (H3N8) viruses apparently diverged from an avian ancestor much earlier and no close relatives have yet been found in any other species. Each of four H3 swine virus isolates analyzed appear to represent independent introductions into pigs, two having been derived from human viruses and two from avian viruses. These last examples provide support for the concept that swine may serve as intermediates in the transmission of avian influenza viruses or their genes to the human virus gene pool.

1.4 Common Ancestry for Human and Classical Swine Viruses

In all of the phylogenies of the internal protein genes and the surface protein H1 HA gene, the human and classical swine virus lineages show a sister group relationship, indicating that they share a common ancestor (Fig. 1). Analyses of amino acid trees of NP, PB2, and M genes show that the common ancestors are all avian like (GORMAN et al. 1990a, b, 1991; ITO et al. 1991). Antigenic similarity of human and classical swine virus N1 NA proteins (e.g., KENDAL and KILEY 1973) predicts the same sister group relationship. The common sister group relationship for all genes of human and classical swine viruses and the closeness of the common ancestors to avian virus proteins suggests that the human and classical swine virus ancestor was not a reassortant virus but an entirely new avian-derived virus (GORMAN et al. 1990b, 1991). It is important to note that the H1N1 human virus as originally constituted prior to 1918 has since been reassorted twice: in 1957 the H1 HA, N1 NA, and the PB1 were replaced with the new avian-like genes, and in 1968 the H2 HA and the PB1 were again replaced with avian-like genes (KAWAOKA et al. 1989; Fig. 1).

2 Differential Evolutionary Rates of Influenza A Viruses

2.1 Evolutionary Rates of Influenza Virus Genes and Proteins

Current paradigms of influenza A virus evolution are based on studies of human viruses where host immune selection pressure is potentially high and virus surface proteins are expected to evolve rapidly. For human influenza viruses, the H3 HA surface protein genes are evolving much more rapidly than the internal protein genes PB1, PB2, PA, NP, and M1 (Table 1). The proportion of silent to total nucleotide changes in surface versus internal protein genes reveals differences in evolution. Among the internal protein genes PB2, NP, and M1, the proportion of silent changes is much higher than for the surface protein H3 HA

Table 1. Nucleotide evolutionary rates for influenza A virus genes based on phylogenetic analyses

Gene segment subtype	Host	Nucleotide evolutionary rate (base/year × 10^{-3})			%nc	N	Period	Source
		tot	c	nc				
PB1	Human	0.87	—	—	—	3	1957–1968	KAWAOKA et al. (1989)
PB2	Human	1.82	0.15	1.67	92	7	1933–1988	GORMAN et al. (1990b)
PA	Human	1.32	—	—	—	4	1934–1968	OKAZAKI et al. (1989)
HA								
H3[a]	Human	7.00	—	—	—	16	1968–1979	BOTH et al. (1983)
H3	Human	4.44	1.91	2.53	57	14	1968–1986	BEAN et al. (1991)
H3[a]	Equine	2.80	—	—	—	2	1963–1979	DANIELS et al. (1985)
H3	Equine	1.74	0.45	1.29	74	13	1963–1986	BEAN et al. (1991)
H1[a]	Human	4.30	—	—	—	14	1977–1983	RAYMOND et al. (1986)
H1	Human	0.61	—	—	—	5	1933–1980	KAWAOKA (unpubl. data)
H1	Swine	1.26	—	—	—	9	1930–1988	KAWAOKA (unpubl. data)
NP	Human	2.20	—	—	—	9	1934–1983	ALTMULLER et al. (1989)
NP	Human	2.18	0.42	1.76	81	16	1933–1983	GORMAN et al. (1991)
NP	Swine	2.12	0.22	1.90	90	11	1930–1988	GORMAN et al. (1991)
NP	Avian-like Swine	2.88	0.47	2.40	83	3	1981–1989	GORMAN et al. (1991)
NP	Equine	0.78	0.21	0.57	73	4	1963–1986	GORMAN et al. (1990a)
NP	Avian	1.21	0.00	1.21	100	19	1927–1982	GORMAN et al. (1991)
M	Human	1.08	—	—	—	13	1933–1988	ITO et al. (1991)
M1		0.83	0.03	0.80	96	13	1933–1988	ITO et al. (1991)
M2		1.36	0.46	0.90	66	13	1933–1988	ITO et al. (1991)
M	Swine	1.30	—	—	—	8	1930–1988	ITO et al. (1991)
M1		1.43	0.05	1.38	97	8	1930–1988	ITO et al. (1991)
M2		0.91	0.48	0.43	47	8	1930–1988	ITO et al. (1991)
NS	Human	1.94	—	—	—	9	1942–1985	BUONAGURIO et al. (1986b)
NS	Human	1.78	—	—	—	14	1933–1977	KAWAOKA et al. (1991)

Evolutionary rates shown are for entire gene segment (tot), coding changes (c), silent or noncoding changes (nc). Coding changes reflect amino acid or protein evolution. % *nc* percent of changes that are silent; *N*, number of virus isolates included in the estimation of evolutionary rates

[a] Based on HA1 subunit sequence

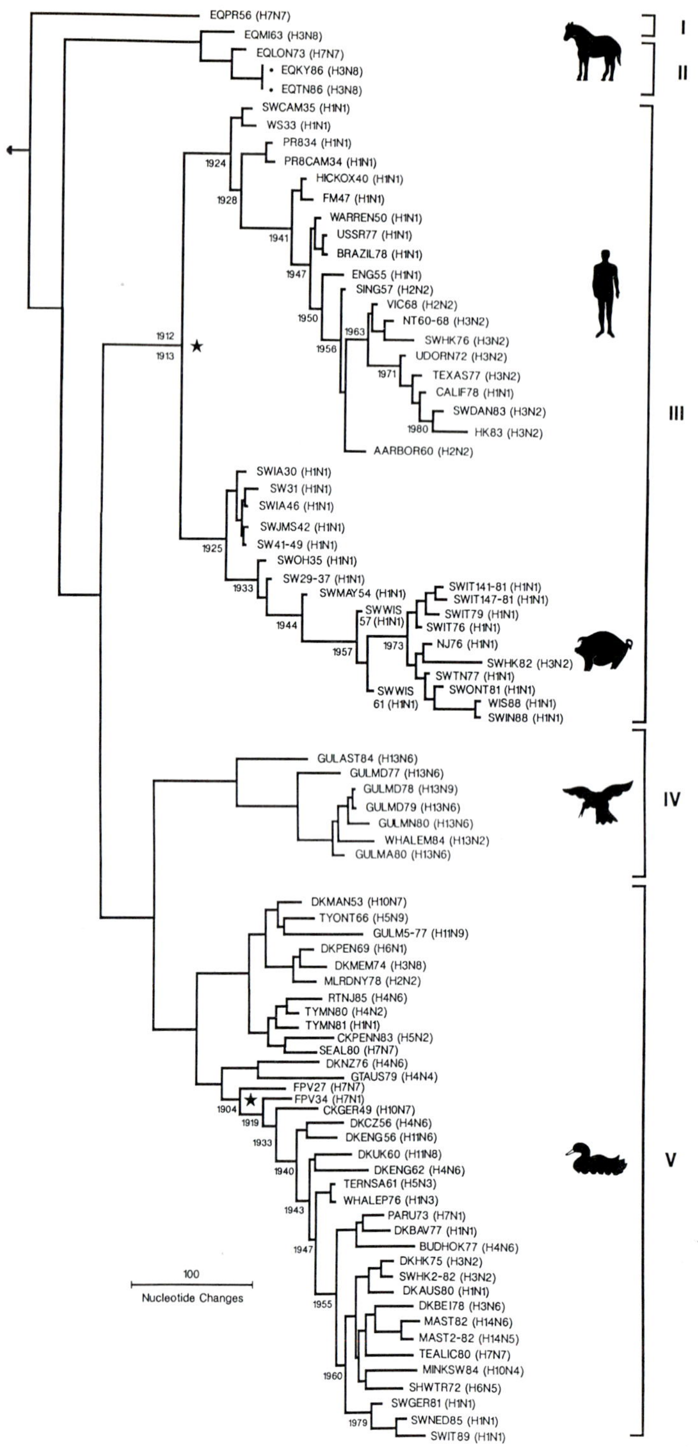

Fig. 2A. For legend see page 84

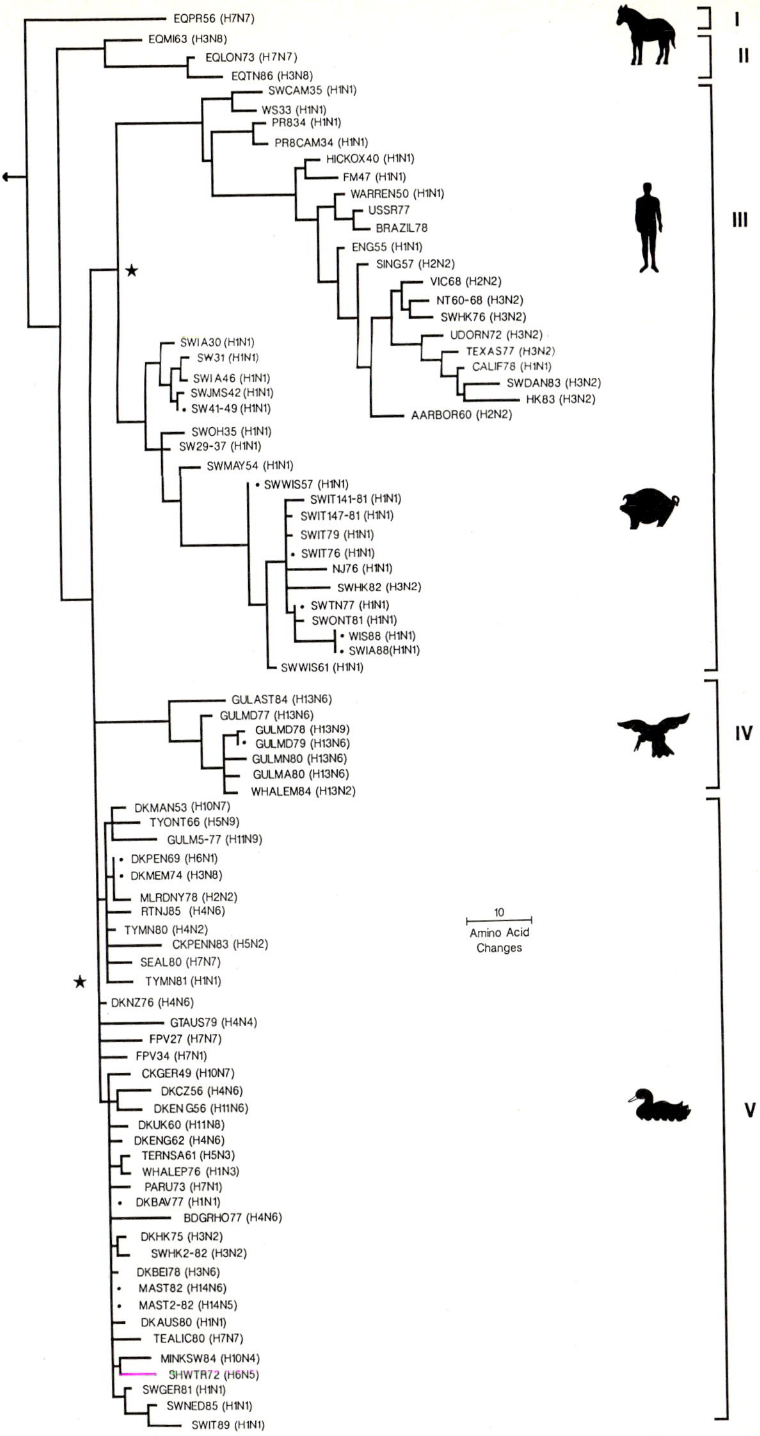

Fig. 2B. For legend see page 84

(81%–96% vs 57%, respectively, Table 1). Furthermore, a comparison of coding and noncoding evolutionary rates for human virus genes shows that they are evolving at different rates. For example, the M1 and M2 genes of the M gene segment are evolving very differently from each other and fit the model of internal versus external protein gene evolution just discussed. M2, a minor influenza virus surface protein gene, is evolving much more rapidly than the internal M1 matrix protein gene and a higher proportion of the nucleotide changes in the M2 gene are nonsilent. M1 is evolving very slowly and shows almost no accumulation of coding changes over a 55-year period (Table 1; ITO et al. 1991).

Homologous genes from host-specific virus strains also evolve at different rates. Recent evolutionary analyses of influenza NP genes demonstrate that avian virus genes are evolving more slowly than those in human viruses (GORMAN et al. 1990a, 1991). Classical swine virus NP genes are evolving similarly to human virus NP genes but at the protein level the swine virus NP genes are more conserved. Genes of H3N8 equine 2 viruses are evolving more slowly than those in human or swine viruses. More astonishing, however, is the lack of evolution observed in avian virus proteins. When the topology of the NP nucleotide phylogenetic tree is used to construct the amino acid tree to evaluate the effect of gene evolution on protein evolution, avian virus proteins show no net evolution over the more than 50 years avian viruses have been isolated (Fig. 2). This indicates that coding changes in avian virus genes are rare (Table 1) and do not show the pattern of cumulative evolution seen in mammalian virus strains (Fig. 2). The same pattern of evolutionary stasis in avian viruses has also been demonstrated for PB2 (GORMAN et al. 1990b), M (ITO et al. 1991), and H3 HA (BEAN et al. 1991) genes.

2.2 Dates of Emergence of Influenza Virus Strains

Evolutionary rates estimated from phylogenetic analyses can be used to estimate dates of emergence or origin of new virus lineages (Table 2). Analyses of NP, PB2, and M gene segments estimate 1905–1914 for the appearance of the common ancestor of human and classical swine H1N1 viruses (Fig. 2; GORMAN

Legend to Fig. 2 (for figure see pp 83 and 84). **A** Phylogenetic tree of 89 influenza A virus NP gene nucleotide sequences rooted to the NP of B/Lee/40. Sequences were analyzed with PAUP software (David Swofford, Illinois Natural History Survey) which uses a maximum parsimony algorithm to find the shortest length trees. The *arrow* indicates the direction of the B/Lee/40 NP from the root node. *Horizontal distance* is proportional to the minimum number of nucleotide changes needed to join nodes and NP sequences. *Vertical lines* are for spacing branches and labels. Roman numerals indicate BEAN'S (1984) RNA NP hybridization groups: *I*, Equine/Prague/56; *II*, recent equine; *III*, human and classical swine; *IV*, H13 gull; *V*, avian. *Animal symbols* indicate host specificities of the lineages. Dates for hypothetical ancestor nodes were derived by dividing branch distance by evolutionary rate estimates. *Stars* indicate the hypothetical ancestors for the human-swine NP lineage (*upper*) and avian NP lineage (*lower*). **B** Phylogenetic tree of influenza A virus NP protein amino acid sequences. The amino acid phylogeny conforms to the topology of the nucleotide tree (**A**) (Sequences represented in these trees are listed in GORMAN et al. 1991)

Table 2. Estimated dates of origin for influenza A viruses[a]

Gene	Host/virus	Date of origin	Source
NP	Human	1914	GORMAN et al. (1990a)
NP	Human	1912	GORMAN et al. (1991)
NP	Classical swine	1913	GORMAN et al. (1991)
NP	Old World avian	1912	GORMAN et al. (1990a)
NP	Old World avian	1904	GORMAN et al. (1991)
NP	Avian-like swine	1979	GORMAN et al. (1991)
PB2	Human	1910	GORMAN et al. (1990b)
NS	Human	1915–20	NAKAJIMA et al. (1984)
NS	Human	1921	KAWAOKA et al. (1991)
NS	Classical swine	1901	KAWAOKA et al. (1991)
M	Human	1915	NAKAJIMA et al. (1984)
M	Human	1905	ITO et al. (1991)
M	Classical swine	1912	ITO et al. (1991)

[a] Dates of origin were estimated from regressions of phylogenetic distances of virus genes against dates of isolation

et al. 1990a, b, 1991; ITO et al. 1991). Estimation of this common ancestor date assumes that the evolutionary rate has remained constant from the origin to the present, which may not be realistic. If the evolutionary rates were somewhat higher during the first few years after the appearance of this avian-like virus in human and swine hosts, the date of origin may be later than 1905–1914. HINI avian-like viruses appeared in swine in Europe in 1979 (SCHOLTISSEK et al. 1983) and have continued to circulate and evolve. The NP genes of these new viruses are evolving at a higher rate than NP genes in human and classical swine viruses over the period 1930–1988. The evolution of these H1N1 avian-like swine viruses may serve as a model for early evolution of H1N1 human and classical swine viruses. By applying the evolutionary rate of the NP genes of H1N1 avian-like swine viruses to pre-1930 human and classical swine virus NP genes the estimated date becomes 1918, which is in closer agreement with historical records and retrospective serological evidence (e.g., MULDER and MASUREL 1958; CROSBY 1989).

Unlike mammalian viruses, estimation of dates of origin for avian virus gene lineages has not been generally successful. In most cases, there is a lack of correspondence between the date of virus isolation and relative position in phylogenetic trees, e.g., North American avian NP (GORMAN et al. 1991), PB2 (GORMAN et al. 1990b), M (ITO et al. 1991), and H3 (BEAN et al. 1991) genes. This situation is probably the result of a combination of an insufficient sample of avian virus isolates, the suspected high diversity of avian virus gene lineages, and the impact of evolutionary stasis on avian virus proteins. Fortunately, NP genes of Old World avian strains show some consistency in dates of isolation versus tree position, thus permitting estimation of an evolutionary rate and date of a common ancestor. The rates of avian virus NP gene evolution is lower than for human and swine viruses and the protein shows no evolution over more than 60 years of avian virus isolates (Fig. 2, Table 1). A minimum estimated date for the common ancestor of Old World avian virus NP genes is 1904 (Fig. 2); severe constraints on avian virus protein evolution results in some back mutations not being reflected in phylogenetic analyses, and as a result, the lengths of the deep internal branches are probably underestimated (GORMAN et al. 1990a). By using 1904 as a reference point, the relative ages of other avian NP gene lineages can be estimated. For example, Australian avian, North American avian, and H13 gull virus NP gene lineages must have diverged from the Old World avian lineage before 1904. Considering the relatively great distance of the isolates from the Old World lineage and the relatively slow rate of evolution in avian virus genes, the H13 gull and North American avian viruses diverged more than a century ago from common ancestors shared with Old World avian viruses.

3 Mechanisms of Evolution in Influenza Viruses

3.1 Evolutionary Stasis in Avian Influenza A Viruses

In contrast to the rapid, progressive changes of both the nucleotide and amino acid sequences of the mammalian virus gene lineages, avian virus genes show far less variation and in most cases there is no clear relationship between dates of isolation and position in the phylogenetic tree. Divergent cumulative evolution observed at the nucleotide level among avian virus genes has been correlated with geographic separation of host populations, e.g., North American avian virus strains versus Old World virus strains (DONIS et al. 1989; GORMAN et al. 1990a; Figs. 1 and 2). The collapse of lineage divergence among avian virus genes at the protein level (e.g., Fig. 2) indicates that the cumulative genetic differences are noncoding changes and also demonstrates a remarkable degree of phenotype stability among geographically separated virus gene pools.

A comparison of patterns of coding and noncoding changes in mammalian and avian virus gene lineages shows fundamental differences in evolution (GORMAN et al. 1990a, b, 1991; BEAN et al. 1991). For example, terminal and internal branches in the mammalian virus NP gene lineages show similar numbers of coding and noncoding changes (compare nucleotide and amino acid trees in Fig. 2). This pattern suggests that mammalian viruses undergo positive directional selection; mammalian hosts continuously select for new phenotypes which results in the continuous elimination of virus predecessors. In contrast, in the avian virus NP gene lineage (Fig. 2), most coding changes occur in the terminal branches while the internal branches show none or few coding changes (as reflected by their collapse in the amino acid tree, Fig. 2B). This pattern suggests that avian viruses are subjected to negative selection in order to maintain the ancestral phenotype. This conservation of phenotype (evolutionary stasis) probably reflects a long-established adaptive optimum for avian virus proteins. A possible mechanism for evolutionary stasis in avian viruses has been proposed (BEAN et al. 1991). If long-term survival favors those virions that have not changed, then virus populations in environments that undergo relatively few replication cycles would be more likely to yield progeny that do not have deleterious mutations. Those replicating in other environments or mutants in the original population might have a temporary selective advantage in a particular host or environment, but the accumulation of mutations in these subpopulations would be deleterious in other circumstances. Thus the original population (perhaps in a very small minority) would have a selective advantage as hosts or environmental conditions change.

3.2 Rapid Evolution in Human Influenza A Viruses

The modes of evolution in avian and human influenza viruses appear to be very different. If as argued below, all influenza A viruses have an avian origin, the rapid cumulative evolution in human virus genes and proteins reflects a lack of equilibrium between virus and host, and significant host-specific differences in the epidemiology and immune responses of avian and human hosts to influenza viruses. The rapid evolution of virus surface proteins of human (as well as those of swine and equine viruses) is undoubtedly driven by immunoselection as the virus circulates in a partially immune population (BOTH et al. 1983). Human influenza A viruses may be viewed as fugitive species, i.e., in order to reinfect the population and thereby avoid extinction, the virus must evolve rapidly enough to evade the immune protection of the host species. As a result of the rapid antigenic evolution of human influenza A viruses, formulation of new vaccines must be changed regularly in order to provide protection.

Phylogenetic analyses have also shown that internal proteins undergo a dramatic increase in evolutionary rate after the introduction of avian virus genes into gene pools of mammalian viruses (e.g., the NP gene, GORMAN et al. 1990a, 1991). One plausible explanation is that evolution of internal proteins is carried by the rapid antigenic evolution of the surface proteins, i.e., following periodic epidemic episodes and subsequent collapses of the virus population, random mutations in internal proteins are fixed by cloning for the next epidemic episode (BUONAGURIO et al. 1986b). Another possibility is that these mutations may be associated with the adaptation of the virus to the new host or are driven by T cell immune selection. All of these mechanisms could be operating simultaneously. However, if the first predominates, the random mutations might be expected to lead to a decrease in the relative fitness of the virus, while the later mechanisms should lead to an increase in the relative fitness of the virus as mutations accumulate.

3.3 Evolution in Influenza B and C Viruses

Patterns of evolution in human influenza B and C viruses do not appear to be extensively driven by antigenic selection, and their rate of accumulative evolution (particularly in influenza C viruses) is slower in comparison to human influenza A viruses (PALESE and YOUNG 1982; BUONAGURIO et al. 1986a, b; YAMASHITA et al. 1988; AIR et al. 1990). Influenza C viruses cause only infrequent outbreaks of mild respiratory disease (KATAGIRI et al. 1983) and occur primarily in young children (O'CALLAGHAN et al. 1980). Similarly, influenza B viruses typically cause milder respiratory illness than influenza A viruses and primarily infect children. Although influenza A viruses infect children and the elderly, this virus differs from the B and C viruses by its continually evolving antigenic character and its ability to reinfect adults and cause symptomatic disease and a renewed immune response. These differences among the A, B, and C viruses have profound effects on their patterns of evolution. Influenza A viruses in humans evolve along a single branch lineage, which indicates that there are no cocirculating strains of the same subtype and the virus evolves by clonal reconstitution following widespread extinction (BUONAGURIO et al. 1985). In contrast, the B and C viruses exhibit multiple lineage evolution which indicates the presence of cocirculating strains within the human population (BUONAGURIO et al. 1985; YAMASHITA et al. 1988). The pattern of epidemiology and evolution of the B and C viruses suggests that they are at or approaching an evolutionary equilibrium with their human hosts whereas the A viruses are not and are prevented from so doing by perturbations arising from reassortment of human virus genomes with those from avian viruses (e.g., PEASE 1987).

Influenza B and C viruses appear to be classical childhood diseases: they primarily infect children and permanent immunity is acquired following an infection. Since children lack previous exposure to influenza viruses they probably do not subject the viruses to strong directional immune selection. Although most adults have immunity to influenza B and C viruses, that immunity may be residual if the individual has not been reexposed regularly to these viruses. Thus, limited virus replication in adults is possible and the infections are probably asymptomatic. In this situation adults are ideal vectors of the virus and can maximize the spread of virus to susceptibles. If the virus were antigenically distinct from previously circulating B and C virus strains, the residual immunity would have been ineffective in preventing symptomatic infection and a full immune response. As a result, an antigenic cycle of selection and evolution as in human influenza A viruses would follow. In contrast to the situation in human influenza A viruses, B and C virus strains which are antigenically more similar to previous strains will have an advantage and continue to circulate within the population. Thus within influenza B and C viruses, the antigenic character of the viruses is expected to converge and remain relatively stable over time. At this point the virus and the host come into evolutionary equilibrium. In this evolutionary model, the stability and convergence of virus phenotype (antigenic character) is dependent on the adult population having previous exposure to the virus and a competent immune response. The evolutionary stasis observed in avian influenza virus proteins may have a similar basis.

How have human influenza B and C viruses escaped the influenza A virus cycle of strong antigenic selection? The answer may lie in understanding the evolution of reemergent human H1N1 influenza A viruses. These viruses remained out of circulation for 20 years before reemerging in 1977 (KENDAL et al. 1978; NAKAJIMA et al. 1978; SCHOLTISSEK et al. 1978). This 20-year hiatus may have broken the cycle of strong antigenic selection and evolution in H1N1 viruses and they now may be evolving similar to influenza B or C viruses. The coexistence of reemergent H1N1 viruses with the H3N2 human influenza A viruses and the lack of persistence of reassorted H1N1-H3N2 viruses suggests that they are antigenically distinct enough not to interfere strongly with each other through the host population immune response (e.g., FRANK et al. 1979, 1973). Thus, the reemergent H1N1 viruses are a distinct human influenza virus species and are evolving independently of their sister H3N2 influenza A viruses.

4 Origin of Influenza Viruses

4.1 Ancestry of Influenza A, B, and C Viruses

The general structural features and genome organization of influenza A, B, and C viruses suggest that they a share common ancestry distinct from other negative-strand RNA viruses (DESSELBERGER et al. 1980; SMITH and PALESE 1989). Of the three virus types, A and B are much more similar to each other in genome organization and protein homology than to C (LAMB 1983; SMITH and PALESE 1989) which suggests that influenza C viruses diverged well before the split between A and B viruses (SMITH and PALESE 1989). The more distant relationship of influenza C virus to the A and B viruses is demonstrated in phylogenetic analyses of NP genes (GAMMELIN et al. 1990). Among the homologous genes that have been compared for influenza A and B viruses, the polymerase genes show the highest level of homology and the organization and size of these genes has remained more similar than that of other genes (Table 3; LAMB 1989). The 60% level of homology between the nucleotide sequences of PB1 genes of A and B viruses is greater than the lowest homologies seen among nucleotide sequences of HA1 subunits of the 14 HA subtypes of influenza A viruses (31.3%–60.6%; KAWAOKA et al. 1990). In comparison, the nucleotide sequences of the HA1 subunits of influenza A and B viruses show a 36% homology (KRYSTAL et al. 1982). The greater range in variation among influenza A HA1 nucleotide sequences than between influenza B HA1 nucleotide sequences and their influenza A counterparts suggests that influenza B viruses diverged from the A viruses after divergence of the early ancestors of present-day HA subtypes. This suggestion is further supported by a phylogenetic analysis of partial HA1 gene

Table 3. Similarities of influenza A and B virus gene sequences[a]

Gene	Sequence similarity (%)		Source
	Nucleotide	Amino acid	
PB1	59.5–60.7	58.3–61.0	SIVASUBRAMANIAN and NAYAK (1982) KEMDIRIM et al. (1986) DEBORDE et al. (1987) KAWAOKA et al. (1989)
PB2	45.4–46.5	37–38	GORMAN et al. (1990b)
PA		38	AKOTO-AMANFU et al. (1987) DEBORDE et al. (1987)
HA[b]	36–48	24–39	KRYSTAL et al. (1982)
NA[c]		35	SHAW et al. (1982)
NP	33.6–35.5	37	LONDO et al. (1983) BRIEDIS and TOBIN (1984) NAKADA et al. (1984) GORMAN et al. (1990a)
M1	33	25	BRIEDIS et al. (1982) ITO et al. (1991)
M2		14	BRIEDIS et al. (1982)
NS	30	9.7–16.2	BRIEDIS and LAMB (1982) KAWAOKA et al. (1991)

[a] Similarities represent percent identity of aligned sequences. No data are available for NA genes

[b] Lower value represents percent identity for HA1 and higher value represents identity for HA2

[c] Comparison is for the region between amino acid residues 116 and 363 of the influenza B virus NA protein sequence

sequences (Fig. 3) which shows the influenza B/Lee/40 HA gene as being more closely related to the HA lineage containing H9, H8, and H12 subtypes than to two other major HA lineages. This analysis suggests that prior to the divergence of influenza B virus, the ancestral avian virus hemagglutinin subtypes had already diverged and that the B virus hemagglutinin and the present 14 avian virus hemagglutinin subtypes were derived from these ancestral subtypes.

Influenza B and C viruses are human viruses and are not found in avian hosts although the C viruses have been isolated from pigs and dogs, which has led to the suggestion that pigs serve as an alternate host reservoir for B and C viruses (GUO et al. 1983). Assuming that the B and C viruses originated from avian viruses they may be viewed as evolutionary relicts of previously widespread avian virus strains. To account for their high degree of divergence from the A viruses and their relative evolutionary equilibrium, they probably diverged many centuries to thousands of years ago from avian influenza virus ancestors. Shared characters between influenza A and B viruses are primitive, i.e., they were derived from a common ancestor. Thus, we expect that older influenza A virus lineages should share more characters with the B viruses than those in more recent lineages. For example, phylogenetic analyses show that the NP, PB2, M,

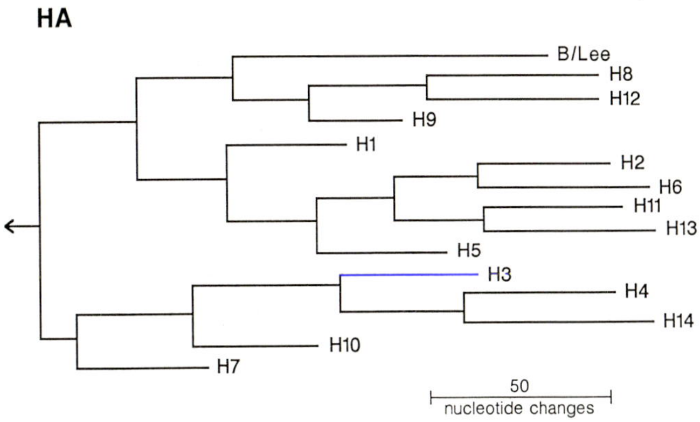

Fig. 3. Phylogeny of influenza virus hemagglutinin (*HA*) gene subtypes. This phylogenetic tree is similar to that in KAWAOKA et al. (1990) except that this tree is unrooted (does not set the B virus HA as an outgroup) and has a different topology. The analysis was based on aligned residues 63–343 (H3 numbering) of HA1 genes and the phylogenetic tree was determined with PAUP software, version 2.4 (David Swofford, Illinois Natural History Survey). The number of variable nucleotides represented is 198, the total tree length is 1021 steps (nucleotide changes) and the consistency index (proportion of changes due to forward mutations) is 0.453. *Horizontal distance* is proportional to the minimum number of nucleotide changes needed to join HA gene sequences. *Vertical lines* are of arbitrary length for spacing branches and labels. The *arrow* indicates the midpoint of the tree

and NS genes of influenza A virus EQPR56 (equine 1) are consistently closer to influenza B virus gene homologues; this pattern suggests that the EQPR56 viruses diverged from avian influenza viruses earlier than other nonavian lineages.

4.2 Evidence for an Avian Origin of Influenza Viruses

The common features of influenza A and B viruses leave little doubt that they share a common ancestor. Although the historical record is incomplete, enough evidence is available to provide some insight into the origin of these viruses. The question of the origin of the influenza viruses actually addresses two related, but distinct questions; (a) In what host did the first influenza virus evolve?; and (b) In what host(s) are the nearest common ancestors of each of the influenza virus gene segments? In the sections that follow we present summaries of phylogenetic analyses that provide strong evidence that all of the current gene segments circulating in both mammals and birds originated from avian influenza viruses.

In any long-continued host-parasite relationship there will be selection in the host to eliminate or lessen the deleterious effects of the parasite. In the parasite, there will be reciprocal selection for mutations that reduce host mortality and for mutations that reduce the deleterious effects of the host on the parasite . At equilibrium, the virus would be expected to replicate efficiently, cause minimal disease to the host, infect a high proportion of the host population, be perpetuated in host populations, and show increased genetic diversity with time. In relationships where the generation time of the parasite is much shorter than the host we can expect the parasite to evolve rapidly towards an adaptive equilibrium or optimum. Failure of this reciprocal host-parasite adaptation process is likely to lead to the extinction of one or the other.

A number of features of avian influenza viruses suggest that waterfowl may be the original hosts. Influenza viruses in wild waterfowl populations are ubiquitous, infection is nearly always asymptomatic, and large amounts of virus are shed by infected birds (WEBSTER et al. 1978). In addition there is considerable genetic diversity in avian viruses; 14 hemagglutinin and 9 neuraminidase subtypes persist and circulate in the avian host reservoir. Each hemagglutinin and neuraminidase subtype appears to be antigenically and genetically homogeneous when compared with the antigenic and genetic distinctness of each subtype. The selective pressure that would have caused diversification and the reasons for the continued coexistence of this array of avian virus subtypes remains unknown. The very high level of conservation observed in proteins of avian viruses suggests that an adaptive optimum has been nearly achieved. The apparent evolutionary stasis of these proteins suggests further that within the normal avian host population, any modification of the protein sequence is likely to prove detrimental in the long run. Therefore, avian influenza viruses and their waterfowl hosts appear to be a classic example of an optimally adapted system. The very low levels of evolution observed for avian virus proteins suggests that many centuries would have been required to generate the current genetic diversity and distinct separation of avian virus hemagglutinin and neuraminidase subtypes.

There is only one known report of a virulent virus causing disease in a wild bird population (Tern/South Africa/61; BECKER 1966). In domestic fowl and mammals outbreaks and epidemics of influenza viruses are relatively frequent but unpredictable and are usually accompanied by disease symptoms and mortality. Only a few of the numerous avian virus subtypes have been observed in nonavian hosts. Evolution of virus proteins in nonavian hosts typically shows a rapid accumulation of mutations away from avian-like forms which indicates an avian origin for these viruses. This is exemplified by evolution of human and classical swine viruses. The high degree of adaptation of avian viruses to their natural hosts, the considerable genetic diversity of avian virus subtypes, and the evolutionary stasis of avian virus proteins suggest that influenza viruses are a long-established pathogen in wild birds and more transient in other hosts.

4.3 Reconstruction of Influenza Virus Phylogenies

Phylogenetic trees represent hypotheses about evolutionary relationships among taxa. The phylogenetic analysis used in these studies (maximum parsimony) makes the assumption that the shortest mutational path connecting the taxa under study will provide a useful hypothetical evolutionary pathway. Thus, our phylogenetic analysis makes no assumptions about relationships based on historical evidence, dates of isolation, or on measures of antigenic and genetic similarity. These other sources of evidence provide independent tests of hypotheses about relationships.

Interpretation of relatively recent events in the evolution of influenza RNA segments is straightforward and the avian origin of some of the genes of current mammalian viruses is easily seen. For example, genetic and phylogenetic analyses have now demonstrated that all genes that have appeared in mammalian virus gene pools over the past century have an avian origin (e.g., KAWAOKA et al. 1989; GORMAN et al. 1990a, b; BEAN et al. 1991; ITO et al. 1991). Each influenza virus gene phylogeny represents only a partial history of virus evolution but consideration of all gene phylogenies together reveals a more complete picture of virus evolution. A comparison of branching patterns among influenza virus gene phylogenies (Fig. 1) demonstrates that reassortment of nonavian with avian viruses has occurred repeatedly over the evolutionary history of influenza viruses. The different relative positions of gene lineages among nonavian viruses indicates that the genes of host-specific viruses are of different relative ages. This suggests that a consequence of the appearance of new reassorted viruses has been the extinction of previous strains or their genes. Finally, these phylogenetic analyses demonstrate that whole avian viruses can be transmitted to new hosts, displace previous strains, and evolve independently from their avian ancestors.

Interpretation of the deeper branches of the trees and speculation on the ultimate origins of a lineage must proceed with caution. Phylogenetic trees generated in this manner have no inherently favored point of origin or direction. The direction of evolution can be inferred by reference to dates of isolation, and hypothetical points of origin can be estimated from the genetic distances on the tree if the rates of mutation have remained constant for all branches within a lineage. Since it is clear that the rates of mutation are greater in mammalian than in avian hosts (Table 1), it is necessary to understand how this may distort phylogenies of virus evolution. All of the phylogenies represented in Fig. 1 show mammalian virus genes branching from the base of the tree. This does not imply that they represent the most primitive forms of the gene, only that they have diverged relatively farther and possibly earlier than other strains analyzed. In all cases the phylogenies are consistent with the hypothesis that influenza viruses have been continuously evolving in waterfowl, and at various times these viruses have been introduced into other avian and mammalian hosts. These introductions are manifested by the formation of new host-specific lineages due to new introductions of influenza viruses or virus genes from avian hosts. This is our current working hypothesis for the origin of influenza viruses (Fig. 4).

4.4 Historical Summary of Influenza Virus Evolution

A historical summary of the major vicariant events (those that lead to lineage divergence) in the evolution of influenza viruses is presented in Fig. 4. Divergence

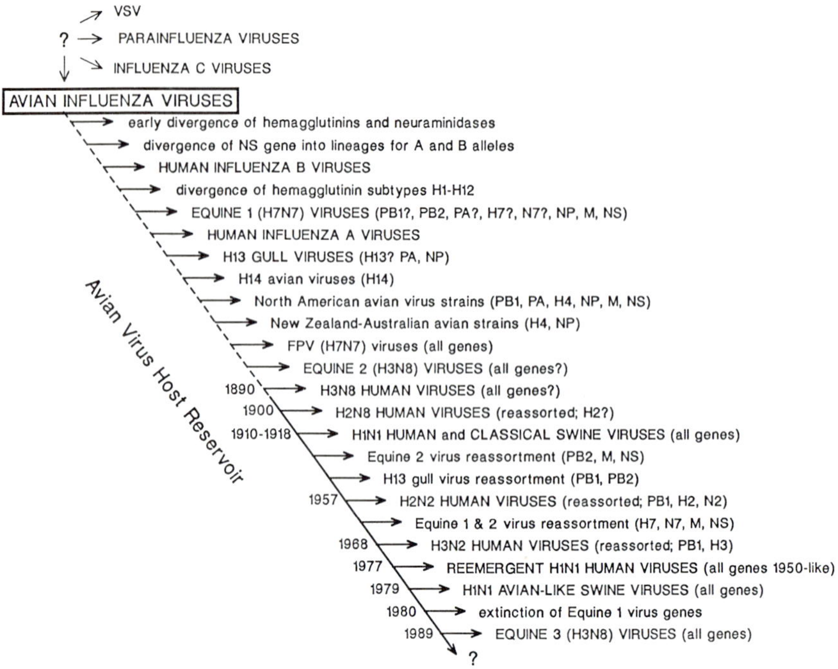

Fig. 4. Historical summary of the evolution of influenza viruses. The vicariant events (those that lead to lineage divergence) depicted in this figure are in rough chronological order and have been deduced from collective analysis of influenza virus gene phylogenies (e.g., Fig. 3), antigenic and genetic data, and historical records. The *dashed line* indicates an indeterminant time frame. The genes involved in evolutionary events are included in parentheses. The Equine 3 viruses at the *bottom* of the figure refer to new avian-like H3N8 viruses that have recently appeared in Northeastern China (GUO et al. 1991). At the top, VSV stands for vesicular stomatitis virus

of the major lineages of HA and NA subtypes and the split between NS "a" and "b" alleles represent possibly the oldest vicariant events in the evolution of influenza A viruses. The diversity of HA and NA subtypes among the older virus isolates (1902–1956) and the distinct pattern of evolutionary divergence among all known HA subtypes (KAWAOKA et al. 1990) indicates that their divergence predates the twentieth century. Moreover, the large differences among some avian virus gene lineages and the apparent slow evolution of avian virus genes (GORMAN et al. 1990a, b, 1991; BEAN et al. 1991) suggests that some HA and NA groups and NS a and b alleles diverged many centuries ago. As previously discussed, the divergence of human influenza B viruses from avian influenza viruses must also be quite old, probably occurring after the divergence of the major avian HA subtypes but before the appearance of more recent HA subtypes (e.g., H13, H4, H14) (Figs. 3, 4).

The oldest vicariant event among mammalian influenza A viruses is the divergence of EQPR56 (equine 1) viruses. GORMAN et al. (1990a) provide 1800 as a latest estimate of the date of the divergence of the EQPR56 virus. The divergence of other host-specific virus gene lineages occurred after this (during the nineteenth century). For example, the origin of the HA, M, NS, NP, and PA genes of present-day H13 gull viruses probably occurred in two separate reassortment events during the nineteenth century. Other major nineteenth century events include the origin of North American avian virus strains, recent equine strains and FPV viruses (Fig. 4).

Present-day human viruses originated in the early twentieth century, just prior to the 1918 pandemic, and classical swine viruses were probably derived from human viruses during the 1918 pandemic (GORMAN et al. 1991). Reassortment in human, recent equine, and possibly H13 gull viruses have occurred since the 1920s. The most recent events have been the appearance of a new avian-derived H1N1 virus in European swine populations in 1979 and the H3N8 virus in horses in Northeastern China in 1989. The new swine influenza virus has continued to evolve and circulate in European swine populations for more than 10 years. The most recent host-specific virus strain to appear is represented by the new avian-like H3N8 equine influenza virus in China (GUO et al. 1991).

Acknowledgements. Work in our laboratory is supported by National Institute of Allergy and Infectious Disease grants AI-29680, AI-08831, AI-20591, and AI-29599 from the National Institutes of Health, Cancer Center Support (CORE) Grant CA-21765, National Research Service Award 5T32-CA09346 to O.T.G., and American Lebanese Syrian Associated Charities.

References

Air GM, Gibbs AJ, Laver WG, Webster RG (1990) Evolutionary changes in influenza B are not primarily governed by antibody selection. Proc Natl Acad Sci USA 87: 3884–3888

Akoto-Amanfu E, Sivasubramanian N, Nayak DP (1987) Primary structure of the polymerase acidic (PA) gene of influenza B virus (B/Sing/22/79). Virology 159: 147–153

Altmuller A, Fitch WM, Scholtissek C (1989) Biological and genetic evolution of the nucleoprotein gene of human influenza A viruses. J Gen Virol 70: 2111–2119

Bean WJ (1984) Correlation of influenza A virus nucleoprotein genes with host species. Virology 133: 438–442

Bean W, Schell M, Gorman O, Kawaoka Y, Katz J, Webster R (1991) Evolution of the H3 influenza virus hemagglutinin from human and non-human hosts. J Virol (in press)

Becker WB (1966) The isolation and classification of tern virus: influenza virus A/Tern/South Africa/61. J Hyg 64: 309–320

Both GW, Sleigh MJ, Cox N, Kendal AP (1983) Antigenic drift in influenza virus H3 hemagglutinin from 1968 to 1980: multiple evolutionary pathways and sequential amino acid changes at key antigenic sites. J Virol 48: 52–60

Briedis DJ, Lamb RA (1982) Influenza B virus genome: sequences and structural organization of RNA segment 8 and the mRNAs coding for the NS1 and NS2 proteins. J Virol 42: 186–193

Briedis DJ, Tobin M (1984) Influenza B virus genome: complete nucleotide sequence of the influenza B/Lee/40 virus genome RNA segment 5 encoding the nucleoprotein and comparison with the B/Singapore/222/79 nucleoprotein. Virology 133: 448–455

Briedis DJ, Lamb RA, Choppin PW (1982) Sequence of RNA segment 7 of the influenza B virus genome: partial amino acid homology between the membrane proteins (M1) of influenza A and B viruses and conservation of a second open reading frame. Virology 116: 581–588

Buonagurio D, Nakada S, Desselberger U, Krystal M, Palese P (1985) Noncumulative sequence changes in the hemagglutinin genes of influenza C virus isolates. Virology 146: 221–232

Buonagurio DA, Nakada S, Fitch WM, Palese P (1986a) Epidemiology of influenza C virus in man: multiple evolutionary lineages and low rate of change. Virology 153: 12–21

Buonagurio DA, Nakada S, Parvin JD, Krystal M, Palese P, Fitch WM (1986b) Evolution of human influenza A viruses over 50 years: rapid, uniform rate of change in NS gene. Science 232: 980–982

Crosby AW (1989) America's forgotten pandemic, the influenza of 1918. Cambridge University Press, New York, pp 337

Daniels RS, Skehel JJ, Wiley DC (1985) Amino acid sequences of haemagglutinins of influenza viruses of the H3 subtype isolated from horses. J Gen Virol 66: 457–464

DeBorde DC, Naeve CW, Herlocher ML, Maassab HF (1987) Nucleotide sequences of the PA and PB1 genes of B/Ann Arbor/1/66 virus: comparison with genes of B/Lee/40 and type A influenza viruses. Virus Res. 8: 33–41

Desselberger U, Racariello VR, Zazra JJ, Palese P (1980) The 3′ and 5′-terminal sequences of influenza A, B and C virus RNA segments are highly conserved and show partial inverted complementarity. Gene 8: 315–328

Donis RO, Bean WJ, Kawaoka Y, Webster RG (1989) Distinct lineages of influenza virus H4 hemagglutinin genes in different regions of the world. Virology 169: 408–417

Frank AL, Taber LH, Glezen WP, Paedes A, Couch RB (1979) Reinfection with influenza A (H3N2) virus in young children and their families. J Infect Dis 140: 829–836

Frank AL, Taber LH, Wells JM (1983) Individuals infected with two subtypes of influenza A virus in the same season. J Infect Dis 147: 120–124

Gammelin M, Altmuller A, Reinhardt U, Mandler J, Harley VR, Hudson PJ, Fitch WM, Scholtissek C (1990) Phylogenetic analysis of nucleoproteins suggests that human influenza A viruses emerged from a 19th-century avian ancestor. Mol Biol Evol 7: 194–200

Gorman OT, Bean WJ, Kawaoka Y, Webster RG (1990a) Evolution of the nucleoprotein gene of influenza A virus. J Virol 64: 1487–1497

Gorman OT, Donis RO, Kawaoka Y, Webster RG (1990b) Evolution of influenza A virus PB2 genes: implications for evolution of the ribonucleoprotein complex and origin of human influenza A virus. J Virol 64: 4893–4902

Gorman OT, Bean WJ, Kawaoka Y, Donatelli I, Guo Y, Webster RG (1991) Evolution of influenza A virus nucleoprotein genes: implications for the origin of H1N1 human and classical swine viruses. J Virol 65: 3704–3714

Guo Y, Yin F, Wang P, Wang M, Zhu J (1983) Isolation of influenza C virus from pigs and experimental infection of pigs with influenza C virus. J Gen Virol 64: 177–182

Guo Y, Wang M, Kawaoka Y, Gorman O, Ito T, Webster RG (1991) Emergence of a new avian-like influenza A virus in horses. Virology (submitted)

Ito T, Gorman O, Kawaoka Y, Bean W, Webster RG (1991) Evolutionary analysis of the influenza A virus M gene with comparison of the M1 and M2 proteins. J Virol 65: 5491–5498

Katagiri S, Ohizumi A, Homma M (1983) An outbreak of type C influenza in a children's home. J Infect Dis 148: 51–56

Kawaoka Y, Gorman OT, Channell DB, Wells KA, Donis RO, Donatelli I, Guo Y, Webster RG (1991) Evolution of the influenza A virus NS gene: Evidence for multiple introductions of human and avian virus genes into pigs. J Virol (submitted)

Kawaoka Y, Webster RG (1991) The evolution of the NS gene of influenza A virus. J Virol (in press)

Kawaoka Y, Krauss S, Webster RG (1989) Avian-to-human transmission of the PB1 gene of influenza A virus in the 1957 and 1968 pandemics. J Virol 63: 4603–4608

Kawaoka Y, Yamnikova S, Chambers TM, Lvov DK, Webster RG (1990) Molecular characterization of a new hemagglutinin, subtype H14, of influenza A virus. Virology 179: 759–767

Kemdirim S, Palefsky J, Briedis DJ (1986) Influenza B virus PB1 protein: nucleotide sequence of the genome RNA segment predicts a high degree of structural homology with the corresponding influenza A virus polymerase protein. Virology 152: 126–135

Kendal AP, Kiley MP (1973) Characterization of influenza virus neuraminidases: peptide changes associated with antigen divergence between early and late N2 neuraminidases. J Virol 12: 1482–1490

Kendal AP, Noble GR, Skehel JJ, Dowdle WR (1978) Antigenic similarity of influenza A (H1N1) viruses from epidemics in 1977–1978 to "Scandinavian" strains isolated in epidemics of 1950–1951. Virology 89: 632–636

Krystal M, Elliott RM, Benz EW, Young JF, Palese P (1982) Evolution of influenza A and B viruses. Conservation of structural features in the hemagglutinin genes. Proc Natl Acad Sci USA 79: 4800–4804

Lamb RA (1983) The influenza virus RNA segments and their encoded proteins. In: Palese P, Kingsbury DW (eds) Genetics of influenza viruses. Springer, Berlin Heidelberg New York, pp 21–69

Lamb RA (1989) Genes and proteins of the influenza viruses. In: Krug RM, Fraenkel-Conrat H, Wagner RR (eds) The influenza viruses. Plenum, New York, pp 1–88

Londo DR, Davis AR, Nayak DP (1983) Complete nucleotide sequence of the nucleoprotein gene of influenza B virus. J Virol 47: 642–648

Mulder J, Masurel N (1958) Pre-epidemic antibody against 1957 strain of Asiatic influenza in serum of older people living in the Netherlands. Lancet 1: 810–814

Nakada S, Creager RS, Krystal M, Palese P (1984) Complete nucleotide sequence of the influenza C/California/78 virus nucleoprotein gene. Virus Res 1: 433–441

Nakajima K, Desselberger U, Palese P (1978) Recent human influenza A (H1N1) viruses are closely related genetically to strains isolated in 1950. Nature 274: 334–339

Nakajima K, Nobusawa E, Nakajima S (1984) Genetic relatedness between A/Swine/Iowa1/5/30 (H1N1) and human influenza viruses. Virology 139: 194–198

O'Callaghan RJ, Gohd RS, Labat DD (1980) Human antibody to influenza C virus: its age-related distribution and distinction from receptor analogs. Infect Immun 30: 500–505

Okazaki K, Kawaoka Y, Webster RG (1989) Evolutionary pathways of the PA genes of influenza A viruses. Virology 172: 601–608

Palese P, Young JF (1982) Variation of influenza A, B, and C viruses. Science 215: 1468–1474

Pease CM (1987) An evolutionary epidemiological mechanism, with applications to type A influenza. Theor Popul Biol 31: 422–452

Raymond FL, Caton AJ, Cox NJ, Kendal AP, Brownlee GG (1986) The antigenicity and evolution of influenza H1 haemagglutinin from 1950–1957 and 1977–1983: two pathways from one gene. Virology 148: 275–287

Scholtissek C, Rohde W, von Hoyningen V, Rott R (1978) On the origin of the human influenza virus subtypes H2N2 and H3N2. Virology 87: 13–20

Scholtissek C, Burger H, Bachmann PA, Hannoun C (1983) Genetic relatedness of hemagglutinins of the H1 subtype of influenza A viruses isolated from swine and birds. Virology 129: 521–523

Scholtissek C, Burger H, Kistner O, Shortridge KF (1985) The nucleoprotein as a possible major factor in determining host specificity of influenza H3N2 viruses. Virology 147: 287–294

Shaw MW, Lamb RA, Erickson BW, Briedis DJ, Choppin PW (1982) Complete nucleotide sequence of the neuraminidase gene of influenza B virus. Proc Natl Acad Sci USA 79: 6817–6821

Sivasubramanian N, Nayak DP (1982) Sequence analysis of the polymerase 1 gene and the secondary structure prediction of polymerase 1 protein of human influenza virus A/WSN/33. J Virol 44: 321–329

Smith FI, Palese P (1989) Variation in influenza virus genes. In: Krug RM (ed) The influenza viruses. Plenum, New York, pp 319–359

Snyder MH, Buckler-White AJ, London WT, Tierney EL, Murphy BR (1987) The avian influenza virus nucleoprotein gene and a specific constellation of avian and human virus polymerase genes each specify attenuation of avian/human influenza A/Pintail/79 reassortant viruses from monkeys. J Virol 61: 2857–2863

Tian SF, Buckler-White AJ, London WT, Reck LJ, Channock RM, Murphy BR (1985) Nucleoprotein and membrane protein genes are associated with restriction of replication of influenza A/Mallard/NY/78 virus and its reassortants in squirrel monkey respiratory tract. J Virology 53: 771–775

Treanor JJ, Snyder MH, London WT, Murphy BR (1989) The B allele of the NS gene of avian influenza viruses, but not the A allele, attenuates a human influenza A virus for squirrel monkeys. Virology 171: 1–9

Webster RG, Laver WG (1975) Antigenic variation of influenza viruses. In: Kilbourne ED (ed) The influenza viruses and influenza. Academic, New York, pp 269–314

Webster RG, Yakhno MA, Hinshaw VS, Bean WJ, Murti KG (1978) Intestinal influenza: replication and characterization of influenza viruses in ducks. Virology 84: 268–278

Webster RG, Kawaoka Y, Bean WJ (1989) What is the potential of avirulent influenza viruses to complement a cleavable hemagglutinin and generate virulent strains? Virology 171: 484–492

Yamashita M, Krystal M, Fitch WM, Palese P (1988) Influenza B virus evolution: co-circulating lineages and comparison of evolutionary pattern with those of influenza A and C viruses. Virology 163: 112–122

Genetic Diversity and Slow Rates of Evolution in New World Alphaviruses

S. C. WEAVER[1,2], R. RICO-HESSE[3], and T. W. SCOTT[2]

1 Introduction

1.1 Alphavirus Replication

Alphavirus is a genus of arthropod-borne viruses (arboviruses) in the family Togaviridae. These viruses have a single-strand messenger or plus-sense RNA genome of ca. 11 700 bases. 42S genomic RNA is found in virions and infected

[1] Department of Biology, The University of California, San Diego, La Jolla, California 92093, USA
[2] Department of Entomology and Center for Agricultural Biotechnology, The University of Maryland, College Park, Maryland 20742, USA
[3] Department of Epidemiology and Public Health, Yale University School of Medicine, New Haven, Connecticut 06510, USA

Current Topics in Microbiology and Immunology, Vol. 176

cells; a subgenomic 26S RNA species, identical to the 3′-third of the 42S genomic messenger RNA (mRNA), is present only in infected cells and codes only for the structural proteins (STRAUSS and STRAUSS 1986; SCHLESINGER and SCHLESINGER 1990).

Alphaviruses replicate in the cytoplasm of infected cells. Entry into vertebrate cells in vitro occurs by receptor-mediated endocytosis, although the receptor(s) have not been definitively identified (KIELIAN and HELENIUS 1986). Following uncoating, 42S RNA serves as mRNA for synthesis of three structural proteins (C, E1, E2) and four nonstructural proteins (nsP1–nsP4); the latter function as the replicase/transcriptase complex. Genomic 42S RNA serves as a template for full length minus-strand synthesis, followed by polymerization of additional plus-strand RNA. Structural proteins are translated from 26S mRNA as a polyprotein. The capsid protein is cotranslationally cleaved and released into the cytoplasm where it interacts with 42S RNA to form icosahedral nucleocapsids. The remaining polyprotein enters the rough endoplasmic reticulum; continued translation is followed by cleavage of p62 and 6K from E1, glycosylation, and oligosaccharide modifications in p62 and E1. Later, p62 is cleaved to yield E3 and E2 (E3 is not found in virions of most alphaviruses). Glycoproteins E1 and E2 are inserted into the plasma membrane via the secretory pathway, and virions mature when nucleocapsids bud through the membrane to acquire their envelope (STRAUSS and STRAUSS 1986; SCHLESINGER and SCHLESINGER 1990).

Replication of alphaviruses in mosquito cells is poorly understood relative to that in vertebrate cells (BROWN and CONDREAY 1986). While vertebrate cell infection generally is cytocidal, infected mosquito cells usually show no cytopathic effects (CPE) in vitro and develop persistent infections. In vivo infection of mosquito vectors is also persistent and proceeds without recognizable CPE in most tissues. However, pathologic changes occur in the midgut of at least two natural alphavirus vectors (WEAVER et al. 1988; WEAVER, unpublished).

1.2 Diversity and Systematics of Alphaviruses

Serologic studies of alphavirus diversity have identified at least 37 members of this genus, which are assigned to seven complexes based on serological cross-reactivity (CALISHER and KARABATSOS 1988). One or more species are found within each alphavirus complex and multiple subtypes and/or varieties exist for several species. In this review we discuss diversity and evolution of New World members of three alphavirus complexes: eastern equine encephalomyelitis (EEE), Venezuelan equine encephalomyelitis (VEE), and western equine encephalomyelitis (WEE). These viruses are epidemiologically important and exhibit considerable natural diversity.

Genetic variability of alphaviruses has only recently been examined at the molecular level. Systematic studies have compared amino acid sequences for representatives of alphavirus complexes, delineating broad evolutionary relationships. Recent dendrograms place the Old World alphaviruses Ross River virus, Semliki Forest virus, and O'nyong-nyong virus in one cluster; New World alphaviruses EEE virus (EEEV), WEE virus (WEEV) and VEE virus (VEEV) occupy a separate cluster along with the Old World Sindbis virus (LEVINSON et al. 1990).

1.3 Alphavirus Transmission Cycles

Most New World alphaviruses are transmitted enzootically by mosquito vectors among avian and small mammal vertebrate hosts (exceptions to mosquito transmission are Fort Morgan virus (FMV) and Bijou Bridge virus (BBV), which are transmitted by a cimicid bug). Humans and domestic animals are only tangentially involved during epizootic/epidemic conditions (SCOTT and WEAVER 1989; PETERS and DALRYMPLE 1990). Except for laboratory infections and horizontal transmission among penned game birds, alphavirus transmission requires the bite of an infected insect. Foci of transmission are therefore defined by habitats that favor survival and reproduction of mosquito vectors. Transovarial transmission in mosquitoes has been suggested for some alphaviruses in Asia and Australia (KAY and AASKOV 1988), but is not believed to occur in the New World (ROSEN 1987). FMV is, however, tansmitted transstadially by its cimicid vectors (WALTON and GRAYSON 1988). Transplacental infection has been reported for VEEV and WEEV in vertebrates, but probably does not contribute to virus amplification (SCOTT 1988). Important gaps in our understanding of the epidemiology of New World alphaviruses include (a) mechanisms for maintenance of interepidemic transmission, (b) factors that contribute to periodic epidemics and epizootics, and (c) mechanisms for alphavirus survival during times when vector mosquitoes are inactive, i.e., winter in temperate regions and the dry season in the tropics.

2 Genetic Diversity and Evolution of New World Alphaviruses

2.1 Eastern Equine Encephalomyelitis Virus

2.1.1 Diversity and Evolution

EEEV is the only species in the EEE complex. CASALS (1964) identified two serologically distinct forms of EEEV; nearly all isolates from North America and the Caribbean belong to the North American variety, while those isolated in Central and South America form the South American variety.

Recent work has demonstrated remarkable antigenic and genetic conservation of EEEV in North America. ROEHRIG et al. (1990) analyzed EEEV isolates using oligonucleotide fingerprinting and monoclonal antibodies. Antigenic conservation was revealed among all North America EEEV isolates examined, while more variation was detected among South than North American strains. Three North American strains isolated over a 49-year period shared over 90% of their T_1-resistant oligonucleotides, suggesting a high degree of conservation in the EEEV 42S genome. These findings have been supported by fingerprinting of additional isolates from North America and the Caribbean (REPIK, personal communication).

Nucleotide sequence data for the 26S genome of four North American EEEV strains, isolated from 1933 to 1985, also revealed remarkable conservation, with only 0.7% sequence divergence over a 52-year period (WEAVER et al. 1991b). The EEEV 26S evolutionary rate was estimated at 0.014% per year, or 1.4×10^{-4} substitutions per nucleotide per year. Deduced amino acid sequences were also highly conserved, with over 99% similarity in pair-wise comparisons. Limited 26S sequences from 13 isolates suggested that EEEV evolves within a single lineage or gene pool in North America, with regular gene flow among transmission foci. All fixations of nucleotide substitutions detected in these limited 26S regions were synonymous changes, suggesting conservation of structural proteins during 55 years of North American transmission (WEAVER et al. 1991b).

The serologic distinction between North and South American variety EEEV isolates (CASALS 1964) is also reflected in genetic analyses. Oligonucleotide fingerprint studies (REPIK, personal communication) indicate that South American strains are genetically distinct from the North American variety, and are more diverse than North American EEEV isolates. Nucleotide sequence data from a Panamanian EEEV isolate showed only 78% similarity to North American strains, supporting this view (WEAVER et al. 1991b). Rates of evolution (nucleotide sequence divergence) in South American EEEV lineages have not been determined.

Few EEEV strains of the South American variety have been isolated; consequently, knowledge of the serological and genetic relationships among these viruses is limited (SCOTT and WEAVER 1989). However, antigenic and genetic diversity of EEEV in Central and South America suggests the possibility of multiple subtypes and/or varieties comparable to those in the VEEV complex.

2.1.2 Transmission Cycles

The distribution of EEEV includes eastern North America, from southern Canada through the Americas, and the Caribbean to central Argentina. In North America, *Culiseta melanura* transmits EEEV among a variety of passerine birds in freshwater swamps along the east coast, and in a few inland locations (SCOTT and WEAVER 1989). Several other mosquito species (genera *Aedes* and *Coquillettidia*) have been implicated as epizootic/epidemic vectors. In Central and South America, mosquitoes in the subgenus *Culex* (*Melanoconion*) are regarded as the principal enzootic vectors, and small mammals are considered vertebrate hosts. In some tropical locations, birds may also be involved in transmission cycles. Very little is known about the natural history of EEEV in the Caribbean, although most EEEV strains isolated there have been of the North American variety.

2.2 Venezuelan Equine Encephalomyelitis Virus Complex

2.2.1 Diversity and Evolution

VEEV is the only species in the VEE complex. The first comprehensive evaluation of VEEV diversity used kinetic hemagglutination inhibition (HI) tests to distinguish multiple subtypes and varieties (YOUNG and JOHNSON 1969); these studies demonstrated that serologically distinct VEE viruses have different geographic distributions. Subsequently, monoclonal antibodies were used to detect variation within the complex, including variation within subtypes (ROEHRIG and MATHEWS 1985; RICO-HESSE et al. 1988).

Currently, six VEEV subtypes (I–VI) are serologically recognized (Table 1) (WALTON and GRAYSON 1988). Subtype I, varieties AB and C have only been isolated during equine epizootics and epidemics, and have therefore been called "epizootic" strains. Subtype I varieties D, E, and F, and subtypes II–VI generally occur in sylvatic transmission foci and are avirulent for equines; they have thus been called "enzootic" strains. However, this usage could be misleading; for example, "enzootic" VEEV strains occasionally cause human illness (WALTON

Table 1. Viruses in the Venezuelan equine encephalomyelitis complex

Subtype	Variety	Pattern of transmission	Location	Vector
I	AB	Epizootic	South, Central, and North America	Various mammalophilic mosquitoes
	C	Epizootic	Northern South America	Various mammalophilic mosquitoes
	D	Enzootic	Ecuador, Panama, Colombia, Venezuela	*Culex* (*Melanoconion*) *ocossa* and *panocossa*
	E	Enzootic	Central America	*Culex* (*Melanoconion*) *taeniopus*
	F	Enzootic	Brazil	Unknown
II (Everglades)		Enzootic	Southern Florida	*Culex* (*Melanoconion*) *cedecei*
III	A			
	Mucambo	Enzootic	South America	*Culex* (*Melanoconion*) *portesi*
	B			
	Tonate	Enzootic	South America,	Unknown
	Bijou Bridge	Unknown	western North America	*Oeciacus vicarius*
	C	Enzootic	Peru	Unknown
IV (Pixuna)		Enzootic	Brazil	Unknown
V (Cabassou)		Enzootic	French Guiana	Unknown
VI		Enzootic	Argentina	Unknown

and GRAYSON 1988), and could cause unrecognized epizootics in rodent or avian host populations.

RNA oligonucleotide fingerprinting studies have revealed considerable genetic diversity among representatives of four VEEV subtypes (TRENT et al. 1979; KINNEY et al. 1983; RICO-HESSE et al. 1988). Subtype I isolates from diverse geographic locations in Central and South America showed less than 50% identity of their T_1-resistant oligonucleotides, and variety ID strains from different locations were also heterogeneous. In contrast, variety IC and ID strains isolated from central Colombia over a 23-year period shared over 85% of their oligonucleotides (RICO-HESSE et al. 1988). This translates to less than 1% divergence of their total genome, or less than 5×10^{-4} substitutions per nucleotide per year. Not only were enzootic variety ID VEEV isolates from a specific geographic region conserved, but a high degree of similarity (over 85% oligonucleotide identity) was observed between ID and epizootic variety IC viruses isolated in the same region. Thus, genetic relatedness within Colombian VEEV strains appears to be a function of geography rather than epidemiological status or serologic grouping. This suggests that epizootic variety IC viruses in Colombia may have originated from enzootic variety ID virus foci (RICO-HESS et al. 1988). These data also support the view the VEEV evolves within multiple genetic lineages in isolated foci of transmission.

2.2.2 Transmission Cycles

Epizootic variety IAB and IC VEEV strains periodically cause extensive equine outbreaks in South and Central America, while humans and other mammals are usually only tangentially involved (WALTON and GRAYSON 1988). Infected equines develop high-titer viremias, facilitating transmission of epizootic VEEV by a variety of mammalophilic mosquito species. Epizootics caused by variety IAB and IC viruses can spread rapidly when large numbers of susceptible equines and vector mosquitoes are available. For example, an outbreak which began near the Guatemala–El Salvador border in 1969 quickly spread north along the west coast of Central America, reaching Texas in 1971. Epizootic/epidemic transmission is often broadly distributed with an irregular pattern of movement along a front of virus activity. Variety IAB and IC VEEV strains have not been isolated in affected regions following the cessation of epizootic activity, and the source of these outbreaks remains an enigma (WALTON and GRAYSON 1988).

Enzootic VEEV complex viruses are widely distributed in the Americas (Table 1; WALTON and GRAYSON 1988); isolations have been made as far south as Argentina and as far north as the southern United States. These VEEV strains circulate in discrete sylvatic transmission foci in tropical and subtropical America and are primarily transmitted among small rodents and birds by mosquitoes. Transmission is nearly continuous within foci, with seasonal expansions and contractions of transmission activity. Four mosquito species are known enzootic VEEV vectors; all belong to the *Culex* (*Melanoconion*) subgenus (Table 1). BBV, a subtype III strain, has been isolated from cliff swallow bugs (*Oeciacus vicarius*) and nestling birds in western North America. It is unknown whether this virus persists in a stable transmission cycle or represents an incidental introduction (WALTON and GRAYSON 1988).

2.3 Western Equine Encephalomyelitis Virus Complex

2.3.1 Diversity and Evolution

The WEE complex contains six species and four subtypes distinguished by neutralization tests; the four New World species are: WEEV, Highlands J virus (HJV), FMV, and Aura virus (REISEN and MONATH 1988). WEE complex viruses isolated in western North America are antigenically distinct from those circulating in eastern North America (HJV) and from one WEEV isolate from Argentina (strain AG80–646). Otherwise, North and South American WEEV isolates are antigenically similar. FMV is sympatric with WEEV (western North America), while Aura virus occurs only in South America.

Among North American WEE complex viruses, WEEV is most often associated with disease (REISEN and MONATH 1988). HJV rarely causes overt illness in humans or domestic animals, and FMV has only been isolated from sick and dead nestling house sparrows.

TRENT and GRANT (1980) examined genetic diversity among 17 WEEV strains isolated from 1941–1975 in North and South America, using oligonucleotide fingerprinting. These isolates shared ca. 75%–100% of T_1-resistant oligonucleotides, representing 8%–9% of the WEEV genome. These data translate to ca. 0.9% nucleotide sequence divergence over a 32-year period, or an estimated 3×10^{-4} substitutions per nucleotide, per year. Fingerprinting of eight isolates of HJV revealed similar genetic conservation. Comparison of 3′-nucleotide sequences of two WEEV strains, isolated 12 years apart in different geographic regions, suggested 0.1%–0.2% divergence per year (HAHN et al. 1988). These data indicate genetic stability and slow evolution, within single genetic lineages, for at least two members of the WEE complex.

2.3.2 Transmission Cycles

Transmission cycles of WEEV are well characterized in North America but essentially unknown in Central and South America (REISEN and MONATH 1988). A WEEV subtype (AG80–646) which is not pathogenic to mammals may be transmitted by *Culex* (*Melanoconion*) mosquitoes among small mammals and birds in subtropical areas of Argentina. Mosquitoes in the genera *Aedes, Anopheles, Mansonia*, and *Psorophora* have been implicated as epidemic/epizootic vectors in Argentina.

The enzootic and epidemic/epizootic mosquito vector of WEEV in western North America is *Culex tarsalis*, which transmits virus among passerine birds in agroecosystems (REISEN and MONATH 1988). At northern latitudes and in the arid southwest, other mosquito species in the genera *Culiseta* and *Aedes*, and mammalian hosts (hares, jackrabbits and ground squirrels) may be involved in WEEV transmission. In North America, most human and equine WEEV infections have been reported from western Canada and north-central United States. HJV is transmitted among passerine birds in eastern North American freshwater swamps by the *Culiseta melanura*; its transmission cycle is nearly identical to that of EEEV in geographic distribution, seasonality, and habitat. FMV occurs in western North America and is transmitted among colonies of nesting songbirds by the cimicid swallow bug, *Oeciacus vicarius*.

3 Factors Regulating Alphavirus Evolution

3.1 Molecular Factors

Antigenic and genetic analyses have revealed considerable diversity among members of New World alphavirus complexes, particularly in the tropics. This supports the view that alphaviruses have undergone adaptive radiation in the New World. However, all evidence obtained by comparison of isolates from individual alphavirus lineages indicates a slow rate of evolution (nucleotide sequence divergence) in nature. Estimates of evolutionary rates range from $1.4–5 \times 10^{-4}$ substitutions per nucleotide per year (see Sect. 2); these rates are ca. ten fold or more lower than those reported for other RNA viruses (WEAVER et al. 1991b). Assuming that alphaviruses form a monophyletic group, these slow rates of evolution suggest that extant species diverged in the distant past. However, slow rates of sequence divergence during this century could reflect a static interval in a punctuated equilibrium pattern of evolution.

Mechanisms responsible for slow evolution in alphaviruses are unknown. However, current knowledge of New World alphavirus transmission cycles and replication may provide insights into this phenomenon. Unlike most viruses which infect a single host taxon, alphaviruses are adapted to efficient replication in both vertebrate and invertebrate hosts. Studies employing host-restricted mutants, host cell transcription and translation inhibitors, and enucleation suggest that different host-specific factors participate in alphavirus replication in vertebrate versus mosquito cells (BROWN and CONDREAY 1986; LEMM et al. 1990). The receptor(s) for alphavirus entry into vertebrate cells is probably common to many taxa, since hosts from several classes are susceptible to infection. In mosquitoes, midgut cell receptors may be virus species or subtype specific, while entry into other cells and tissues probably involves a more generalized, distinct mechanism. This implies alphavirus interaction with several distinct receptors and/or multiple entry modes during natural replication. Broad conservation in multiple envelope glycoprotein determinants would be predicted if several domains participate in entry into various cell types during the transmission cycle. One or more specific sorting signals may also be required for targeting of alphavirus envelope proteins to specific membranes of polarized cells during mosquito infection (WEAVER et al. 1990, 1991b).

Selection for optimum codon usage may play a role in constraining RNA sequences of alphaviruses (STRAUSS and STRAUSS 1986). Codon usage is nonrandom in all alphaviruses sequenced to date, including EEEV (CHANG and TRENT 1987) and VEEV (KINNEY et al. 1986). Codon usage may differ in vertebrate versus mosquito genes due, in part, of differences in usage of the dinucleotide CG (the C is methylated in vertebrate but not invertebrate DNA, leading to evolutionary CG loss in vertebrates). Alphavirus codon usage may be tightly regulated and balanced to permit efficient translation of highly expressed genes in both vertebrate and mosquito cells.

Taken together, these considerations imply distinct structural and genetic requirements, or different evolutionary constraints on alphavirus replication in vertebrate versus mosquito hosts.

Many other vector-borne viruses are also believed to evolve slowly in nature. Rates of nucleotide substitution, deduced from oligonucleotide fingerprint analyses of individual arbovirus lineages including Old World alphaviruses Sindbis virus (OLSON and TRENT 1985), and Getah virus (MORITA and IGARASHI 1984), and flaviviruses Kunjin virus (FLYNN et al. 1989), Murray Valley encephalitis virus (COELEN and MACKENZIE 1988), Saint Louis encephalitis (SLE) virus (TRENT et al. 1981), dengue 2 virus (TRENT et al. 1989), and yellow fever virus (DEUBEL et al. 1985) range from $4\text{–}9 \times 10^{-4}$ substitutions per nucleotide per year. These estimates are similar to those for New World alphaviruses, supporting the hypothesis that alteration of vertebrate and invertebrate hosts constrains the evolution of arboviruses. This hypothesis could be tested by comparing evolutionary rates of two-host versus single-host viruses. For example, in the Flaviviridae, California isolates of the arbovirus SLE virus could be compared with sympatric Modoc and Rio Bravo viruses, which are not vector-borne.

3.2 Recombination

Although intramolecular genetic recombination could occur during dual infection of vertebrate hosts by alphaviruses, the possibility of recombination is heightened during persistent replication within mosquito vectors. Dual infection of mosquitoes may occur in nature as a consequence of multiple viremic host contacts during a genotrophic cycle (e.g., two or more partial blood meals) or during sequential cycles. Laboratory studies demonstrating lack of alphavirus interference with mosquito superinfection (CHAMBERLAIN and SUDIA 1957) suggest that recombination among alphaviruses could occur in dually infected mosquitoes (in locations where sympatric distribution of viruses occurs). Recombination with endogenous mosquito viruses, although not yet documented, could also add to alphavirus diversity.

Among single-stranded, unsegmented RNA viruses, recombination in nature was first described for polioviruses, in vaccinated individuals (KEW and NOTTAY 1984) and in wild viruses isolated in the field (RICO-HESSE et al. 1987). Alphavirus recombination was recently implicated in the evolution of WEEV: a 1953 strain isolated in California appears to have arisen by recombination between EEEV- and Sindbis-like viruses; WEEV thus has encephalogenic properties of EEEV, but antigenic specificity of Sindbis virus (HAHN et al. 1988). The WEEV prototype strain (McMillan), isolated in 1941 in Canada, shares these characteristics, placing the recombination event before 1941 at an unknown location. Sequence data for Aura, FMV and HJV are needed to determine if these WEE complex viruses descended from the recombinant ancestor of WEEV, or diverged prior to the recombination event. The potential exists for increasing alphavirus diversity through recombination, and it may just be a matter of time before other examples of this phenomenon are detected. Recombination might be expected among viruses which share vectors and vertebrate hosts, such as FMV and BBV, or EEEV and HJV.

3.3 Mosquito and Vertebrate Host Ecology

In this section we discuss patterns of alphavirus transmission based on concepts of parasite evolution (PRICE 1980). We begin by considering diversity of alphaviruses in the New World tropics and end by addressing the lack of diversity in temperate regions of North America.

Diversity and variation in VEEV throughout its range, and in EEEV in tropical America, are consistent with the tendency for parasites to (a) be adapted for taking advantage of small, disjointed environments, (b) become specialized for exploiting resources that are important for survival and reproduction, and (c) exist in conditions of nonequilibrium because tenure within a host is ephemeral, and colonization of a new host can be risky with a significant change of failure. In other words, extinction rates can be high. The significance of these concepts is supported by the short replication time and high fecundity of alphaviruses. In fact, the founder effect may be an important process for alphavirus diversification (Sect. 4.4).

VEEV transmission cycles provide examples of these characteristics of parasite ecology. The distribution of enzootic VEEV transmission is patchy and highly focal. Different subtypes and varieties are transmitted by different mosquito species in the subgenus *Culex* (*Melanoconion*) (Table 1; WALTON and GRAYSON 1988). These well-established observations are consistent with the notion that VEEV has diversified by mechanisms that capitalize on its ability to occasionally establish new foci of transmission in disjointed habitats. Mechanisms for dispersal could include the flight of viremic, secondary vertebrate hosts (birds or bats) or transport of infected mosquitoes in air currents. Because maintenance of transmission requires a series of finely tuned events that consistently overlap in time and space (SCOTT and WEAVER 1989), establishing a new focus of transmission is probably a rare event. However, after colonization, an alphavirus' rapid replication rate and high mutation frequency would facilitate swift adaptation to a new niche; colonist viruses could thus become distinct from their progenitor. Once new sites of transmission are established, restricted movement patterns of enzootic vertebrate and mosquito hosts in tropical America (rodents and *Culex* (*Melanoconion*) mosquitoes) may allow VEEV subtypes and varieties to maintain their physical and genetic isolation. These factors may thereby facilitate genetic divergence and adaptive radiation of VEE complex viruses.

An alternative explanation for tropical diversity of VEEV and EEEV is diversification in concert with mosquito vectors (coevolution). It should be noted, however, that colonization and coevolution are not necessarily mutually exclusive processes. The remarkable diversity of *Culex* (*Melanoconion*) mosquitoes (>150 species in the subgenus) and the consistent and sometimes highly specialized association of enzootic VEEV strains with mosquitoes in this subgenus (WEAVER et al. 1984; WALTON and GRAYSON 1988) superficially support the notion of coevolution. A rigorous analysis of virus and mosquito phylogenies should be carried out to test this hypothesis (MITTER and BROOKS 1983). Although coevolution of arboviruses and mosquito vectors has recently been discussed (ELDRIDGE 1990), conclusions are premature pending appropriate phylogenetic analyses.

In sharp contrast to the diversity of EEEV and VEEV in South and Central America is the extreme homogeneity of EEEV in North America and of WEEV throughout its range. Ecological factors that could contribute to the slow rate of evolution for these viruses are a slower virus replication rate, lack of vector diversity, and mobility of avian hosts. The replication rate of viruses in exothermic vectors is reduced in a seasonal temperate climate, compared to the tropics. Reduction in replication cycles per unit time should diminish the potential for virus diversification. In this regard, the unknown overwintering mechaism(s) for these viruses might constitute a significant selective pressure against variation.

Low vector diversity in temperate locations may also favor virus homogeneity, since parasite and host diversity tend to be positively correlated. In North America, EEEV is transmitted enzootically by *Culiseta melanura*, which unlike tropical *Culex* (*Melanoconion*) species, belongs to a species-poor taxon and has few competitors for virus transmission. Competitors would be species that are consistently found in large numbers in freshwater swamps during the virus transmission season, and that blood feed preferentially on the avian hosts of EEEV (SCOTT and WEAVER 1989).

Post-breeding random wanderings of viremic birds during the late summer and fall may constitute and efficient mechanism for exchange of virus genotypes (gene flow) among geographically isolated transmission foci minimizing isolation of EEEV populations. On the other hand, virus in temperate foci may undergo annual winter extinction, followed by summertime reintroduction via viremic birds arriving from southern foci of continuous transmission. These dispersal mechanisms may help to explain results from molecular studies indicating that North American EEEV evolves within a single gene pool with frequent gene flow among transmission foci (WEAVER et al. 1991b).

Homogeneity of WEEV may similarly be maintained by gene flow provided by infected birds flying between North and South America. However, lack of information concerning South American WEEV transmission cycles precludes evaluation of mobile birds versus sedentary rodents as tropical vertebrate hosts. An alternative hypothesis for WEEV conservation is its recent origin, following recombination between EEEV- and Sindbis-like viruses (HAHN et al. 1988). If WEEV only recently established ifself in South America, it may simply be a matter of time before it invades additional available niches, like the Argentinean strain (AG80–646) of WEEV (REISEN and MONATH 1988). WEEV might eventually diversify in a way similar to VEEV and EEEV in South America, while retaining genetic homogeneity in North America.

4 Adaptive Landscape Model for Alphavirus Evolution

The "adaptive landscape" developed by WRIGHT (1932), as part of his shifting balance theory of evolution, is conceptually useful in modeling virus evolution. In the adaptive landscape, a two-dimensional field of all possible genetic combinations, or genotypes (the field is actually N-dimensional) is graded with respect to adaptive fitness (Z axis). The landscape consists of a number of adaptive peaks separated by valleys of low fitness; natural selection drives a population up the nearest adaptive peak. For a virus to evolve within a fixed landscape, it usually must traverse a valley of low fitness to reach a higher fitness peak. In the absence of disruptive influences, and if distances between peaks are great, natural selection will favor remaining on the current fitness peak. We use the adaptive landscape here as a model for explaining constraints on alphavirus evolution (see Fig. 1).

A growing body of molecular and epidemiological evidence (see Sect. 3.1) suggests different genetic requirements for optimal alphavirus replication in mosquito versus vertebrate portions of the transmission cycle. This implies that distinct adaptive landscapes exist for mosquito versus vertebrate infections. It is unlikely that virus populations can alternate between separate, nonoverlapping vertebrate and mosquito peaks during each transmission cycle because of the difficulty in regularly traversing the low-fitness valley between peaks. Therefore, an alphavirus should evolve within intersecting peaks which include an overlap saddle of adequate fitness (height) to prevent extinction during host alternation (Fig. 1C). Within the limited landscape occupied by a current alphavirus genotype, independent adaptive peaks for mosquito and vertebrate landscapes may rarely overlap, and probably never completely coincide. Therefore, the two-host landscape (Fig. 1C) contains overlapping peaks which are more widely separated than those on either single-host landscape. This relative increase in

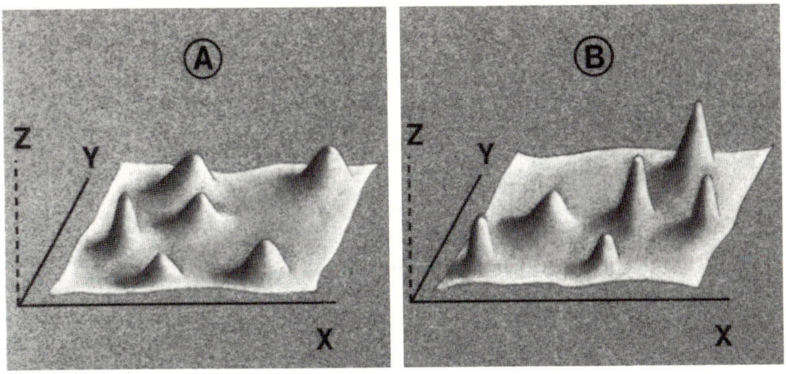

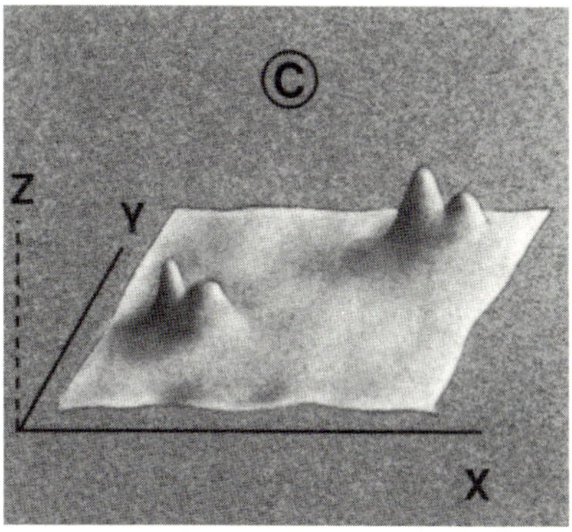

Fig. 1 A–C. Limited two-dimensional region of a highly schematic adaptive landscape for alphavirus evolution. *X* and *Y* axes represent two dimensions in an N-dimensional field of possible genetic combinations; *Z* axis (height) indicates relative fitness of genotypes defined by X and Y axes. **A** Landscape representing alphavirus fitness for vertebrate host infection, containing randomly distributed peaks. **B** Distinct, random landscape for mosquito host infection. **C** Alternating host landscape showing only overlapping mosquito and vertebrate peaks

the separation of peaks decreases the opportunity for movement across a low-fitness valley to another peak (genetic change within the population, or evolution). However, in these regions of partial peak overlap, the virus population may undergo subtle genetic shifts from mosquito to vertebrate peak during transmission cycles.

Ignoring other considerations, the two-host landscape model therefore predicts slower evolution in alphaviruses than in single-host viruses. This prediction is consistent with genetic and phenotypic conservation, or slow evolution in New World alphaviruses.

Several other factors discussed by Wright (1982) affect evolution within the adaptive landscape model and thus warrant discussion with regard to alphavirus evolution. In the interest of brevity, and because the epidemiology and patterns of EEEV evolution are better understood than those of other New World alphaviruses, we restrict our discussion of these factors to EEEV evolution in North America.

4.1 Gene Flow

Under conditions of adaptive landscape stability, WRIGHT (1932, 1982) predicted that species with efficient gene flow among populations undergo "mass selection" and remain on the fitness peak which they have historically reached. Gene flow contributes to genetic stasis by causing species divided into small, discrete populations to evolve as a single, effectively panmictic population of homogeneous genetic composition. Gene flow thereby increases the effective population size, minimizing founder effects and the impact of population partitioning (see Sects. 4.4, 4.5). Thus, gene flow can restrain evolution by preventing natural selection and genetic drift from establishing and maintaining regional genetic differences (SLATKIN 1987). Repeated extinction of isolated populations can also lead to higher effective rates of gene flow when a new population is established from mixed colonist genotypes (FUTUYMA 1986).

Nucleotide sequence analysis of EEEV isolates indicates regular gene flow among transmission foci sampled, presumably due to virus transport by infected birds during migration or postbreeding random wandering (WEAVER et al. 1991b). According to Wright's model, gene flow contributes to North American EEEV genetic stability and slow evolution by ensuring that viruses of maximum fitness (individuals occupying the current fitness peak) are always represented in isolated populations (transmission foci). Seasonal EEEV extinction in temperate foci (EEEV overwintering has not been documented) and annual reintroduction from southern regions could effectively increase gene flow and contribute to genetic stability.

Intuitively, it is attractive to assume that efficient gene flow via infected birds limits EEEV evolution to a single genetic lineage in North America (WEAVER et al. 1991b). However SLE virus, which is also transmitted by mosquitoes among avian hosts, evolves in several distinct North American lineages (TRENT et al. 1981). Factors responsible for differing patterns of evolution of these two arboviruses are unknown.

4.2 Landscape Stability

Stability of the adaptive landscape minimizes evolutionary change or favors genetic conservation. However, if the topography (location of fitness peaks) changes, a species will move across the landscape along with the fitness peak currently occupied (WRIGHT 1982). Stability of the EEEV landscape is promoted by several epidemiological features including a single enzootic mosquito vector and minimal immune selection by passerine birds (WEAVER et al. 1991b). These factors may promote genetic conservation of EEEV in nature.

The appearance of defective interfering (DI) virus within a population can destabilize the adaptive landscape by introducing new selective pressure on the standard virus, effectively lowering the fitness of its historically occupied peak. Previously unfit mutants, which are resistant to interference, can arise and displace previously fit genotypes. This process can promote rapid evolution of RNA viruses in vitro (STEINHAUER and HOLLAND 1987). Persistent alphavirus infections of mosquito vectors could facilitate DI-generated landscape changes and rapid arbovirus evolution. DI virus is known to accompany persistent alphavirus infections of mosquito cells in vitro (BROWN and CONDREAY 1986) but has not been studied in vivo. However, conditions accompanying natural alphavirus infections of mosquitoes may minimize the effects of DI virus. For example, during dissemination within *Culiseta melanura*, movement of EEEV from the midgut epithelium to salivary glands includes passage through basal lamlna surrounding the midgut, fat body and salivary glands. Ultrastructural studies showing large concentrations of virions adjacent to these basal lamina suggest that they may limit virus movement during sequential infection of mosquito tissues (WEAVER et al. 1990). This may reduce multiplicities of infection, delaying DI virus appearance. Natural mortality of *Culiseta melanura* (SCOTT and WEAVER 1989) and reductions in EEEV titer in mosquito saliva during persistent infection (undetectable levels after 21 days of infection) (WEAVER et al. 1990) may also minimize transmission of virus from persistently infected mosquitoes. Potential evolutionary consequences of DI virus during in vivo mosquito infections deserve further attention.

4.3 Mutation Frequency

For a population occupying a fitness peak, a high mutation frequency increases the area of the peak occupied, similar to the effect of a decrease in selective pressure (WRIGHT 1982). High polymerase error frequencies (on the order of 10^{-4}) inherent in RNA virus replication (STEINHAUER and HOLLAND 1987) can therefore increase the area of a peak occupied by RNA viruses; this could expedite movement across the landscape, facilitating rapid virus evolution.

A few temperature-sensitive mutants of Sindbis virus, believed to involve single base substitutions, revert to wild type at frequencies of 10^{-8}–10^{-9}, suggesting high-fidelity replication of some portions of the viral genome. However, most data suggest a high mutation frequency in most regions of the alphavirus genome (reviewed by HAHN et al. 1989). Genetic and phenotypic diversity within natural EEEV isolates (S.C.W. REPIK and P. REPIK, unpublished), and antigenic variation within clones of the WEEV McMillan strain (HENDERSON 1964) imply alphavirus quasispecies populations consistent with high mutation frequencies. Thus, although alphaviruses are probably capable of rapid evolution under appropriate circumstances they appear to be highly conserved in nature. This is consistent with the adaptive landscape model's prediction that a high mutation frequency can increase the area of a fitness peak occupied by a population, but cannot allow movement to another peak in the absence of other mitigating factors. Under conditions of strong selective pressure and a stable landscape, alphavirus evolution apparently proceeds slowly despite a high mutation frequency.

4.4 Founder Effects

In the adaptive landscape model, founder effects promote evolutionary change when populations become very small, permitting stochastic sampling accidents to overcome selective pressure; this results in random fixation of genotypes (WRIGHT 1982). Efficient gene flow and strong selection for a consensus genotype are probably important in minimizing founder effects on EEEV evolution. Also, a high mutation frequency may provide genetic diversity sufficient for movement of small populations across the landscape, and encounters with high-fitness peaks.

For EEEV in North America, founder effects could be realized at several levels: (a) a single infected, migratory bird or wind-borne mosquito could initiate transmission within an isolated focus (lack of information as to the mechanism of EEEV overwintering or reintroduction into temperate foci precludes evaluation of this scenario), or (b) a virus population could be reduced to small numbers during various stages of the mosquito-bird transmission cycle. For example, during early seasonal, low-level enzootic transmission activity, a mosquito could become infected after engorging on a bird with a low-titer viremia; one or a few virus particles could thus establish a mosquito infection which might later become amplified within the transmission focus. However, experimental studies have shown that, for many alphaviruses including EEEV, vertebrate host viremias are very high in magnitude and vector midguts are extremely susceptible to oral infection. This implies that virus populations typically remain relatively large during initial midgut infection (WEAVER et al. 1991a), and subsequently during virus dissemination to salivary glands. Similarly, infected *Culiseta melanura* transmit ca. 100–1000 pfu of EEEV to vertebrate hosts during the first 2 weeks of infection (WEAVER et al. 1990). Since survival of infected mosquitoes beyond 2 weeks is probably rare in nature (SCOTT and WEAVER 1989) avian infections may typically include relatively large numbers of founder EEE virions. Thus, founder effects, which could promote rapid evolution, may be minimized during natural EEEV transmission.

4.5 Population Partitioning

Partitioning of a species into small, isolated populations can permit accidents of sampling to overcome selection pressures, promoting genetic change in a manner similar to that resulting from founder effects (WRIGHT 1982; Sect. 4.4). Partitioning also increases the probability that one population will encounter a gradient leading to another fitness peak. Thus, individual populations undergo a "trial and error mechanism," and genetic change is inversely related to population sizes, but directly related to the number of independent demes (WRIGHT 1982). Evolution of EEEV, which is partitioned into many discrete foci of transmission in North America, could be favored by this reasoning. However, it is unclear whether virus persists throughout the year in temperate foci (SCOTT and

WEAVER 1989). EEEV may be annually reintroduced from southeastern sites of year-round transmission into northern locations, without temperate overwintering. Thus, partitioning in northern foci may not augment EEEV evolution unless accompanied by regular southward gene flow (e.g., via migratory birds) during the transmission season (otherwise, temperate virus populations would meet an evolutionary dead-end following annual winter extinction). Efficient gene flow can also counteract partitioning effects (WRIGHT 1982), and population sizes within individual EEEV foci may be large enough to negate the influence of partitioning. Furthermore, strong selective pressures acting within a stable landscape (consistent with patterns of nucleotide substitution in the EEEV structural genome) may suppress genetic change even in small, partitioned populations (WRIGHT 1982).

Acknowledgments. We thank David Clarke, Esteban Domingo, John Holland, Charles Mitter, Thomas Monath, George Roderick and Robert Tesh for informal review of the manuscript. This work received financial support from National Institutes of Health grant AI26787.

References

Brown DT, Condreay LD (1986) Replication of alphaviruses in mosquito cells. In: Schlesinger S, Schlesinger M (eds) The togaviruses and flaviviruses. Plenum, New York, pp 171–207

Calisher CH, Karabatsos N (1988) Arbovirus serogroups: definition and geographic distribution. In: Monath TP (ed) The arboviruses: epidemiology and ecology, vol 1. CRC, Boca Raton, pp 19–57

Casals J (1964) Antigenic variants of eastern equine encephalitis virus. J Exp Med 119: 547–565

Chamberlain RW, Sudia WD (1957) Dual infections of eastern and western equine encephalitis virus in *Culex tarsalis*. J Infect Dis 101: 233–236

Chang G-JJ, Trent DW (1987) Nucleotide sequence of the genome region encoding the 26S mRNA of eastern equine encephalomyelitis virus and the deduced amino acid sequence of the viral structural proteins. J Gen Virol 68: 2129–2142

Coelen RJ, Mackenzie JS (1988) Genetic variation of Murray Valley encephalitis virus. J Gen Virol 69: 1903–1912

Deubel V, Pailliez JP, Cornet M, Schlesinger JJ, Diop M, Diop A, Digoutte JP, Girard M (1985) Homogeneity among Senegalese strains of yellow fever virus. Am J Trop Med Hyg 34: 976–983

Eldridge B (1990) Evolutionary relationships among California serogroup viruses (Bunyaviridae) and *Aedes* mosquitoes (Diptera: Culicidae). J Med Entomol 27: 738–749

Flynn LM, Coelen RJ, Mackenzie JS (1989) Kunjin virus isolates of Australia are genetically homogeneous. J Gen Virol 70: 2819–2824

Futuyma DJ (1986) Evolutionary biology. Sinauer, Sunderland

Hahn CS, Lustig S, Strauss EG, Strauss JH (1988) Western equine encephalitis virus is a recombinant virus. Proc Natl Acad Sci USA 85: 5997–6001

Hahn CS, Rice CM, Strauss EG, Lenches EM, Strauss JH (1989) Sindbis virus ts103 has a mutation in glycoprotein E2 that leads to defective assembly of virions. J Virol 63: 3459–3465

Henderson JR (1964) Immunologic characterization of western equine encephalomyelitis virus strains. J Immunol 93: 452–461

Kay BH, Aaskov JG (1988) Ross River virus (epidemic polyarthritis). In: Monath TP (ed) The arboviruses: epidemiology and ecology, vol 4. CRC, Boca Raton, pp 93–112

Kew OM, Nottay BK (1984) Evolution of the oral poliovaccine strains in humans occurs by both mutation and intramolecular recombination. In: Canock R, Lerner R (ed) Modern approaches to vaccines. Cold Spring Harbor Laboratory, Cold Spring Harbor, pp 357–362

Kielian M, Helenius A (1986) Entry of alphaviruses. In: Schlesinger S, Schlesinger M (eds) The togaviruses and flaviviruses. Plenum, New York, pp 91–119

Kinney RM, Trent DW, France JK (1983) Comparative immunological and biochemical analysis of viruses in the Venezuelan equine encephalitis complex. J Gen Virol 64: 135–147

Kinney RM, Johnson BJB, Brown VL, Trent DW (1986) Nucleotide sequence of the 26S mRNA of the virulent Trinidad donkey strain of Venezuelan equine encephalitis virus and deduced sequence of the encoded proteins. Virology 152: 400–413

Lemm JA, Durbin RK, Stollar V, Rice CM (1990) Mutations which alter the level of nsP4 can affect the efficiency of Sindbis virus replication in a host-dependent manner. J Virol 64: 3001–3011

Levinson RS, Strauss JH, Strauss EG (1990) Complete sequence of the genomic RNA of O'nyong-nyong virus and its use in the construction of alphavirus phylogenetic trees. Virology 175: 110–123

Mitter C, Brooks DR (1983) Phylogenetic aspects of coevolution. In Futuyma DJ, Slatkin M (eds) Coevolution. Sinauer, Sunderland, pp 65–98

Morita K, Igarashi A (1984) Oligonucleotide fingerprint analysis of strains of Getah virus isolated in Japan and Malaysia. J Gen Virol 65: 1899–1908

Olson K, Trent DW (1985) Genetic and antigenic variations among geographical isolates of Sindbis virus. J Gen Virol 66: 797–810

Peters CJ, Dalrymple J (1990) Alphaviruses. In: Fields BN, Knipe DM (eds) Virology, 2nd edn. Raven, New York, pp 713–761

Price PW (1980) Evolutionary biology of parasites. Princeton University Press, Princeton

Reisen WK, Monath TP (1988) Western equine encephalitis. In: Monath TP (ed) The arboviruses: epidemiology and ecology, vol 1. CRC, Boca Raton, pp 89–137

Rico-Hesse R, Pallansch MA, Nottay BK, Kew OM (1987) Geographic distribution of wild poliovirus type 1 genotypes. Virology 160: 311–322

Rico-Hesse R, Roehrig JT, Trent DW, Dickerman RW (1988) Genetic variation of Venezuelan equine encephalitis virus strains of the ID variety in Colombia. Am J Trop Med Hyg 38: 195–204

Roehrig JT, Mathews JH (1985) The neutralization site on the E2 glycoprotein of Venezuelan equine encephalomyelitis virus is composed of multiple conformationally stable epitopes. Virology 142: 347–356

Roehrig JT, Hunt AR, Chang G-J, Sheik B, Bolin RA, Tsai TF, Trent DW (1990) Identification of monoclonal antibodies capable of differentiating antigenic varieties of eastern equine encephalitis viruses. Am J Trop Med Hyg 42: 394–398

Rosen L (1987) Overwintering mechanisms of mosquito-borne arboviruses in temperate climates. Am J Trop Med Hyd 37: 695–765

Schlesinger S, Schlesinger MJ (1990) Replication of togaviridae and flaviviridae. In: Fields BN, Knipe DM (eds) Virology, 2nd edn. Raven, New York, pp 697–711

Scott TW (1988) Vertebrate host ecology. In: Monath TP (ed) The arboviruses: epidemiology and ecology, vol 1. CRC, Boca Raton, pp 257–280

Scott TW, Weaver SC (1989) Eastern equine encephalomyelitis virus: epidemiology and evolution of mosquito transmission. Adv Virus Res 37: 277–328

Slatkin M (1987) Gene flow and the geographic structure of natural populations. Science 236: 787–792

Steinhauer DA, Holland JJ (1987) Rapid evolution of RNA viruses. Annu Rev Microbiol 41: 409–433

Strauss EG, Strauss JH (1986) Structure and replication of the alphavirus genome. In: Schlesinger S, Schlesinger M (eds) The togaviruses and flaviviruses. Plenum, New York, pp 35–90

Trent DW, Grant JA (1980) A comparison of New World alphaviruses in the western equine encephalitis virus complex by immunochemical and oligonucleotide fingerprint techniques. J Gen Virol 47: 261–282

Trent DW, Clewey JP, France JK, Bishop DHL (1979) Immunochemical and oligonucleotide fingerprint analysis of Venezuelan equine encephalomyelitis complex viruses. J Gen Virol 43: 365–381

Trent DW, Grant JA, Vorndam AV, Monath TP (1981) Genetic heterogeneity among Saint Louis encephalitis virus isolates of different geographic origin. Virology 114: 319–332

Trent DW, Grant JA, Monath TP, Manske CL, Corina M, Fox GE (1989) Genetic variation and microevolution of dengue 2 virus in southeast Asia. Virology 172: 523–535

Walton TE, Grayson MA (1988) Venezuelan equine encephalomyelitis. In: Monath TP (ed) The arboviruses: epidemiology and ecology, vol 1. CRC, Boca Raton, pp 59–85

Weaver SC, Scherer WF, Cupp EW, Castello DA (1984) Barriers to dissemination of Venezuelan encephalitis viruses in the Middle American enzootic vector mosquito, *Culex* (*Melanoconion*) *taenio pus*. Am J Trop Med Hyg 33: 953–960

Weaver SC, Scott TW, Lorenz LH, Lerdthusnee K, Romoser WS (1988) Togavirus-associated pathologic changes in a natural mosquito vector. J Virol 62: 2083–2090

Weaver SC, Scott TW, Lorenz LH (1990) Patterns of eastern equine encephalomyelitis virus infection in *Culiseta melanura* (Diptera: Culicidae). J Med Entomol 27: 878–891

Weaver SC, Scott TW, Lorenz LH, Repik PR (1991a) Detection of eastern equine encephalomyelitis virus deposition in *Culiseta melanura* following ingestion of radiolabeled virus in blood meals. Am J Trop Med Hyg 44: 250–259

Weaver SC, Scott TW, Rico-Hesse R (1991b) Molecular evolution of eastern equine encephalomyelitis virus in North America. Virology 182: 774–784

Wright S (1932) The roles of mutation, inbreeding, crossbreeding and selection in evolution. Proceedings of the Sixth International Congress of Genetics 1, pp 356–366

Wright S (1982) Character change, speciation, and the higher taxa. Evolution 36: 427–443

Young NA, Johnson KM (1969) Antigenic variants of Venezuelan equine encephalitis virus: their geographic distribution and epidemiologic significance. Am J Epidemiol 89: 286–307

Emergence and Transmission of Influenza A Viruses Resistant to Amantadine and Rimantadine

F. G. HAYDEN[1] and A. J. HAY[2]

1 Introduction

Many clinical studies have documented the efficacy of amantadine and rimantadine for prophylaxis and treatment of influenza A virus infections (DOUGLAS 1990; TOMINACK and HAYDEN 1987). Antiviral activity has been demonstrated in various animal models of influenza (HAYDEN 1986) and during clinical use in humans (DOUGLAS 1990). Amantadine- and rimantadine-resistant mutants have been recovered during studies in mice (OXFORD et al. 1970, OXFORD and POTTER 1972), birds (WEBSTER et al. 1985; BEARD et al. 1987; BEAN et al. 1989), and

[1] Departments of Internal Medicine and Pathology, University of Virginia Health Sciences Center, Charlottesville, Virginia, USA
[2] Virology Division, National Institute for Medical Research, The Ridgeway, Mill Hill, London, England

Current Topics in Microbiology and Immunology, Vol. 176

recently in children and adults treated with these drugs (HALL et al. 1987; THOMPSON et al. 1987; BELSHE et al. 1988; HAYDEN et al. 1989). The impact of drug resistance on the clinical usefulness of these drugs is thus of obvious concern. Factors which may influence the clinical importance of drug-resistant viruses include their frequency and rapidity of emergence, genetic stability, transmissibility, pathogenicity, and ability to compete epidemiologically with wild-type viruses (BEAN et al. 1989). The following sections review the limited information available from animal and human studies that address these characteristics and the correlation of these factors with particular resistance mutations.

2 Genetic Basis of Resistance

Drug-resistant variants are estimated to occur with a frequency of 1 in 10^3–1 in 10^4 in egg or cell culture-grown virus populations (APPLEYARD 1977; LUBECK et al. 1978) and can be selected by passage in cell culture in the presence of either drug. Resistance is transferable by genetic reassortment of the gene segment 7 between sensitive and resistant strains (HAY et al. 1979; LUBECK et al. 1978; BELSHE et al. 1988), indicating that the M gene is the major determinant of drug susceptibility. Most resistant variants are totally insensitive to the specific anti-influenza A action of micromolar concentrations of these drugs (described below), although they remain susceptible to the nonspecific action of higher drug concentrations ($\geqq 10\,\mu g/ml$) in cell culture (HAY et al. 1986). Viruses exhibit either a strict cross-susceptibility or cross-resistance to amantadine, rimantadine, and related drugs.

RNA sequence analyses of more than 140 isolates of resistant influenza A viruses, recovered either during cell culture passage or during administration of the drugs in vivo, have identified the resistance determinants as point mutations resulting in substitutions in amino acids 26, 27, 30, 31, or 34 of the M2 protein, the product of a spliced messenger RNA (mRNA) of the M gene (HAY et al. 1991; BELSHE et al. 1988; HAYDEN et al. 1989; BEAN et al. 1989; MAST et al. 1989; ROUMILLAT et al. 1990). Most resistant isolates contain a single amino acid change, although mixed populations with independent resistance mutations and variants with dual mutations have been described (BELSHE et al. 1988; BEAN et al. 1989). Several different amino acid changes have been recognized at certain positions (e.g., alanine→valine or threonine at position 30). M2 RNA sequence analysis of resistant variants has served to verify biological assay results and to provide a genetic marker for epidemiologic studies of virus transmission. Enzyme-linked immunoassays (ELISA) which measure expression of viral hemagglutinin (BELSHE et al. 1988) or broader type-specific antigens (KENDAL 1990) provide a sensitive assay for resistance which correlates well with the presence of specific M2 mutations.

3 Mechanisms of Antiviral Action

The replication of the susceptible influenza A viruses is specifically inhibited in cell culture by low concentrations (0.01–1.0 μg/ml) of amantadine hydrochloride or rimantadine hydrochloride (BELSHE and HAY 1989). Such concentrations are achievable in blood and respiratory secretions during clinical use (TOMINACK and HAYDEN 1987). Depending on the influenza A virus subtype, the major antiviral action is directed against either of two stages in the replicative cycle. Most human strains are susceptible to a block in virus uncoating by an as yet undefined mechanism (HAY 1989; HAY et al. 1991). In contrast, certain avian strains (e.g., H7 subtype) show impairment of virus maturation as a consequence of drug-induced inhibition of an M2-mediated alteration in hemagglutinin structure (SUGRUE et al. 1990). It has been proposed that the drugs block the function of M2 involved in regulating the pH within vesicles of the post-Golgi transport pathway by interacting directly with the transmembrane domain of M2 (SUGRUE and HAY 1991). The observation that the same amino acid substitutions render viruses resistant to both antiviral actions implies a common function of M2. It has been postulated that the tetrameric M2 protein may form a proton-selective channel which is blocked by adamantamines in an analogous manner to their anticholinergic, and possibly antiparkinsonian, actions (HAY 1989; SUGRUE and HAY 1991).

4 Emergence of Resistant Viruses

4.1 Surveillance of Epidemic Strains

During more than two decades of limited amantadine and rimantadine use in humans, naturally occurring epidemic strains of influenza A viruses have remained sensitive to the antiviral action of these drugs (OXFORD and POTTER 1973; HAYDEN et al. 1980; BELSHE et al. 1989; HAY, unpublished observations). Strains representing all three human influenza A subtypes and viruses infecting a variety of species have been shown to be sensitive. Reports of resistance in viruses recovered from nondrug-exposed persons have not been substantiated by RNA sequence analysis (HEIDER et al. 1980; PEMBERTON et al. 1986). The mechanism by which certain highly passaged laboratory strains of H1N1 subtype virus (e.g., R/PR/8/34, A/WSN/33) have acquired resistance is unclear, since the parental strains were initially isolated before the use of the drugs. Since resistant variants occur within genetically heterogeneous virus populations, the failure to recover naturally occurring, drug-resistant strains indicates that drug resistance does not confer any selective advantage.

4.2 Treatment Studies

Several studies have assessed the frequency of recovering drug-resistant virus from individuals receiving rimantadine treatment for H3N2 subtype infection (Table 1). HALL et al. (1988) found that 27% of all rimantadine-treated children and 45% of those who were virus positive after the fourth treatment day shed a resistant virus. In a family-based study, HAYDEN et al. (1989) found that in similar proportions of adults or children receiving rimantadine therapy, drug-resistant virus was recovered on the fifth day of treatment (Table 1). In elderly institutionalized adults, 11% of all rimantadine recipients and 27% of those shedding virus 4 days or longer into therapy had drug-resistant isolates (R. BETTS, personal communication). It is evident that the recovery of resistant viruses is frequently associated with therapeutic use of these drugs in both children and adults.

The time course for emergence of drug-resistant variants during therapy has not been well characterized. Resistant isolates obtained after four or more days of therapy have been fully resistant, although some have contained mixtures of sensitive and resistant viruses (BELSHE et al. 1988). In an avian model of H5N2 subtype infection, BEAN et al. (1989) found that drug-resistant virus was shed in respiratory secretions at 2 days and in feces by 3 days after initiating amantadine treatment. A small study of ambulatory adults with uncomplicated influenza found that shedding of resistant virus was often detectable by the 3rd day of rimantadine treatment (HAYDEN et al. 1991). These findings emphasize the rapidity with which resistant variants can replace sensitive strains during therapeutic use of these drugs.

Consistent with the observations in experimental avian influenza (BEAN et al. 1989), once shedding of resistant virus develops, subsequent isolates from the same individual remain resistant. In children HALL et al. (1987) found that shedding of resistant virus may continue for up to 7 days, while HAYDEN et al. (1989) found that those who shed resistant virus on the fifth treatment day were

Table 1. Frequency of recovering drug-resistant influenza A (H3N2) virus during rimantadine treatment

Reference	Year of study	Patient group	Patients treated (*n*)	Patients shedding resistant virus (*n*)	Patients shedding resistant virus (%)
HALL et al. (1987)	1983	Children	37	10	27
HAYDEN et al. (1989)	1988	Children	21	6	29
HAYDEN et al. (1989)	1988	Adults	7	2	29
HAYDEN et al. (1991)	1988	Adults	6	3	50
BETTS (personal communication)	1986	Elderly	26	3	11

negative for virus by the tenth treatment day. However, the limited follow-up in these trials has not allowed a definite assessment of the duration of resistant virus shedding and hence the potential risk period for transmitting infection due to such strains.

It is unknown which virus, host, and possibly drug factors are important in regard to the emergence of drug-resistant viruses. Higher levels of viral replication may enhance the likelihood of selecting resistant variants. For example, it remains to be determined whether the frequency of recovering resistant virus will be lower in those treated for H1N1 subtype infection, since viral titers are generally lower in such individuals compared to H3N2 subtype infection (THOMPSON et al. 1987). One study in experimental murine influenza found that high drug doses led to more rapid selection of resistant virus (OXFORD and POTTER 1973). However, the effect of dose has not been studied in clinical trials, and no direct comparisons of the frequency of resistance emergence have been made between amantadine and rimantadine. Although most of the data comes from studies involving rimantadine, there is no evidence that any difference exists between amantadine and rimantadine with respect to the generation of drug resistance.

4.3 Prophylaxis Studies

The high level of protective efficacy observed with seasonal chemoprophylaxis (DOUGLAS 1990) suggests that it is associated with a lower risk of resistance emergence than treatment. However, it is currently unknown whether some persons failing prophylaxis develop naturally occurring infections due to de novo emergence of drug-resistant virus. Resistant virus has been recovered from volunteers with experimentally induced H3N2 subtype influenza who were taking amantadine both before and after challenge with large viral inocula (SCHIFF and HAYDEN, unpublished observations).

5 Transmissibility of Resistant Viruses

5.1 Experimental Avian Influenza

Under conditions modelling virus transmission in flocks, WEBSTER et al. (1985) found that birds receiving amantadine or rimantadine prophylaxis and remaining in close contact with drug-treated, H5N2 subtype-infected birds developed infections caused by drug-resistant virus. The possible importance of drug administration to contact birds was not assessed independently, nor were the specific mutations accounting for resistance in the isolates from the index and infected contact birds determined. The ability of drug-resistant virus to compete with sensitive wild-type virus for transmission was assessed in the absence of selective drug pressure (BEAN et al. 1989). Birds shedding resistant virus were mixed with those shedding wild-type and with noninfected, untreated contact birds. After 3 days the latter group was removed and housed with noninfected contacts, and this process was repeated for three passages extending over a 2 week period. In three of four experiments, resistant virus could still be recovered from some or all of the final group of contact birds. Neither wild-type nor resistant virus had an obvious selective advantage for transmission in the absence of the drug (BEAN et al. 1989).

5.2 Human Influenza

The transmission of resistant influenza virus was assessed in a multicenter family-based trial in the United States (HAYDEN et al. 1989). Once an influenzal illness was recognized in the household, all of the eligible family members, including the ill index case and healthy contacts, were assigned as a block to treatment with rimantadine or placebo for 10 days. The development of illness in a contact which was proven to be due to influenza A virus infection occurred in about one-third of either placebo or rimantadine households and in about one-fifth of contacts in such households. Consequently, the calculated efficacy of rimantadine for postcontact prophylaxis was low in this study (Table 2). Secondary illnesses caused by apparent transmission of drug-resistant virus were found in five rimantadine-treated families, and in each instance the M2 protein changes detected in multiple isolates from one person or within a household were the same. In four of the five implicated households the ill index case was a young child.

Three other family-based studies have assessed the usefulness of postexposure prophylaxis with amantadine or rimantadine administered for 10-day periods (Table 2). During an H2N2 subtype epidemic in the United Kingdom, GALBRAITH et al. (1969a) found complete protection of household contacts against influenza A illness with amantadine. The same investigators found much

Table 2. Placebo-controlled trials of postexposure prophylaxis in families

Reference	Virus subtype year of study	Drug	Index case treated	Efficacy in contacts (%)
GALBRAITH et al. (1969a)	H2N2 1967	Amantadine	No	100*
GALBRAITH et al. (1969b)	H3N2 1968	Amantadine	Yes	20*
BRICAIRE et al. (1990)	H1N1 1988	Rimantadine	No	69**
HAYDEN et al. (1989)	H3N2 1988	Rimantadine	Yes	3*

* Reduction in laboratory documented influenza A illness compared to placebo;
** reduction in influenzal illness compared to placebo

lower levels of efficacy during a H3N2 subtype outbreak in the following year (GALBRAITH et al. 1969b). In addition to the change in the epidemic strain, against which most contacts had low antibody titers, the study design was altered in that the index cases were not treated in the first trial but were treated in the second one (Table 2). A recent French study conducted with rimantadine found significant protection of contacts, when the study did not involve treatment of the ill index cases (BRICAIRE et al. 1990). The findings indicate that both amantadine and rimantadine are effective for postexposure prophylaxis in families when index cases are not treated.

Although these studies are not directly comparable, the results suggest that the presence of a treated index case may be important with respect to reduced prophylactic efficacy in contacts, and support the conclusion that transmission of resistant virus can occur when rimantadine or amantadine is used for both treatment of ill index cases and prophylaxis of contacts. COUCH et al. (1986) found that treatment of ill index cases with amantadine or rimantadine appeared to reduce the likelihood of secondary illness in untreated family contacts, but it has not been determined whether those family members not receiving drug prophylaxis develop infections due to resistant virus shed by treated index cases. Similarly, no studies to date have directly tested the effect of randomization of index cases to drug or placebo on the efficacy of drug prophylaxis in contacts.

Recently, transmission of resistant influenza virus was also implicated by the recovery of drug-resistant virus from prophylaxis failures in nursing homes in which amantadine had been used during outbreak control (MAST et al. 1989; ROUMILLAT et al. 1990). In one home, MAST et al. (1989) described three patients residing in contiguous rooms who developed illnesses over a 5-day period, from which resistant viruses with the same mutation in position 27 were recovered. Thus, transmission of resistant virus, based on resistance markers and on epidemiologic evidence, appears to occur in circumstances of close contact between treated ill patients and those receiving drug prophylaxis.

6 Pathogenicity of Resistant Viruses

6.1 Virulence in Animals

Drug-resistant viruses appear to retain virulence in animal model studies involving direct inoculation of resistant strains. OXFORD and POTTER (1973) found that a mouse-adapted H2N2 subtype virus which was resistant to amantadine induced lung lesions in mice in the presence or absence of the drug to a similar degree as parental, sensitive virus did in untreated mice. BEAN et al. (1989) assessed the virulence of resistant avian strains by inoculating selected sensitive and resistant isolates into birds receiving no treatment. All passages of resistant or sensitive strains caused infection and illness, and some resistant strains appeared fully virulent. Mortality was not affected by amantadine administration

(BEAN et al. 1989). SWEET et al. (1991) assessed the virulence in ferrets of human H3N2 subtype resistant isolates with defined changes at positions 27, 30, or 31 of M2. When inoculated intranasally into ferrets, the drug-resistant viruses induced the same magnitude of fever and nasal cellular inflammatory responses as their drug-sensitive parental strains.

6.2 Virulence in Humans

Patients receiving chemoprophylaxis who have developed influenza associated with the recovery of resistant virus (i.e., prophylaxis failures) have generally had typical influenzal illness (BELSHE et al. 1989; HAYDEN et al. 1989; MAST et al. 1989). This may in part reflect an ascertainment bias since those with milder degrees of illness may not have been cultured for virus in some studies. In the family-based study described above (HAYDEN et al. 1989), the contact cases with drug-resistant infection experienced illnesses that were influenzal in character and associated with bed confinement or restricted activity. No obvious difference in viral pathogenicity has yet been found for drug-resistant human influenza viruses. Importantly, no evidence suggests that infections related to resistant viruses are more severe than that caused by wild-type strains.

Another issue regarding the pathogenicity of resistant viruses is the possible effect of resistance emergence on illness resolution in treated patients. HALL et al. (1987) found that rimantadine-treated children experienced significantly greater reductions in fever and illness severity during the first 3 days of treatment compared with those receiving acetaminophen. Compared to rimantadine recipients who did not shed resistant virus, the illness severity scores tended to be higher later in therapy in those shedding resistant virus, but the differences were too small to be clinically significant. HAYDEN et al. (1991) confirmed that rimantadine was associated with a net therapeutic benefit despite the recovery of resistant virus from one-third of treated patients. In the subgroup of patients shedding resistant virus, illness appeared to be somewhat more prolonged than rimantadine-treated patients who did not shed resistant virus, but no late increases in illness severity were observed. It remains unclear whether a causal relationship exists between recovery of resistant virus and prolongation of illness. The possibility that an abbreviated course of treatment, such as 1–2 days, might provide clinical benefit and reduce the likelihood of selecting resistant virus has not been studied.

7 Replication and Genetic Stability of Resistant Viruses

No apparent differences in growth characteristics in eggs or cell culture have been observed between sensitive parental viruses and their resistant variants selected in vivo (OXFORD et al. 1970; BELSHE et al. 1988). Similarly, limited studies indicate that resistant viruses replicate as well as wild-type ones in experimental infections of mice (OXFORD and POTTER 1973), birds (BEAN et al. 1989), and ferrets (SWEET et al. 1991).

Resistance also appears to be a stable property, since human variants remain resistant after multiple passages in vitro in the absence of the drugs. However, studies of drug-resistant variants of certain H7 avian viruses have found that mutations in M2 (e.g., alanine 30 → threonine or serine 31 → asparagine). which do not affect the growth properties of resistant variants of human H3 or avian H5 subtype viruses, do affect replication in cell culture to the extent of being associated with reversion to wildtype or selection of a compensatory M2 mutation during extended passage in the absence of the drug (HAY et al. 1991). Thus, particular resistance mutations are not equally tolerated by different influenza A strains under in vitro conditions. As described above, drug-resistant H5N2 subtype avian strains rëtained resistance during multiple in vivo passages in the absence of amantadine (BEAN et al. 1989). Comparable in vivo data is not available for humans at present.

8 Influence of M2 Changes

The relationship between particular mutations in M2 and the biologic characteristics of drug-resistant human influenza viruses has received very limited study. Table 3 shows the number of isolates with particular resistance mutations which

Table 3. Recovery of drug-resistant influenza A (H3N2) viruses and relationship to M2 protein substitutions

Residue no.	Amino acid change	Patients shedding drug-resistant viruses		
		During treatment (*n*)	During prophylaxis	
			Family contacts (*n*)	Nursing home residents (*n*)
26	Leu→Phe	0	0	2
27	Val→→Ala	1	0	3
30	Ala→→Val	3	1	1
30	Ala→→Thr	1	0	1
31	Ser→→Asn	13	4	3

The patients shedding resistant isolates during treatment were receiving rimantadine (BELSHE et al. 1988; HAYDEN et al. 1989; HAYDEN et al. 1991). The prophylaxis failures occurred in family members receiving rimantadine (HAYDEN et al. 1989) or in nursing home patients receiving amantadine (MAST et al. 1989; ROUMILLAT et al. 1990)
Leu, leucine; phe, phenylalanine; val, valine; ala, alanine; thr, threonine; ser, serine; asn, asparagine

have been recovered from individuals receiving rimantadine treatment and from those who were prophylaxis failures, that is, those who developed illness during chemoprophylaxis either with rimantadine in families or with amantadine during the nursing home outbreaks. The most common mutation detected in vitro during therapeutic use has been at position 31 (serine → asparagine). Not unexpectedly, such isolates have been found to be the commonest ones recovered in the small number of family contacts studied to date. The nursing home studies have found that prophylaxis failures have been associated with recovery of viral isolates with resistance mutations at other positions in M2. Changes at each of the four positions in M2 have been associated with influenza-like illness, but insufficient data exists to determine whether any particular type of mutation is associated with a lower risk of transmission or reduced pathogenicity. Whether there is particular significance in the first clinical isolates of resistant variants of H3N2 with a substitution in residue 26 (leucine → phenylalanine) during the 1989–1990 epidemic (ROUMILLAT et al. 1990) is not known. It is possible that differences in the hemagglutinin or other viral proteins between successive epidemic strains may predispose the virus to particular drug resistance changes in M2. One corollary is that drug resistance changes in M2 may become less tolerable to subsequent epidemic strains and thereby reduce their ability to compete with wild-type virus in the absence of selective drug pressure.

9 Summary

Amantadine- and rimantadine-resistant viruses have been recovered from approximately 30% of patients treated for acute H3N2 subtype influenza and less often from their close contacts receiving drug prophylaxis. The limited data suggest that resistant viruses can emerge rapidly during drug therapy, as early as 2–3 days into treatment. These viruses retain their resistance phenotype during multiple passages in the laboratory and appear to be genetically stable in this regard. Studies in families and in nursing homes indicate that resistant isolates appear to be transmissible from treated patients and cause typical influenza in contacts receiving drug prophylaxis. It is unknown whether resistant human viruses are capable of competing with wild-type ones during multiple cycles of infection in the absence of the drug. These viruses appear to be pathogenic, and no evidence indicates that they differ from wild-type strains.

Thus, these viruses clearly possess the biologic properties that are associated with clinically important drug resistance. However, limited information is available to assess their actual impact. It is unknown what degree of selective drug pressure would be required to cause substantial transmission of resistant viruses during community outbreaks. Natural selection of antigenic variants and disappearance of previous variants may prevent the emergence of viruses that have been altered in the genes coding both for the surface glycoproteins and for the M2 protein. However, the emergence of drug-resistant influenza viruses appears to pose potential clinical problems in certain epidemiologic situations involving close contact with treated patients.

References

Appleyard G (1977) Amantadine-resistance as a genetic marker for influenza viruses. J Gen Virol 36: 249–255

Bean WJ, Threlkeld SC, Webster RG (1989) Biologic potential of amantadine-resistant influenza A virus in an avian model. J Infect Dis 159: 1050–1056

Beard CW, Brugh M, Webster RG (1987) Emergence of amantadine-resistant H5N2 avian influenza virus during a simulated layer flock treatment program. Avian Dis 31: 533–537

Belshe RB, Hay AJ (1989) Drug resistance and mechanisms of action on influenza A viruses. J Respir Dis 10: S52–S61

Belshe RB, Smith MH, Hall CB, Betts R, Hay AJ (1988) Genetic basis of resistance to rimantadine emerging during treatment of influenza virus infection. J Virol 62: 1508–1512

Belshe RB, Burk B, Newman F, Cerruti RL, Sim IS (1989) Resistance of influenza A virus to amantadine and rimantadine: results of one decade of surveillance. J Infect Dis 159: 430–435

Bricaire AF, Hannoun C, Boissel JP (1990) Prévention de la gripple A. Efficacité et tolérance du chlorhydrate de rimantadine. Presse Med 19: 69–72

Couch RB, Kasel JA, Glezen WP, Cate TR, Six HR, Taber LH, Frank AL, Greenberg SB, JM Zahradnik, Keitel WA (1986) Influenza: its control in persons and populations. J Infect Dis 153: 431–440

Douglas RG (1990) Prophylaxis and treatment of influenza. N Engl J Med 322: 443–450

Galbraith AW, Oxford JS, Schild GC, Watson GI (1969a) Protective effect of 1-adamantanamine hydrochloride on influenza A2 infections in the family environment. A controlled double-blind study. Lancet 2: 1026–1028

Galbraith AW, Oxford JS, Schild GC, Watson GI (1969b) Study of 1-adamantanamine hydrochloride used prophylactically during the Hong Kong influenza epidemic in the family environment. Bull WHO 41: 677–682

Hall CB, Dolin R, Gala CL, Markovitz DM, Zhang YQ, Madore PH, Disney FA, Talpey WB, Green JL, Francis AB, Pichichero ME (1987) Children with influenza A infection: treatment with rimantadine. Pediatrics 80: 275–282

Hay AJ (1989) The mechanism of action of amantadine and rimantadine against influenza viruses. In: Notkins AL, Oldstone MBA (eds) Concepts in viral pathogenesis III. Springer, Berlin Heidelberg New York, pp 561–567

Hay AJ, Kennedy NTC, Skehel JJ, Appleyard G (1979) The matrix protein gene determines amantadine-sensitivity of influenza viruses. J Gen Virol 44: 807

Hay AJ, Zambon HC, Wolstein Holme AJ, Skehel JJ, Smith MH (1986) Molecular basis of resistance of influenza A viruses to amantadine. J Antimicrob Chemother [Suppl B] 18: 19–29

Hay AJ, Grambas S, Bennett MS (1991) Resistance of influenza A viruses to amantadine and rimantadine. In: Kumar A (ed) Advances in molecular biology and targeted treatment for AIDS. Plenum, New York (in press)

Hayden FG, Cote KM, Douglas RG Jr (1980) Plaque inhibition assay for drug susceptibility testing of influenza viruses. Antimicrob Agents Chemother 17: 865–870

Hayden FG (1986) Animal models of influenza virus infection for evaluation of antiviral agents. In: Zak O, Sande MA (eds) Experimental models in antimicrobial chemotherapy, Academic, Orlando, pp 353–371

Hayden FG, Belshe RB, Clover RD, Hay AJ, Oakes MG, Soo W (1989) Emergence and apparent transmission of rimantadine-resistant influenza A virus in families. N Engl J Med 321: 1696–1702

Hayden F, Sperber SJ, Belshe R, Clover R, Hay A, Pyke S (1991) Recovery of drug-resistant influenza A virus during therapeutic use of rimantadine. Antimicrob Agents Chemother 35: 1741–1747

Heider H, Adamczyk B, Presber HW, Schroeder C, Feldblum R, Indulen MK (1981) Occurrence of amantadine- and rimantadine-resistant influenza A virus strains during the 1980 epidemic. Acta Virol (Praha) 25: 395–400

Kendal A (1990) A prototype kit for amantadine sensitivity testing of influenza viruses (Abstract P 34–021). 8th International Congress of Virology, Berlin

Lubeck MD, Schulman JL, Palese P (1978) Susceptibility of influenza A viruses to amantadine is influenced by the gene coding for M protein. J Virol 28: 710–716

Mast EE, Davis, JP, Harmon MW, Arden NH, Circo R, Tyszka GE (1989) Emergence and possible transmission of amantadine-resistant viruses during nursing home outbreaks of influenza A (H3N2) (Abstr 65). In: 29th Interscience Conference on Antimicrobial Agents and Chemotherapy. American Society for Microbiology, Washington, p 111

Oxford JS, Potter CW (1973) Aminodamantane-resistant strains of influenza A2 virus. J Hyg (Camb) 71: 227–236

Oxford JS, Logan IS, Potter CW (1970) Passage of influenza strains in the presence of aminoadamantane. Ann NY Acad Sci 173: 300–313

Pemberton RM, Jennings R, Potter CW, Oxford JS (1986) Amantadine resistance in clinical influenza A (H_3N_2) and (H_1N_1) virus isolates. J Antimicrob Chemother [Suppl] 18: 135–140

Roumillat F, Rocha E, Regnery H, Wells D, Cox N (1990) Emergence of amantadine-resistant influenza A viruses in nursing homes during the 1989–1990 influenza season (Abstr P34–42). 8th International Congress of Virology, Berlin

Sugrue RJ, Hay AJ (1991) Structural characteristics of the M2 protein of influenza A viruses: evidence that it forms a tetrameric channel. Virology 180: 617–624

Sugrue RJ, Bahadur G, Zambon MC, Hall-Smith M, Douglas AR, Hay AJ (1990) Specific structural alteration of the influenza haemagglutinin by amantadine. EMBO J 9: 3469–3476

Sweet C, Hayden FG, Jakeman KJ, Grambas S, Hay AJ (1991) Virulence of rimantadine-resistant human influenza A (H3N2) viruses in ferrets. J Infect Dis 164: 969–972

Thompson J, Fleet W, Lawrence E, Pierce E, Morris L, Wright P (1987) A comparison of acetaminophen and rimantadine in the treatment of influenza A infection in children. J Med Virol 21: 249–255

Tominack RL, Hayden FG (1987) Rimantadine hydrochloride and amantadine hydrochloride use in influenza A virus infections. In: Knight V, Gilbert B (eds) Infectious disease clinics of North America. Saunders, Philadelphia, pp 459–478

Webster RG, Kawaoka Y, Bean WJ, Beard CW, Brugh M (1985) Chemotherapy and vaccination: a possible strategy for the control of highly virulent influenza virus. J Virol 55: 173–176

Selection of Zidovudine-Resistant Variants of Human Immunodeficiency Virus by Therapy*

D. D. RICHMAN

1 Introduction

The likelihood of emergence of drug resistance is a function of mutation rate and the number of replicative events. The mutation rate of human immunodeficiency virus (HIV) is presumed to be at least as high as any virus with a single-stranded RNA genome. The number of replicative events in a host infected with HIV are incalculably high as a result of years of persistent replication that is poorly restricted by immune surveillance. Viral chemotherapy in humans has selected for drug-resistant variants of influenza A virus, herpes simplex virus, varicella zoster virus, cytomegalovirus and rhinovirus (RICHMAN 1990). The prospect of

Departments of Pathology and Medicine, University of California San Diego and VA Medical Center, Infectious Diseases-111F, 3350 La Jolla Village Drive, San Diego, CA 92161, USA
* This work was supported by grants HB-67019, AI-27670, AI-30457, AI-29164 from the National Institutes of Health and by the Research Center for AIDS and HIV Infection of the San Diego Veterans Affairs Medical Center

Current Topics in Microbiology and Immunology, Vol. 176

drug resistance to zidovudine (AZT) therefore did not appear as a surprise to many.

2 The Phenotype of Reduced Susceptibility

2.1 The Initial Report

In the initial study of HIV susceptibility to AZT (LARDER et al. 1989), isolation of HIV was attempted with 186 peripheral blood mononuclear cell specimens from subjects at different stages of infection who had received therapy with AZT for various periods. A total of 46 isolates were obtained from 33 individuals. The use of MT2 lymphoblastoid cells for the isolation procedure permitted the preparation of large stocks of virus that could be frozen in aliquots and titrated. Susceptibility to AZT with these low-passage clinical isolates of HIV could not be tested reliably with the described assays of inhibition of cytopathology or production of p24 antigen (LARDER et al. 1990). This dilemma was resolved by the use of a CD4-expressing HeLa cell line (obtained from B. Chesebro, National Institute of Allergy and Infectious Diseases, Rocky Mountain Laboratories, Hamilton, Mont.) that readily permitted plaque reduction assays with all isolates tested (CHESEBRO and WEHRLY 1988). In addition, this system permitted assay of a wide range of compounds, including nucleosides, interferons, and recombinant soluble CD4.

Study of these original isolates permitted several conclusions:

1. Isolates from subjects not treated with AZT display a narrow range of susceptibility to AZT, with the 50% inhibitory concentration (IC_{50}) ranging from 0.01 to 0.05 μM (Table 1).
2. This narrow range of susceptibility is seen with isolates from subjects at all stages of HIV infection from asymptomatic through advanced acquired immunodeficiency syndrome (AIDS).
3. This narrow range of susceptibility is observed with isolates displaying both cytopathic and noncytopathic phenotypes in vitro.
4. Isolates from patients with AIDS or advanced AIDS-related complex (ARC) display no detectable reduction in susceptibility during the first 6 months of AZT treatment; almost all isolates from such individuals display some reduction in susceptibility after 6 months of therapy (Table 1).
5. Sequential isolates from individual patients receiving AZT therapy may display progressive, stepwise increases in resistance.
6. Several isolates with >100-fold increases in the IC_{50} of AZT have been identified.

An additional observation suggested by the original study was the presence of a "shoulder" on the syncytial focus inhibition curve that was consistent with a more highly resistant subpopulation. Unfortunately the focus assay does not

Table 1. Sensitivity of HIV isolates to AZT, by duration of therapy

Duration of therapy (months)	No. of isolates	IC_{50} (μM)		
		Mean	Median	Range
0	18	0.03	0.03	0.01–0.05
1–5	6	0.03	0.03	0.007–0.05
6–11	8	1.0	0.6	0.06–4.0
12–17	8	1.0	0.07	0.04–6.0
$\geqq$ 18	3	3.0	2.0	0.1–6.0

IC_{50} values were determined directly from plots of percentage plaque reduction vs. zidovudine concentration ($\log_{10}$). All isolates obtained during therapy and 15 of 18 isolates obtained in the absence of therapy were from patients with AIDS-related complex or AIDS. Reprinted with permission from *Science* (LARDER et al. 1989). Copyright 1989 by the American Association for the Advancement of Science

permit the retrieval of infectious virus from foci to clone phenotypically distinct virus. More recently additional inhibition curves even more suggestive or phenotypic mixtures have been observed and these virus stocks have been confirmed to be genotypic mixtures (see below).

2.2 Other Assays and Reports of Reduced Susceptibility

A distinct advantage of the syncytial focus assay in CD4 HeLa cells is that it generates a monotonic sigmoid curve that is highly reproducible when focus number is plotted against the log of the concentration of drug. The assay thus permits reproducible results, quantitative susceptibilities, easy detection of spurious single values and the detection of phenotypic mixtures. A disadvantage of the assay however is that it requires high-titer virus stocks which in practice can only be obtained from approximately one-third of specimens from seropositive individuals. Other assays have used the inhibition of production of supernatant reverse transcriptase or p24 antigen in the presence of various concentrations of drug. These assays have also documented the selection of isolates of HIV with reduced susceptibilities to AZT after prolonged therapy (ROOKE et al. 1989; LAND et al. 1990).

2.3 Cross-Resistance to Other Antivirals

With regard to resistance to other antiretroviral compounds, the five highly AZT resistant isolates have been shown to display cross-resistance to nucleosides containing a 3′-azido moiety including 3′-azido-2′,3′-dideoxyuridine (AZdU), 3′-

azido-2′,3′-dideoxyguanosine (AZG) and 3′-azido-2′,3′-dideoxyadenosine (AZA) (LARDER et al. 1990; RICHMAN, unpublished observations). No cross-resistance to other nucleosides, including several thymidine analogues, has yet been documented (LARDER et al. 1990), although this possibility is at least theoretically conceivable. In addition no cross-resistance to other nonnucleoside reverse transcriptase inhibitors or of compounds acting at other sites of HIV replication have been documented (LARDER et al. 1990; RICHMAN et al. 1991a). These observations are encouraging with regard to the use of other nucleosides such as ddC or ddI and of drug combinations.

2.4 Effect of Stage of Disease and Drug Dose on AZT Resistance

An extension of the original studies to a total of 97 isolates from 73 individuals has provided information regarding the effects of disease stage and drug dose on the rates of emergence of resistance (RICHMAN et al. 1990). For baseline data, 42 isolates were examined from subjects who denied any history of prior AZT therapy. Forty-one of these displayed IC_{50} values to AZT of $< 0.045\ \mu M$. One displayed an IC_{50} of $0.17\ \mu M$. Upon investigation this individual had developed macrocytosis and had measurable serum levels of AZT on multiple-stored serum specimens obtained prior to the development of the drug-resistant isolate.

Susceptibilities to AZT were determined in 55 isolates from 31 patients receiving AZT (RICHMAN et al. 1990). Patients with late-stage HIV infection (AIDS or advanced ARC) developed resistance significantly sooner than those with early-stage disease ($p = 0.0002$). By 12 months after initiation of AZT therapy, as estimated 89% (95% confidence interval, CI = 64%–99%) of persons with late-stage HIV infection have developed resistance, compared with 31% (95% CI = 16%–56%) of those with early-stage infection (Fig. 1). It is possible that the clinical significance of resistance could be a function of the degree of drug susceptibility. All six subjects who developed highly resistant virus were from among the 14 with late-stage HIV infection. For this population, the estimated proportion that develops highly resistant virus within 1 year after initiation of AZT is 33% (95% CI = 16%–59%), while no high-level resistance was documented in the first 18 months of therapy among earlier stage patients (Fig. 1).

Lower initial CD4 lymphocyte counts were also predictive of increased likelihood of the emergence of resistant isolates ($p = 0.004$). The estimated rates of resistance at 1 year were 89%, 41% and 27% for baseline CD4 cell counts < 100, 100–400, and > 400 CD4 cells/mm^3 (95% CIs = 63%–99%, 18%–75%, and 11%–59%, respectively).

Development of resistance occurred somewhat sooner among individuals assigned to higher daily doses of AZT (1200–1500 mg) than those assigned to lower doses (500–500 mg), although this difference did not attain statistical significance ($p = 0.18$ without controlling for stage and $p = 0.06$ after controlling for stage). Baseline positivity (> 37 pg/ml) for serum HIV p24 antigen, which occurred in five of the late-stage subjects and none of the early-stage subjects,

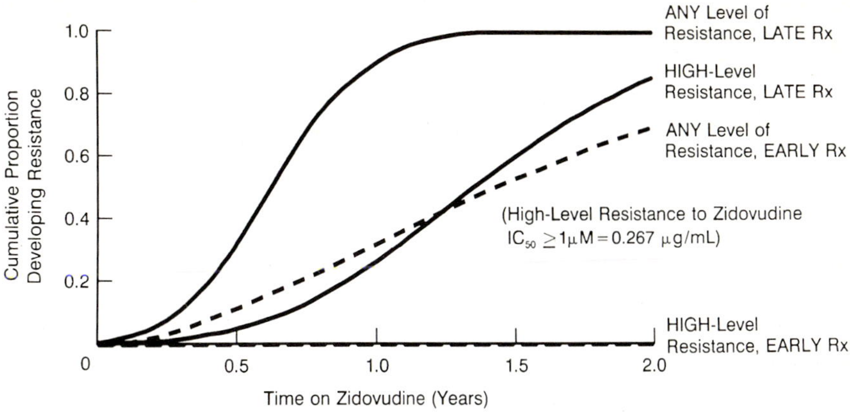

Fig. 1. Estimated cumulative proportion of persons developing resistant isolates as a function of time since initiation of AZT by stage of HIV infection. Patients with late-stage infection had less than 200 CD4 lymphocytes and HIV-related symptoms. Patients with early-stage disease had 200–500 CD4 lymphocytes and mild or no symptoms. Any level resistance is defined as an IC_{50} of $> 0.05\ \mu M$. High-level resistance is defined as an IC_{50} of $> 1.0\ \mu M$. No high-level resistance was seen in the early-stage patients during this interval. (From RICHMAN et al. 1990)

was not significantly correlated with the development of resistance ($p = 0.2$). These results are encouraging based upon the studies and recommendations that a 500-mg daily dose of AZT is indicated (VOLBERDING et al. 1990; FISCHL et al. 1990; CARPENTER et al. 1990).

2.5 Enzymologic Basis of Resistance

The antiviral effect of AZT is conferred by the triphosphate that is generated by anabolic phosphorylation by host cell thymidine kinase and other enzymes (FURMAN et al. 1986). AZT triphosphate inhibits the reverse transcriptase of HIV in cell free enzyme assays and also acts as a terminator of DNA chain elongation because the 3′-azido group prevents the formation of 3′,5′-phosphodiester bonds. It was not surprising therefore when mutations in the gene for the resistant viral reverse transcriptase were documented (see below). What remains puzzling, however, has been the inability to demonstrate an enzymologic difference in the mutant reverse transcriptase (LARDER et al. 1989). Utilizing enzyme extracted either from AZT-sensitive and -resistant virions or prepared from enzyme expressed in *Escherichia coli* after molecular cloning from these viruses, no differences in inhibition by AZT triphosphate has been demonstrated in cell free enzyme assays. Because the genetics are definitive, these observations would suggest that cell free enzyme assays do not reflect the mechanism of inhibition of AZT triphosphate upon the transcription complex in the cell.

2.6 Clinical Significance of AZT Resistance

The clinical importance of AZT-resistant HIV has been difficult to document. There are several reasons for this difficulty. First the development of resistance is not abrupt. It occurs slowly and progressively. It is possible that the significance of different levels of susceptibility could be quite different clinically. These different levels appear over periods of months to years, and recent observations with assays for the presence of mutations in clinical specimens suggest that mixtures of viruses with different resistance genotypes may be circulating simultaneously in the same individual. Moreover clinical endpoints in HIV disease are often neither clear-cut nor the immediate consequence of a change in virus replication, but rather the result of an opportunistic consequence of immunosuppression. Nevertheless it seems probable to many that replication in vitro in the presence of concentrations of AZT that are clinically unattainable will prove to be important.

One approach that may prove informative is the selection of AZT-resistant mutants of feline immunodeficiency virus (FIV) (REMINGTON et al. 1991). AZT-resistant mutants of HIV have been difficult to select in cell culture (SMITH et al. 1987). In contrast, resistant mutants of FIV have been readily selectable, perhaps because growth and plaquing is possible in a cat monolayer cell culture system. The resistant isolates have cross-resistance to other compounds identical to the resistant isolates of HIV (LARDER et al. 1990). The mutant and parental strains of FIV may provide information regarding both drug susceptibility in vivo and virulence.

3 Genetics of AZT Resistance

3.1 Mutations Associated with Resistant Isolates

The mechanism of resistance to AZT is attributable not surprisingly to mutations in the viral reverse transcriptase. Sequencing the reverse transcriptase gene of five pairs of isolates that displayed more than 100-fold reductions in susceptibility during the course of therapy documented multiple mutations, four of which appeared common (LARDER and KEMP 1989). When these four mutations at codons 67, 70, 215, and 219 were inserted by site-directed mutagenesis into the susceptible, infectious molecular clone pHXB2, a greater than 100-fold reduction in AZT susceptibility resulted. Sequential isolates from the same individual that displayed progressive, stepwise increments in resistance were associated with the sequential cumulative acquisition of these four mutations (LARDER and KEMP 1989). Cumulative mutations thus contribute additively or synergistically to stepwise reductions in susceptibility. Mutations at the four identified codons are among the most important, but almost certainly not the exclusive, contributors to the resistance phenotype.

Several investigators have developed assays utilizing sequence amplification methodologies to assay for these point mutations. BOUCHER et al. (1990) utilizing primer pairs for the polymerase chain reaction (PCR) that include the wild-type or mutant sequence for codon 215 demonstrated the appearance of mutant sequence at codon 215 is asymptomatic patients receiving chronic therapy with AZT. Mutations gradually appeared over a 2-year period with therapy and correlated with the phenotype of resistance. Mitsuya and colleagues have discriminated wild-type or mutant sequences with restriction endonucleases after PCR of the reverse transcriptase gene to identify the appearance of mutations at codon 215 with therapy (MITSUYA, personal communication). LÓPEZ-GALÍNDEZ et al., have utilized patterns of susceptibility to ribonuclease A to discriminate wild-type or mutant sequence at codon 215 (LÓPEZ-GALÍNDEZ et al. 1991). Although isolates from California and Spain had very distinctive digestion patterns, the pattern characteristic of a mutation at codon 215 occurred only in patients from either area receiving chronic AZT therapy.

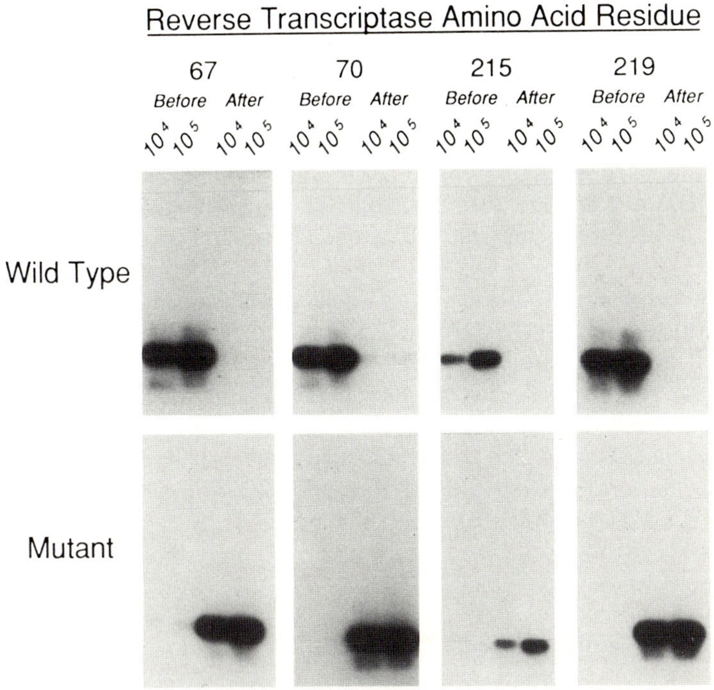

Fig. 2. Detection of genotype of HIV reverse transcriptase sequence directly in the peripheral blood mononuclear cells from a patient during therapy with AZT. The peripheral blood mononuclear cells of patient A012 were probed for wild-type or mutant genotype at the four codons of interest. The five dates of collection of the lymphocytes are indicated as are the AZT susceptibilities of three of the corresponding virus isolates. AZT therapy was initiated on 26 March 1986 (From RICHMAN et al. 1991b)

RICHMAN et al. (1991b) have utilized a PCR technique with primer pairs that generate a 535 base pair sequence that spans all four codons of interest in the reverse transcriptase. Four pairs of oligonucleotide probes that are specific for wild-type or mutant sequence at each of the codons are then used to characterize the sequence at each codon utilizing as target either patient peripheral blood mononuclear cells or virus isolates on which AZT susceptibility has been performed (Fig. 2). The results generated with this assay are summarized below.

GINGERAS et al. have utilized an isothermal, single-cycle amplification technique (GUATELLI et al. 1990), termed the self-sustained sequence replication (3SR) system, that can discriminate wild-type or mutant sequence at each of the four codons. Because this amplification method generates a predominance of one strand of single-stranded RNA, direct sequencing is possible, thus permitting a number of additional issues to be investigated (GINGERAS et al. 1991).

3.2 Time Course and Sequence of Appearance of Mutations

A total of 304 independent specimens (virus stocks or peripheral blood mononuclear cells) from 168 individuals have been genotypically characterized utilizing the PCR method (RICHMAN et al. 1991b). Sixty-seven specimens have been obtained prior to AZT therapy, all of which have displayed wild-type genotype. Sixty specimens obtained from individuals receiving AZT therapy have contained a mutant sequence at a single codon: 5 at codon 67, 23 at codon 70, 31 at codon 215, and 1 at codon 219. Thus a mutation may first appear at any codon but the selection for some mutations occurs far more readily than for others.

The cumulative proportion of individuals with a mutation at each codon has also been determined. These overall rates do not indicate the sequence of appearance of mutations in all individuals, as is demonstrated by the data already presented regarding the first mutation to develop. In addition, because of the number of specimens tested, the 95% confidence limits of the values for each curve are relatively wide. The proportion of specimens with mutations at 1 year were 33% for codon 67 (95% CI = 20%–51%) 59% for codon 70 (95% CI = 44%–75%), 63% for codon 215 (95% CI = 48%–78%), and 13% for codon 219 (95% CI = 1%–31%).

3.3 Correlation of Genotype with Phenotype

Highly resistant virus contains mutant sequence in the codons under consideration and when these mutations were placed in a infectious DNA construct, the resulting virus was converted from sensitive to highly resistant. Nevertheless it has not been clearly established to what extent each mutation contributes to reduced AZT susceptibility and what proportion of AZT resistance can be attributed to these four codons. All isolates obtained prior to AZT therapy were previously shown to have an IC_{50} of $< 0.045\ \mu M$ (LARDER et al. 1989; RICHMAN et al. 1990). Isolates with a single mutation at codons 70 or 215 were examined for drug susceptibility. Most isolates with a single mutation had a susceptibility that fell within the range of sensitive isolates, although the susceptibilities ranged over a more than tenfold range for isolates with mutations at codons 70 or 215. This observation suggests that a mutation may have a variable impact in a different genetic context or that additional mutations, not at one of the four codons, also contribute to reduced susceptibility. This hypothesis is supported by the observation in a patient whose isolate with a single mutation at codon 215 changed from sensitive ($IC_{50} = 0.02\ \mu M$) to resistant ($IC_{50} = 0.17\ \mu M$) over a 2-month period (RICHMAN et al. 1991b).

The results of logistic regression analyses have shown that phenotypic resistance is statistically related to site 215 ($p = 0.003$), site 70 ($p = 0.006$), site 219 ($p = 0.04$), and marginally associated with site 67 ($p = 0.084$) (RICHMAN et al. 1991b). However, the best fitting model includes the total number of mutant sites among sites 70, 215, and 219 ($p < 0.0001$). In fact, when all three sites were mutant, the probability of resistance was 100%; if two of the three sites were mutant, the probability of resistance was 90%; if one of the three sites was mutant, the probability of resistance was 45%; and if none of the sites were mutant, the probability of resistance was 0% (Fig. 3). The results of the linear regression analyses on the continuous log-transformed IC_{50} were consistent with those from the logistic regression analyses. The most predictive model includes the total number of mutant sites among 70, 215, and 219 (Fig. 3). Mutation

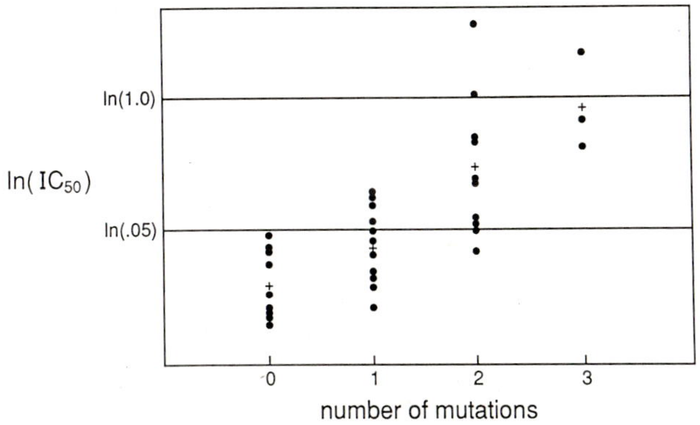

Fig. 3. Relation of susceptibility of isolates of HIV to number of mutations at codons 70, 215, and 219 of the reverse transcriptase gene. The natural log of the IC_{50} of virus isolates is indicated with the number of mutations at codons 70, 215, and 219. All values are graphed for virus stocks on which both AZT susceptibility testing and genotypic analysis was performed. Sequential specimens from the same patient with the same values were excluded. Values for individual virus stocks are depicted with ●. The cutoff for sensitive virus has been defined as $0.05\ \mu M$. The geometric means (+) of each set of values was $0.02\ \mu M$ for no mutations, $0.04\ \mu M$ for one mutation, $0.21\ \mu M$ for two mutations, and $0.88\ \mu M$ for three mutations. (From RICHMAN et al. 1991b)

information from site 67 did not add any additional information, and adjusting for time on study had no effect on the estimates in either analysis.

3.4 Evidence for the Existence of Genotypic Mixtures in Patients on Therapy

The suggestion of mixed populations of virus with different AZT susceptibilities has been confirmed with genotypic analysis. BOUCHER et al. (1990) documented several individuals with the simultaneous presence of both wild-type and mutant sequence at codon 215. LÓPEZ-GALÍNDEZ et al. (1991) documented by sequencing of clones the simultaneous presence in the same individuals of both the phenylalanine and tyrosine mutations at codon 215. RICHMAN et al. (1991b) have demonstrated mixtures at each of the codons, occasionally several simultaneously, during the transition from pure wild type to pure mutant sequences in that individual.

3.5 Selection with a Subpopulation with Passage In Vitro

A small proportion of virus isolates have been documented to change susceptibility pattern or genotype with passage in vitro in the absence of drugs (RICHMAN et al. 1991b; GINGERAS et al. 1991). This phenomenon occurs more frequently if a mixed population is present in the original mononuclear cell specimen. Shifts to either more- or less-sensitive populations have been documented.

3.6 Nonreactivity with Either Wild-Type or Mutant Probes

The PCR assay described by RICHMAN et al. (1991b) did not fail to amplify and detect at least one codon in any of the 67 clinical samples obtained from seropositive individuals prior to AZT therapy. With AZT therapy, however, 222 in 237 peripheral blood cell or virus stock specimens failed to react with either wild-type or mutant probe for one or more of the codons. Preliminary sequencing studies suggest that the appearance of additional mutations either with the codon in question or in adjacent codons accounts for this diminished probe affinity. This problem will presumably affect most such assays with this highly mutable virus. It is important to appreciate that a mutation in the reverse transcriptase could affect drug susceptibility, have a neutral effect on drug susceptibility, or confound assays to detect other specific sequences.

4 Conclusions

The development of reduced susceptibility to AZT in vitro has been described by several laboratories using isolates from patients receiving prolonged drug therapy. The likelihood of developing resistance increases with advanced disease stage and with lower CD4 lymphocyte counts but appears not to be related to drug doses with daily doses of AZT at 500 mg or more. Mutations at four codons of the reverse transcriptase have been associated with the resistance phenotype. Assays to detect these mutations directly in the peripheral blood mononuclear cells of treated patients have confirmed the development of these mutations in association with reduced susceptibility in epidemiologically unrelated study populations in the Netherlands, Spain, and California.

Several approaches to reduce the rate of emergence of drug resistance clinically are under investigation. Alternating regimens, for example of AZT and ddC (YARCHOAN et al. 1988; SKOWRON and MERIGAN 1990; BOZZETTE and RICHMAN 1990) would be expected to ameliorate drug toxicity with two drugs with nonoverlapping toxicities. An alternating regimen would also be predicted to at least double the interval before resistance developed, because the selective pressure of therapy with any one drug is present only one-half of the time. AZT and ddC in combination are also in clinical trial (MENG et al. 1990). Combination chemotherapy, by analogy with bacteria and tumor cells, would be predicted to select for resistance with a probability that is the product of the probabilities of each drug alone. These hypotheses are currently under investigation.

Assuming that the importance of drug resistance will be documented, all future in vitro and in vivo evaluation of candidate drugs must contend with the prospect of drug resistance. Studies of candidate drugs in vitro must include the assessment of in vitro selection for resistance, of cross-resistance with other compounds, and of drug interactions with regard to synergy, antagonism and toxicity. The evaluation of drugs in the clinic must be designed with the prospect that the future of chemotherapy for HIV, as for tuberculosis and most malignancies, will be with combination regimens.

References

Boucher CAB, Tersmette M, Lange JMA, Kellam P, de Goede REY, Mulder JW, Darby G, Goudsmit J, Larder BA (1990) Zidovudine sensitivity of human immunodeficiency viruses from high-risk, symptom-free individuals during therapy. Lancet 336: 585–590.

Bozzette SA, Richman DD (1990) Salvage therapy for zidovudine-intolerant HIV-infected patients with alternating and intermittent regimens of AZT and ddC. Am J Med [Suppl 5B] 88: 24S–26S

Carpenter CCJ et al. (1990) State-of-the-art conference on azidothymidine therapy for early HIV infection. Am J Med 89: 335–344

Chesebro B, Wehrly K (1988) Development of a sensitive quantitative focal assay for human immunodeficiency virus infectivity. J Virol 62: 3779–3788

Fischl MA, Parker CB, Pettinelli C, Wulfsohn M, Hirsch MS, Collier AC, Antoniskis D, Ho M, Richman DD, Fuchs E, Merigan TC, Reichman RC, Gold J, Steigbigel N, Leoung GS, Rasheed S, Tsiatis A, AIDS Clinical Trials Group (1990) A randomized controlled trial of a reduced daily dose of zidovudine in patients with the acquired immunodeficiency syndrome. N Engl J Med 323: 1009–1014

Furman PH, Fyfe JA, St Clair MH, Weinhold KJ, Rideout JL, Nusinoff-Lehrman S, Bolognesi DP, Broder S, Mitsuya H, Barry DW (1986) Phosphorylation of 3′-azido-3′deoxythymidine and selective interaction of the 5′-triphosphate with human immunodeficiency virus reverse transcriptase. Proc Natl Acad Sci USA 83: 8333–8337

Guatelli JC, Whitfield KM, Kwoh DY, Barringer KJ, Richman DD, Gingeras TR (1990) Isothermal, in vitro amplification of nucleic acids by a multi enzyme reaction modeled after retroviral replication. Proc Natl Acad Sci USA 87: 1874–1878

Gingeras TR, Prodanovich P, Latimer T, Guatelli JC, Richman DD, Barringer KJ (1991) Use of self-sustained sequence replication (35R) amplification reaction to analyze and detect mutations in zidovudine-resistant human immunodeficiency virus. J Infect Dis (in press)

Land S, Treloar T, McPhee D, Birch C, Doherty R, Cooper D, Gust ID (1990) Decreased in vitro susceptibility to zidovudine of HIV isolates obtained from patients with AIDS. J Infect Dis 161: 326–329

Larder BA, Kemp SD (1989) Multiple mutations in HIV-1 reverse transcriptase confer high-level resistance to zidovudine (AZT). Science 246: 1155–1158

Larder BA, Darby G, Richman DD (1989) HIV with reduced sensitivity to zidovudine (AZT) isolated during prolonged therapy. Science 243: 1731–1734

Larder BA, Chesebro B, Richman DD (1990) Susceptibilities of zidovudine-susceptible and -resistant human immunodeficiency virus isolates to antiviral agents determined by using a quantitative plaque reduction assay. Antimicrob Agents Chemother 34: 436–441

López-Galindez C, Rojas JM, Nájera R, Richman DD, Perucho M (1991) Characterization of genetic variation and AZT resistance mutations of HIV by the RNAs A mismatch cleavage method. Proc Natl Acad Sci USA 88: 4280–4284

Meng TC, Fischl MA, Richman DD (1990) ACTG 106: phase I/II study of ddC and AZT: combination in patients with AIDS and advanced ARC. Am J Med [Suppl 5B] 88: 27S–30S

Remington KM, Chesebro B, Wehrly K, Pedersen NC, North TW (1991) Mutants of feline immunodeficiency virus resistant to 3′-azido-3′-deoxythymidine. J Virol 65: 308–312

Richman DD (1990) Viral drug resistance. Curr Opin Infect Dis 3: 819–823

Richman DD, Grimes JM, Lagakos SW (1990) Effect of stage of disease and drug dose on zidovudine susceptibilities of isolates of human immunodeficiency virus. J AIDS 3: 743–746

Richman DD, Rosenthal AS, Skoog M, Eckner RJ, Chou T-C, Sabo JP, Merluzzi VJ (1991a) BI-RG-587 is active against zidovudine-resistant human immunodeficiency virus type 1 and synergistic with zidovudine. Antimicrob Agents Chemother 35: 305–308

Richman DD, Guatelli JC, Grimes J, Tsiatis A, Gingeras TR (1991b) The detection of mutations associated with zidovudine resistance in human immunodeficiency virus utilizing the polymerase chain reaction. J Infect Dis (in press)

Rooke R, Tremblay M, Soudeyns H, DeStephano L, Yao X-J, Fanning M, Montaner JSF, O'Shaughnessy M, Gelmon K, Tsoukas CD, Gill J, Ruedy J, Wainberg MA, Canadian Zidovudine Multi-Centre Study Group (1989) Isolation of drug-resistant variants of HIV-1 from patients on long-term zidovudine therapy. AIDS 3: 411–415

Skowron G, Merigan TC (1990) Alternating and intermittent regimens of zidovudine (3′-azido-3′-deoxythymidine) and dideoxycytidine (2′,3′-dideoxycytidine) in the treatment of patients with acquired immunodeficiency syndrome (AIDS) and AIDS-related complex. Am J Med [Suppl 5B) 88: 20S–23S

Smith MS, Brian EL, Pagano JS (1987) Resumption of virus production after human immunodeficiency virus infection of T lymphocytes in the presence of azidothymidine. J Virol 61: 3769–3773

Volberding PA, Lagakos SW, Koch MA, Pettinelli C, Myers MW, Booth DK, Balfour DH, Reichman RC, Bartlett JA, Hirsch MS, Murphy RL, Hardy WD, Soiero R, Fischl MA, Bartlett JG, Merigan TC, Hyslop NE, Richman DD, Valentine FT, Corey L, AIDS Clinical Trials Group (1990) Zidovudine in asymptomatic human immunodeficiency virus infection. A controlled trial in persons with fewer than 500 CD4-positive cells per cubic millimeter. N Engl J Med 322: 941–949

Yarchoan R, Perno CF, Thomas RV, Klecker RW, Allain JP, Wills RJ, McAtee N, Fischl MA, Dubinsky R, McNeely MC, Mitsuya H, Pluda JM, Lawley TJ, Leuther MD, Safai B, Collins JM, Myers CE, Broder S (1988) Phase studies of 2′,3′-dideoxycytidine in severe human immunodeficiency virus infection as a single agent and alternating with zidovudine (AZT). Lancet 1: 76–81

Genetic Diversity and Evolution of Retroviruses

J. M. Coffin

1 Introduction

Retroviruses are one of the most widespread and probably the most biologically diverse group of infectious agents of vertebrates. Virtually all mammals—as well as some birds, reptiles, and fish—have yielded infectious retroviruses when examined sufficiently closely. Within a species, the viruses isolated can display considerable diversity of biological properties. For example, within the group of closely related murine leukemia viruses are found agents which differ in receptors used for infection; in mode of transmission for genetic (as endogenous germline proviruses) to horizontal and vertical (via milk or infection in utero); in pathogenicity from benign to highly virulent; and in disease spectrum from a variety of malignancies of varying latency to immunodeficiencies, anemias, neurological diseases, and others.

Two fundamental aspects of retrovirus biology form the basis of the generation of this diversity. First, the mechanism of replication of retroviruses from an RNA genome through an integrated proviral DNA intermediate inherently empowers a wide variety of virus cell interactions. For example, it permits

Tufts University School of Medicine, 136 Harrison Avenue, Boston, Massachusetts 02111, USA

Current Topics in Microbiology and Immunology, Vol. 176

(but does not require) stable long-term "latent" association of the virus and host genetic information. Also, it allows the virus to adapt readily to the transcriptional characteristics of a particular cell type. Furthermore, it tolerates the generation and maintenance of defective genomes like those that contain oncogenes, or pathogenic variants of virion proteins. Second, the same replication mechanism carries with it the mechanism for generation of diversity: an enzyme system prone to misincorporation errors (although not exceptionally so), and a DNA synthetic mechanism that requires the system to be capable of frequent recombination and rearrangement of genetic information.

In this brief, but opinionated, review, I will discuss the mechanisms by which errors are introduced during retrovirus replication, the principles of mutation and selection in the generation of retroviral diversity, some specific examples that illuminate these principles, and how these might play out in the evolution of retrovirus genomes over the long term.

2 Mechanisms of Variation

Retroviruses are unique in that three enzyme systems (reverse transcriptase, cellular DNA polymerase, and RNA polymerase) figure in the replication of their genomes (Coffin 1990b; Varmus 1987, 1988; Varmus et al. 1984, 1985). The error rate of cellular DNA replication systems is quite low; the rate of error in transcription and processing during genome synthesis, with a few exceptions described later, has not yet been assessed. Most attention has been paid to the reverse transcriptase process, which has two relevant properties. First, like virtually all replication systems encoded by simple viruses, reverse transcriptase lacks a proofreading or error-correcting activity. Second, a more unique aspect is its ability to transfer a growing chain from one template to another during DNA synthesis. Such strand transfers or "jumps" must occur twice during reverse transcription to generate long terminal repeats (LTRs) at each end of the viral DNA. A similar process of strand transfer between the two copies of the diploid genome template also seems to provide a mechanism for repair of damage such as breaks in the RNA (Coffin 1979; Hu and Temin 1990a). The consequence of such a mechanism is a high rate of recombination—both "legitimate" to rearrange viral sequences between related viruses and "illegitimate" to delete or duplicate viral sequences or incorporate nonviral sequences into the genome.

2.1 Point Mutation

Most studies of misincorporation rates by reverse transcriptase have been done using in vitro systems which contain purified enzymes and substrates, and a wide range of values has been obtained, ranging from 10^{-2} to less than 10^{-4} errors per base incorporated (Gopinathan et al. 1979; Preston et al. 1988; Roberts et al.

1988, 1989). These values are interesting, and imply that reverse transcriptase ranks with RNA replicases (BATSCHELET et al. 1976; J. J. HOLLAND et al. 1989, 1990; PARVIN et al. 1986) in error frequency, but are difficult to apply to the real world since they are certain to be dependent on experimental parameters such as ion concentrations and conformation of the template within the infected cell, which are presently impossible to determine, much less duplicate.

More useful values for mutation rates should come from direct measurements during virus infection of cells, but relatively few studies have been reported. Error rates of around 10^{-4} (plus/minus a factor of 3 or so) per base per replication have been reported for avian retroviruses on passage through chicken cells (COFFIN et al. 1980; LEIDER et al. 1988), with correction for selective effects. These studies are based on measuring the most frequent errors and might overestimate the rate if, as suggested by the in vitro studies, the error rate is strongly dependent on sequence context. More valuable are single-step experiments, in which multiple progeny of a single round of infection are cloned, selected for a specific change (such as reversion of a nonsense mutation selectable in bacterial cloning vectors) and analyzed. Until the recent development of retroviral vectors and packaging cell lines (DANOS and MULLIGAN 1988; DOUGHERTY et al. 1989; LINIAL and MILLER 1990; MILLER and BULTIMORE 1986), it was impossible to maintain adequate control over replication cycles in order to perform such experiments. Experiments of this sort have yielded somewhat lower rates—on the order of 10^{-5} misincorporation errors per base pair per replication (DOUGHERTY and TEMIN 1988; PATHAK and TEMIN 1990b). The difference in rates compared to the population studies could reflect the different experimental system, the different virus, or the fact that the latter study examined a specific site rather than the entire genome.

A similar analysis, in which the nature and frequency of the mutations which inactivate an inserted gene was studied, revealed that an occasional viral DNA had suffered from more mutations than expected on a random basis (PATHAK and TEMIN 1990b). This phenomenon—called "hypermutation"—seems to be the consequence of some aberration in the particular virion that gave rise to this particular DNA molecule, such as a mutant or improperly processed reverse transcriptase. In one study, it was observed that hypermutation tended to change GA to AA sequences and it was proposed that the mutation might be due to slippage and realignment during reverse transcription (VARTANIAN et al. 1991). Genomes which have suffered a similar sort of hypermutation have also been found in surveys of viral DNA populations in HIV-infected individuals (VARTANIAN et al. 1991), and similar phenomena have been reported for other RNA viruses (BASS et al. 1989).

2.2 Rearrangement

In addition to misincorporation errors, retroviruses are also subject to a high frequency of errors due to sequence rearrangements, such as insertions or deletions of small numbers of bases and deletions or reduplications of larger amounts of sequence. Certain sequences are particularly prone to such rearrangements. For example, regions flanked by short repeated sequences tend to be either deleted or reduplicated as a consequence of homologous recombination between the repeats (PATHAK and TEMIN 1990a). Also, runs of identical bases seem to be particularly unstable. In one study, it was found that a sequence of ten identical residues had a 40% probability of being extended or shortened by a base during a single round of replication (PATHAK and TEMIN 1990b).

Most of the time, rearrangements of this sort will be lethal to the virus, producing frameshift mutations and other serious problems. Nevertheless, there are a number of examples of important variation by such mechanisms. For example, some strains of HIV are distinguished from all others by a perfect reduplication of short sequences in *gag* and *pol* (MYERS et al. 1990). Also in HIV, duplication of short sequence in *env* followed by divergence of the duplications by point mutations seems to have been an important mechanism for generation of sequence variants in the env proteins (COFFIN 1986; MYERS et al. 1990). Finally, reduplications in the enhancer region of the LTR of murine leukemia viruses are important in the evolution of pathogenic variants during lymphomagenesis (GOLEMIS et al. 1990; STOYE et al. 1991a).

A special class of rearrangements of retroviral sequences includes those involving the ends of the DNA molecule. Since the ends of each LTR contain sequences necessary to specify integration, aberrations in their structure often lead to DNA molecules which are incapable of integration and therefore do not contribute significantly to progeny virus. By the same token, however, unintegrated molecules—particularly circular forms—are readily cloned and therefore many cloning strategies tend to select strongly for molecules in which such aberrations have occurred. Such molecules have been intensively studied, and include several types. Autointegration—the joining of the ends of a DNA molecule to an internal site in the same molecule—results in a rearranged circle or two small circles (LEE and COFFIN 1990; SHOEMAKER et al. 1980). Other kinds of errors detectable in cloned circular forms include a variety of rearrangements of sequence at the joint between the LTRs (OLSEN et al. 1990), many of which probably result from improper sites of initiation or strand transfer during reverse transcription.

2.3 Recombination

Retroviruses exhibit extraordinarily high rates of recombination—both homologous, joining one genome to another at the corresponding sequences, or illegitimate, joining viral to nonviral sequences or rearranging viral sequences at unrelated sites. Both of these are quite important to the biology of the virus. Homologous recombination allows the rapid exchange of traits (such as host range) among related viruses as well as the acquisition of sequences from endogenous proviruses, and probably helps the evolution of viruses. Illegitimate recombination has given rise to viruses containing cellular sequences, such as oncogenes.

While it is possible that some recombination events of both types take place at the level of viral DNA (indeed, some workers still argue that most illegitimate events do; GOODRICH and DUESBERG 1990), the bulk of evidence as well as the weight of opinion favor the reverse transcription process (COFFIN et al. 1980; HU and TEMIN 1990a, b; SWAIN and COFFIN 1991). Homologous recombination is a consequence of the dimeric viral genome and the ability of reverse transcriptase to switch templates while elongating a growing DNA chain. It is sufficiently frequent that even closely spaced markers on the genome can behave as if genetically unlinked in experiments where distinctly marked viruses are grown together (COFFIN et al. 1980). In the one reported experiment in which the appearance of recombinants in a single cycle of infection was measured and a measurement of frequency was possible, it was estimated that some 40% of genomes at risk had undergone at least one crossing-over during DNA synthesis (HU and TEMIN 1990a, b).

Two distinct (but not exclusive) models for recombination have been proposed, which differ at the step in reverse transcription where recombination occurs (Fig. 1). In the "forced copy choice" model, the synthesis of a minus

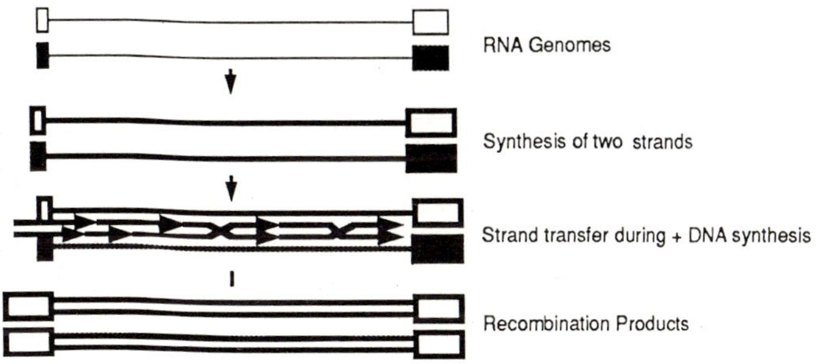

a

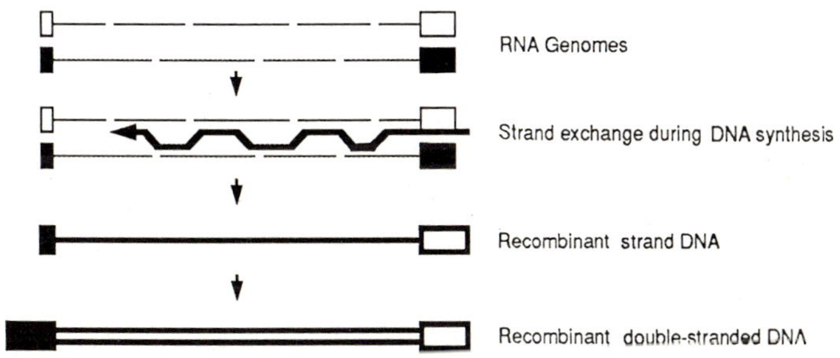

b

Fig. 1 a, b. Models for retroviral recombination. **a** Strand aggression. **b** Forced copy choice. Note that the two models are not mutually exclusive. (HU and TEMIN 1990b)

strand (i.e., one complementary to the genome RNA) is interrupted when the enzyme encounters a break in the RNA, forcing it to transfer elongation to the other genome in the same virion and continue synthesis (COFFIN et al. 1980). Alternatively, the "strand aggression" model posits that, if two complete minus strands are made, then the possibility of exchange of plus strands (which are sometimes fragmentary) also exists (JUNGHANS et al. 1982). The debate on this issue has gone on for years. Modern technology should provide the tools for finally settling the issue. In the study of HU and TEMIN (HU and TEMIN 1990a, b) cited above, two classes of recombinants were found; those which had a single detectable crossover, and those which had more than one crossover. The suggestion by these authors that the single crossovers might have occurred during negative strand synthesis and the multiple crossovers during synthesis of positive strands remains to be tested. An intriguing aspect of this study was the linkage of LTR exchanges (caused by a first jump from the 5′ end of one genome molecule to that 3′ end of the other) to the crossover frequency. Proviruses with a single crossover tended to have recombinant LTRs while proviruses with multiple crossovers more commonly had nonrecombinant LTRs. These differences may reflect differences in the organization of the genome RNA within the virion and their influence on the recombination process in ways that are still unclear.

2.4 Nonhomologous Recombination

The best studied case of nonhomologous recombination in retroviruses is the acquisition of oncogenes—a rare event, and one that leads to a highly virulent, usually defective, virus which is probably incapable of surviving more than a short time in the wild, but which can find a good niche in the laboratory if discovered and brought to culture by the inquisitive scientist. To date, some 30 or so oncogenes—cell-derived sequences which have been acquired by retrovirus genomes and usually subject to additional mutations—have been described, and have formed the basis for most modern research on the molecular basis of cancer (BISHOP 1983, 1991; BISHOP et al. 1982).

Two somewhat different scenarios for the "capture" of oncogenes by retroviruses have been proposed (Fig. 2). In boh models, the initial event would be integration of a provirus into a protooncogene leading to its conversion (or "activation") to oncogene status and overgrowth of the infected cell. The illegitimate recombination would then ensue. In one scheme (GOLDFARB and WEINBERG 1981; SWANSTROM et al. 1983), the first event would be deletion of a region encompassing the 3′ end of the provirus and neighboring cell sequence. Transcription of the resulting defective provirus would give rise to hybrid virus-oncogene transcripts, which, after processing, would be packaged into virions. An illegitimate recombination event during reverse transcription would then form the 3′ joint of oncogene to virus sequence. In the second model, copackaging of virus and flanking cellular sequence into virions does not require a deletion, but occurs as a consequence of inefficient 3′ end formation (HERMAN and COFFIN

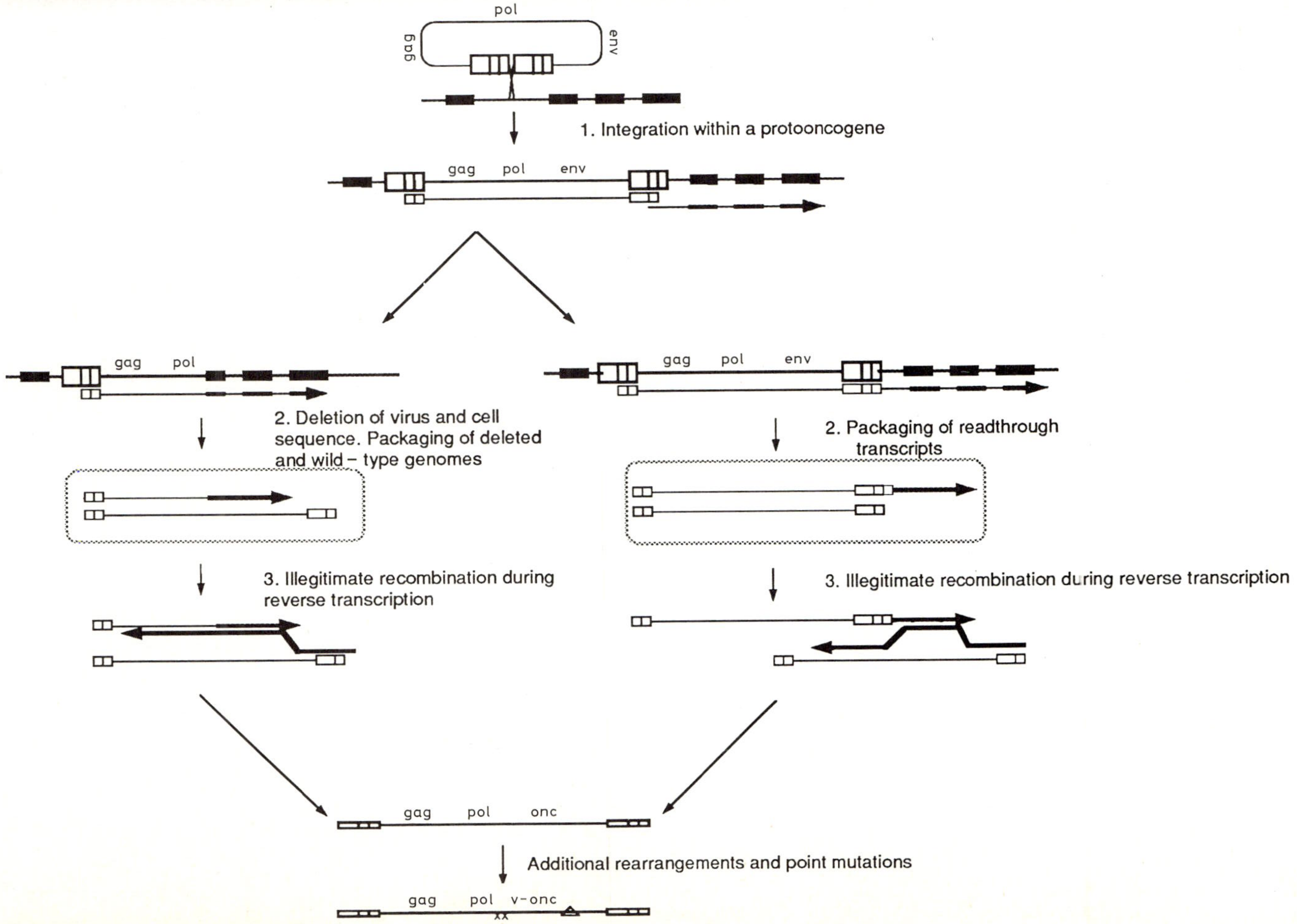

Fig. 2. Models for oncogene capture

1986) leading to the generation of copackaging of hybrid "readthrough transcripts" which will be substrates for reverse transcriptase-mediated illegitimate recombination (HERMAN and COFFIN 1987).

Note that the initial integration within a protooncogene is not an essential step, since illegitimate recombination could also join sequences in RNA molecules which happened to be copackaged as accidental inclusions within virions, or even were present in the infected cell. Indeed, there is evidence for occasional incorporation of random cell-derived sequences into viral DNA molecules (OLSEN et al. 1990; PATHAK and TEMIN 1990a). However, the formation of hybrid transcripts greatly increases the frequency of packaging of cellular sequences, and the activation of protooncogenes provides an additional strong level of selection of an otherwise very rare event.

A recent study in our laboratory supports the "readthrough" model of oncogene capture. We introduced into cells a DNA molecule consisting of a provirus followed by a selectable (*neo*) marker, and varied the frequency of readthrough transcripts by varying the total number of polyadenylation signals from 0 to 2. Transfer of the *neo* marker to fresh cells by infection with the virus produced was directly related to the frequency of readthrough transcripts and, presumably, unrelated to mutations at the DNA level (SWAIN and COFFIN 1991). Detailed analysis of the proviruses obtained demonstrated illegitimate recombination during reverse transcription: several proviruses contained long (up to 40-base) poly(dA) stretches obviously derived from the 3′ poly(A) of the hybrid transcript. Analysis of the crossover sites of these and prior studies from a number of laboratories show that there are no obvious preferred sites and that there is no particular requirement for sequence similarity at the crossover site: the modal number of matching basis is one, probably reflecting a requirement for priming of synthesis following a strand transfer which itself seems to have no particular requirement for accurate base pairing. In some cases, common short sequences (4–6 bases) in the vicinity of crossover sites have been noted (DOGGETT et al. 1989), but are of uncertain significance.

3 Variability of Virus Populations

As the preceding discussion shows, the retrovirus life-style contains the capacity for extensive variation, both mutational and recombinational. Accumulation of mutations in a virus population at each cycle of replication is determined by three factors: the acquisition of new mutations; their loss by reversion; and the relative growth rate of mutant versus wild-type virus (selective advantage or disadvantage). The accumulation of mutants in a population can be modelled as a function of these. Relatively few formal studies on this subject have appeared (see BATSCHELET et al. 1976 for one example), and we have used a simplified approach (COFFIN 1990a; COFFIN et al. 1980). Figure 3 shows how the variables

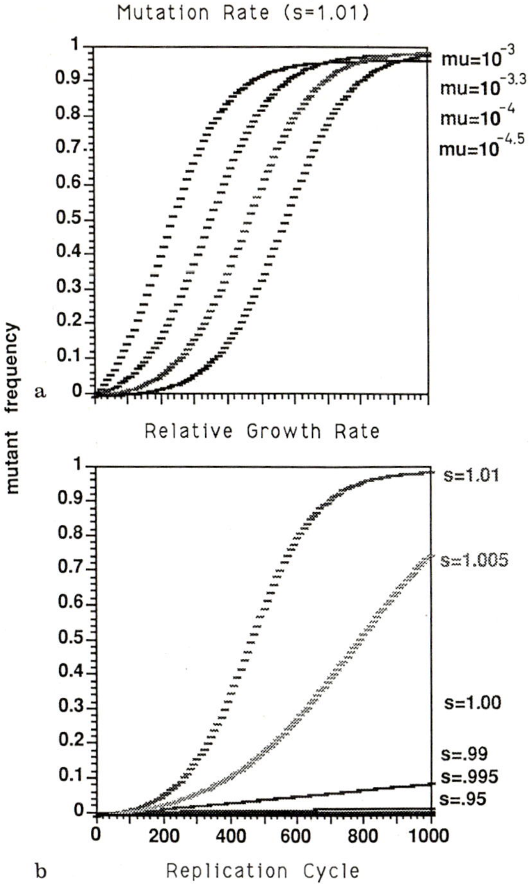

Fig. 3 a, b. Predicted variation as a function of mutation frequency (**a**) calculated assuming a relative growth rate(s) of mutant to wild-type virus of 0.01 or of relative growth rate, calculated assuming a mutation rate of 10^{-4} (**b**). Calculations were done using an iterative application of the formula in COFFIN (1990a)

affect the accumulation of mutations in a virus population at some representative values for mutation frequency (mu) and relative growth rate (S), iterated through a thousand cycles of replication, assuming a single large virus population and constant replication rate and selective conditions.

It should be apparent that under these conditions, even large changes in mutation rate (30-fold in the example shown) have a relatively small influence on the rate of appearance of mutations as compared to small differences in relative growth rate.

For example, at a mutation rate of 10^{-4} per base per replication, a mutation with a 1% advantage (i.e., relative growth rate of 1.01) becomes 50% of the population in about 400 cycles. A ten fold increase in mutation rate only halves the number of cycles necessary, while a 0.5% decrease (from 1.01 to 1.005) in selective advantage more than doubles the number of cycles. Thus, under the conditions modelled here (i.e., a sufficiently large population replicating for a sufficient number of cycles), subtle selective influences can be the most important determinants of change of virus populations.

With increasing time, this model predicts that the mutant frequency at any one position will approach an asymptote at which the contributions or forward and reverse mutations and relative growth rates will exactly balance. For example, if the net mutation rate is 10^{-4} and a given mutation gives a relative growth of 0.99, then its frequency in the population will stabilize at (roughly) 1% and remain at that value through all subsequent cycles. At this level, mutations appear at $(0.99) \times (10^{-4}) \cong 10^{-4}$ and are lost from the population at $0.01 - (0.99 \times 0.01) \cong 10^{-4}$.

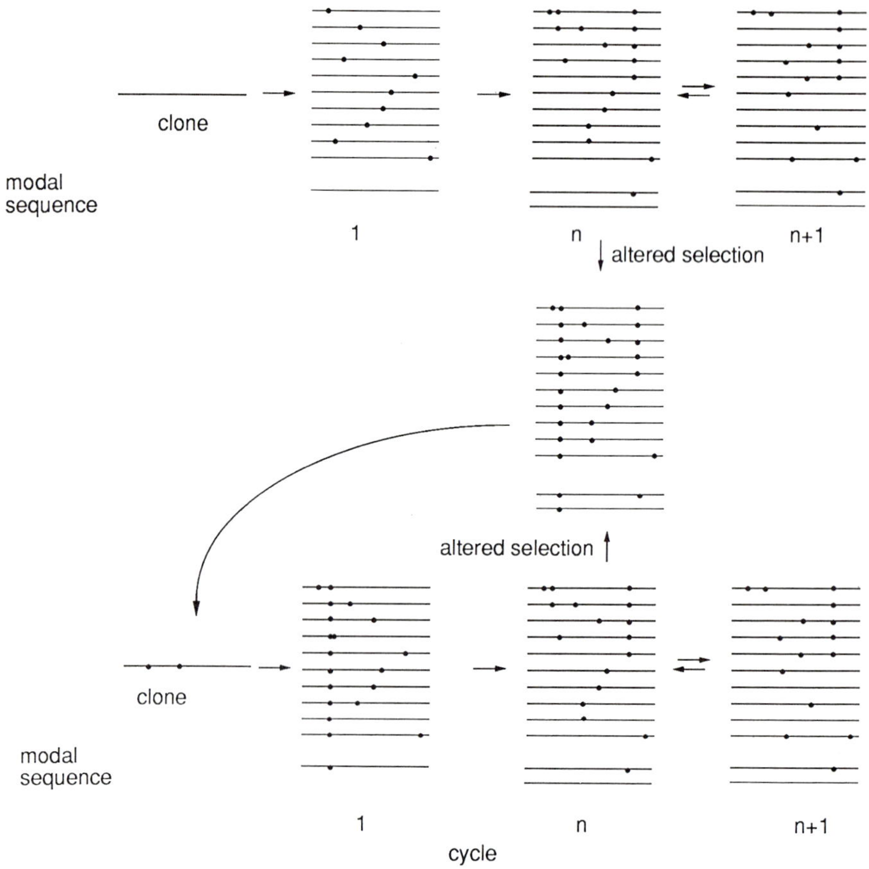

Fig. 4. Viral quasispecies evolution and selection. The distribution in genes of mutations under the mutation-selection models is illustrated, showing how the population can respond by changing the balance of mutants to altered selective pressure with reversion to populations even after "fixation" of variants by recloning

Thus, given sufficient time, the viral "quasispecies" approaches a steady state at which all mutations are present at a characteristic and stable frequency (Fig. 4). Cloning of a virus genome from such a quasispecies (as by passage of virus from one individual to another) will "fix" a specific set of mutations, each with a probability equal to its frequency in the population. If growth is continued under the same selective conditions, then mutation and selection can conspire to recreate the same or a very similar quasispecies. Conversely, if a quasispecies is subjected to altered selective influences, as might happen if an antibody appears, or the virus infects another tissue, then the quasispecies allows rapid selection from the pool of preexisting mutations and thus rapid adaptation of the virus to new conditions.

Note that the recloning step introduces a random element into the picture in that any mutation—even a strongly counterselected one—has a finite probability of being fixed. The more frequent the recloning, the less chance for restoration of the quasispecies, and the more the population will seem to drift genetically. This consideration highlights two features necessary for a virus population to behave as described above: the number of replication cycles as a population must be large; and the changes in most bases should be subject to selection. In other words, there should be relatively few neutral mutations. In the following sections, I will present several specific examples which present evidence that these conditions hold for several important retrovirus models.

3.1 In Vitro Passage

To test the roles of mutation and selection in molding retrovirus populations, we performed a simple experiment in which an avian retrovirus (Rous sarcoma virus) was passaged repeatedly and rapidly from one culture to the next at relatively high multiplicity, and changes in the genomes were monitored using both fingerprinting techniques and polymerase chain reaction (PCR) amplification of a specific region of interest. The rationale for this study was that tumor viruses arise and are grown under selection conditions that promote the survival of the infected cell, most likely at the expense of the most rapid possible virus replication. By releasing the virus from this constraint, one should see the evolution of the virus to a more rapidly replicating, but more cytopathic, lifestyle. The results of this study bear out the rationale: the oncogene *src* was rapidly lost from the genome and the virus became significantly more cytopathic with passage. As happens with many viruses under these conditions, highly defective genomes with a large deletion removing all of *pol* and parts of *gag* and *env* via a nonhomologous recombination event (VOYNOW and COFFIN 1985a, b) were also strongly selected.

Of greatest interest for our present purposes, however, was a set of point mutations in a region of *env* encoding about 100 amino acids in the amino terminal half of the SU protein (BOVA et al. 1986, 1988; DORNER and COFFIN 1986; DORNER et al. 1985), which includes both highly conserved sequences and a short region (Vr2; DORNER et al. 1985) that varies somewhat among avian leukosis virus (ALV) isolates. Initial analysis revealed several strongly selected changes within this region, and the kinetics of one of these matched a theoretical mutation-selection curve with a mutation frequency of 3×10^{-4} changes per base per passage (or about $1-1.5 \times 10^{-4}$ per replication cycle) and a relative growth rate of 1.05. PCR amplification and sequence analysis of 30–40 genomes from this region at virus passage levels revealed the following (J. COFFIN, C. BARKER, D. FIORE, and C. NAUGLE, in preparation):

1. One of the strongly selected changes affects an amino acid which is identical and lies in a strongly conserved region in all related retroviruses. The amino acid change is a nonconservative one (Arg–Gln), consistent with the altered selection.
2. Another, equally strongly selected change was a noncoding mutation of one highly conserved base to any of the three others. This makes the important point that *noncoding* changes cannot be equated with *neutral* ones. Strong selective influences can act on the genome itself as well as on its product. Such influences could be at the level of efficiency of reverse transcription, codon usage, interaction with processing signals (e.g., splicing), or packaging into virions. In this instance, we suspect that this mutation is coselected with a coding change to maintain RNA structure. In any case, it is important to bear in mind that selection can operate at levels other than amino acid sequence, particularly in viruses with RNA genomes.
3. To estimate the contribution of "neutral" mutations to the overall genetic diversity, we assessed their accumulation over the course of the experiment by counting the number of idiosyncratic mutations, i.e., those mutations seen only once in the entire experiment. Since neutral mutations will accumulate in the population at a rate approximately equal to the mutation rate, this analysis should provide an upper bound estimate for the number of changes not subject to significant selection. At most, such mutations appeared at a rate of about 4×10^{-6} per passage or perhaps 100-fold less than our estimate of the mutation rate. Thus only a very small fraction of changes in the region examined (about 25% of which would be noncoding) are without significant effect on growth.

In sum, this experiment shows that highly conserved sequences can be rapidly altered by changes in selective environment, that selection operates on coding and noncoding sequences, and that no mutation can be considered to be neutral.

3.2 Mouse Lymphoma Viruses

Several strains of inbred mice, including AKR, C58, and HRS/J, succumb to T-cell lymphoma by 1 year of age. It has long been recognized that the disease, which resembles the one induced by some exogenous viruses, has a basis in the endogenous viruses inherited by these strains of mice (CHATTOPADHYAY et al.

1982; GROSS 1951; HARTLEY et al. 1977; TAYLOR et al. 1985). Individually, however, these viruses are benign: they are either incapable of replicating in mouse cells, or, if able to replicate, unable to replicate efficiently in the target organ (the thymus). A series of studies from our laboratory and others has revealed the following sequence of events (CHATTOPADHYAY et al. 1989; HARTLEY et al. 1977; HOGGAN et al. 1986; C. A. HOLLAND et al. 1989; STOYE and COFFIN 1987; STOYE et al. 1991):

1. Shortly after birth, the product of an ecotropic (Emv) provirus appears and replicates in the animal, leading to viremia. This virus, although capable of infecting and replicating in many tissues, does not replicate efficiently in the thymus and does not itself induce malignant transformation. Like most endogenous proviruses, the inherited Emv provirus is extensively methylated at CpG sequences and therefore not expressed. Once an initial expression event occurs, most likely as a chance event in one or a few cells, this inhibition is lost and subsequent replication is quite efficient.
2. A recombination event leads to acquisition of LTR sequences from a closely related provirus of the Xmv group (STOYE et al. 1991). The effect of these new sequences is to provide a somewhat altered U3 region which confers a higher level of expression (and thus replication) in thymocytes (C. A. HOLLAND et al. 1989; THOMAS and COFFIN 1982). In some strains of mice, a mutational event substitutes for the recombination (MASSEY et al. 1990).
3. A second recombination event with the progeny of yet another (polytropic or Pmv) provirus leads to acquisition of an altered *env* gene, whose product recognizes a different receptor (REIN 1982). By chance, the species distribution of receptors for the Pmv type envelope is broader than for the Emv, and these recombinant viruses were first identified by their ability to form cytopathic foci on a mink lung cell line. Viruses of this sort are still called MCF (mink cell focus-forming) viruses for this reason. Until recently, the role of the altered *env* gene in promoting oncogenesis was unclear. Recent evidence (J. P. LI and BALTIMORE 1991) suggests that the Pmv type *env* protein interacts with the interleukin-2 (IL-2) receptor to stimulate growth of infected cells, an interaction which could enhance both virus replication and oncogenesis in the target cells.
4. A mutation occurs in the LTR, duplicating (or triplicating) a 60–100 base central region of the enhancer domain which includes binding sites for several transcription factors known to be important in determining expression and pathogenicity (GOLEMIS et al. 1990; Y. LI et al. 1987; SPECK and BALTIMORE 1987; SPECK et al. 1990). The duplication most likely increases the efficiency of interaction of the LTR with these factors and enhances replication still more.

Viruses with all these changes are the ultimate transforming agents, and the mechanism of oncogenesis also requires activation of one of a number of protooncogenes by insertion of provirus in their vicinity. In the usual case, MCF viruses are found only in the thymus and appear in high amount (one provirus per cell) well before the occurrence of visible tumor (STOYE et al. 1991). Thus, these viruses are selected on the basis of their ability to replicate, and the ability of their virions to transform is a side effect due to an integration event which is very rare on a per cell basis, but virtually certain when a whole organ is infected.

There is no reason to believe that the recombination events that generate MCF viruses are specific in any particular way, so the frequency of these events is certainly extremely low. Furthermore, all MCF viruses isolated from one animal have identical recombination crossover points, but those from different animals differ, again supporting the conclusion that the appearance of these viruses is the result of an evolutionary process in which very rare, sequential, recombination events are selected as a result of increased ability to replicate in a specific target organ.

3.3 Genetic Variation in Human Immunodeficiency Virus

Given the above discussion, it is instructive to consider the well-studied example of human immunodeficiency virus (HIV) and related lentiviruses. Once the first few nucleotide sequences of different HIV isolates were published, it became apparent that natural isolates of HIV were subject to considerable genetic variation (ALIZON et al. 1986; COFFIN 1986; HAHN et al. 1985; WONG-STAAL et al. 1985). Indeed, this variation could be used to develop trees relating HIV-1 and HIV-2 isolates to one another and to collections of related viruses from several primate species (HUET et al. 1990; MYERS et al. 1990) (Fig. 5). More recently, similar kinds of population analyses have been applied directly to clinical samples, most commonly by PCR amplification of selected regions of viral RNA or DNA from infected tissue (or cell culture) and sequence analysis of a number of clones. Such analyses have been done comparing virus populations in an individual as a function of time (DELASSUS et al. 1991; HAHN et al. 1986; MEYERHANS et al. 1989), of target organ (CORDONNIER et al. 1989; O'BRIEN et al. 1990; SHIODA et al. 1991), of

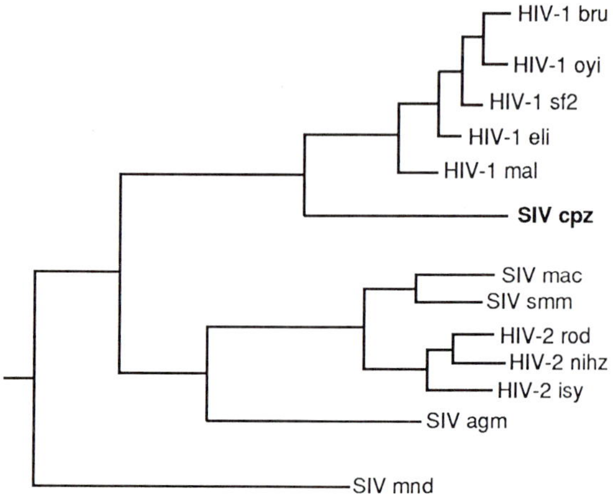

Fig. 5. Sequence relationships of HIV and SIV isolates. (Redrawn from HUET et al. 1990)

drug therapy (D. D. RICHMAN, this volume), or of removal of virus to cell culture (KODAMA et al. 1989; MEYERHANS et al. 1989). The cumulative results of these studies support the general conclusion that HIV in infected individuals behaves like the sort of evolving quasispecies discussed above:

1. The virus population is genetically quite disperse and becomes more so with time.
2. The diversity is not randomly distributed, but rather concentrated in certain regions—most prominently the hypervariable (V) regions of *env* previously identified by comparison of different isolates.
3. The distribution of variants in the populations changes rapidly in response to altered conditions such as growth in different organs, or removal to cell culture.
4. Particularly noteworthy is the appearance of large proportions of virus with increased resistance to azidothymidine (AZT) following therapy (JAPOUR et al. 1991; LARDER et al. 1989; LARDER and KEMP 1989). This result means that even after years of infection, the virus population in an infected individual is still actively replicating, as opposed to being produced from a preinfected population of surviving cells with resident (and unchanging) proviruses. Thus, the number of replication cycles in HIV between transmission to another individual may be very large (perhaps in the thousands), an important condition for development of a quasispecies of the sort discussed above.
5. Some of the variation observed is in the V3 region previously identified as a major site of interaction with neutralizing antibodies (GRIFFITHS et al. 1991; NARA et al. 1990) and is thus likely to be the result of selective pressure exerted by the immune response. It is, however, naive to treat all the variation observed as being due to immune selection, as some workers have tried to do. The *env* proteins are the major site of interaction between the virus and the outside world, and variation could be selected for any number of reasons. For example, sequences involved in interaction with various cell types (monocytes, neurons, and others) are also found in *env* (O'BRIEN et al. 1990; SHIODA et al. 1991). Other aspects that might be important and variable include extent of sensitivity to superinfection resistance (mediated by loss of receptor due to preinfection of the cell with the same virus) (WEISS 1982); the pressure of nonantibody neutralizing factors; the ability of the virus to cause cell fusion (FREED et al. 1991; HELSETH et al. 1990); and others. Given the multiyear replication course of the virus in the face of a changing environment as the infected individual gradually progresses to acquired immunodeficiency syndrome (AIDS), the opportunity for selected genetic variation in many respects is clear and the virus obviously takes it.

3.4 Reprise

All of these examples should serve to drive home the important lesson of retrovirus genetic variation: the mechanism of replication both creates the means of variation and provides a life-style that permits the virus the ability to take advantage of the opportunities provided by this variation. The strongest force driving the variation observed, however, is selection. To repeat:

1. It is clearly fallacious to assume that any mutation seen is "neutral".
2. Selective forces do not need to be large to mold a virus population. In most cases, the advantage of a selected sequence can be too small to measure in any conceivable experiment. For example, all retroviruses contain in their LTRs sequences which specify cleavage and poly(A) addition to the end of the genome. However, if such a sequence is inactivated, the resulting virus replicates only slightly less well than the wild-type virus (SWAIN and COFFIN 1989).
3. Selective forces may well change during the course of an infection cycle. In HIV, for example, the virus that passes from individual to individual may have certain selected properties (organ specificity of replication, for example) that are counterselected in the whole organism. In this way, a cyclic pattern of variation could be set up.
4. Another sort of cyclic pattern can arise from the difference in environment in one infected individual as compared to the next. An immune escape variant selected to ward off a specific antibody in one individual will be inappropriate (and probably counterselected) when the virus is passed to another individual who will not, of course, develop the same antibodies. Similar situations have been seen in the rapid appearance of certain mutations in viruses taken from the clinic to cell culture (HIRSCH et al. 1989; KODAMA et al. 1989) and their subsequent reversion when reintroduced into experimental animals.
5. There can be no such thing as a "rate of variation". Every base is subject to different selective forces which themselves may vary (sometimes cyclically) with time. Furthermore, the curves relating variation to time are sigmoidal, not linear. To attempt such a calculation is to fall into the obvious trap of assuming that one can extend from any one base to any other, and to risk making huge errors.

4 Implications for Viral Evolution

Retroviruses have evolved into several distinct genera that share similar life-styles and overall genome organization, although differing considerably in nucleotide sequence as well as other important features such as the presence of additional "regulatory" genes (COFFIN 1990a, b). Within this diversity, however, is sufficient shared amino acid sequence in several proteins, such as reverse transcriptase (DOOLITTLE et al. 1989, 1990; MCCLURE et al. 1988; XIONG and EICKBUSH 1990) (R. DOOLITTLE, this volume), to detect and trace the relationship among the virus group (Fig. 6). These traces can even be extended to include

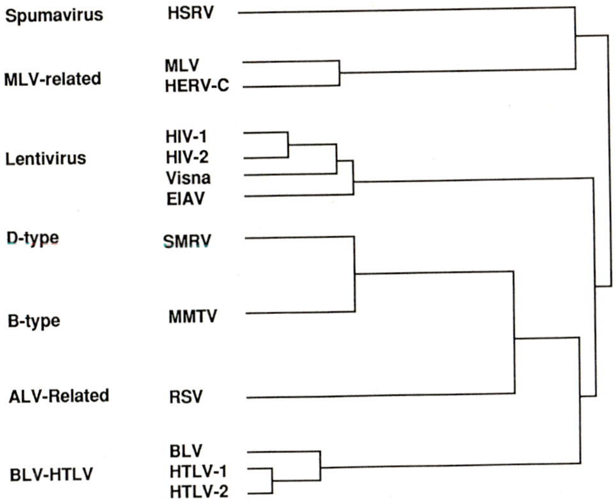

Fig. 6. Relationships of retrovirus genera as revealed by the amino acid sequence of reverse transcriptase. *MLV*, Murine leukemia virus; *EIAV*, equire infectious anemia virus; *MMTV*, mouse mammary tumor virus; *RSV*, respiratory syncytial virus; *BLV*, bovine leukemia virus, *HTLV*, human T-cell lymphotrophic virus. (Redrawn from DOOLITTLE et al. 1989, 1990)

nonviruses, such as the retrotransposable elements of yeast and other species (McCLURE 1991).

Examination of these trees in the light of known modern-day sequence variation (in lentivirus, for example) has seemed to workers to provide something of a paradox: recent variation is so rapid that one would have expected all relationships between groups to have been completely lost in a short period of time. Two explanations have been raised. First, that retroviruses have, in fact appeared only very recently, and all have diverged from a common ancestor within the last few thousand years (D. B. SMITH and JUGLIS 1987; T. T. SMITH et al. 1988). Second, that all retroviruses have an alternative, endogenous (germline) phase in which they are very stable, and they differ from one another by far fewer cycles of reverse transcription than would appear (DOOLITTLE et al. 1989, 1990).

Clearly neither of these is correct. The species distribution of exogenous and endogenous retroviruses is highly incompatible with a recent origin of this group. For example, several proviruses are known to have been inserted in the primitive germline more than 5×10^6 years ago, and one of these is very closely related to a modern-day virus of mice (REPASKE et al. 1985). It is far more probable that retroviruses have coexisted with vertebrates throughout their evolution.

The endogenous virus hypothesis is not tenable either. Endogenous viruses are often closely related to exogenous viruses of the same host, but clearly represent a distinct evolutionary lineage. While recombination between the two can readily be detected (when strongly enough selected, COLICELLI and GOFF 1987), there is no reason to suppose the sort of direct back and forth movement

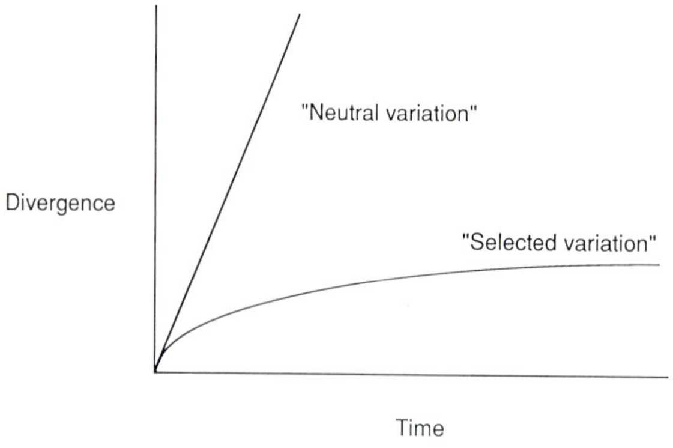

Fig. 7. Time scales of evolution. The two curves show the relationships of sequence diversity with time assuming that all positions vary in the absence of "neutral" variation

that would maintain sequence identity. Furthermore, at least three genera of retroviruses do not have any related endogenous proviruses, yet do not seem to have varied at a significantly greater rate.

Clearly, the fallacy—as previously mentioned and cartooned in Fig. 7 lies in the fact that one cannot assume "neutrality" of any mutation or a constant "rate" of change. Rather, more recent variation most likely represents selected variation. To extrapolate from selected variation to sequences selected for constancy is to risk very large errors. Indeed, much of the evolutionary divergence observed may well be selected by environmental change—particularly adaptation of virus to new host species.

To conclude: While it is important to know how and why these viruses vary, in order to understand both diversity and evolution, it is at least equally important to understand and describe the selective forces that act on virus populations and shape these changes.

References

Alizon M, Wain-Hobson S, Montagnier L, Sonigo P (1986) Genetic variability of the AIDS virus: nucleotide sequence analysis of two isolates from African patients. Cell 46: 63–74
Bass BL, Weintraub H, Cattaneo R, Billeter MA (1989) Biased hypermutation of viral RNA genomes could be due to unwinding/modification of double-stranded RNA. Cell 56: 331
Batschelet E, Domingo E, Weissmann C (1976) The proportion of revertant and mutant phage in a growing population, as a function of mutation and growth rate. Gene 1: 27–32
Bishop JM (1983) Cellular oncogenes and retroviruses. Annu Rev Biochem 52: 301–354
Bishop JM (1991) Molecular themes in oncogenesis. Cell 64: 235–248
Bishop JM, Varmus HE (1982) Functions and origins of retroviral transforming genes. In: Weiss R, Teich N, Varmus H, Coffin J (eds.) RNA tumor viruses. Cold Spring Harbor Laboratory, Cold Spring Harbor, pp 999–1108

Bova CA, Manfredi JP, Swanstrom R (1986) *env* Genes of avian retroviruses: Nucleotide sequence and molecular recombinants define host range determinants. Virology 152: 343–354

Bova CA, Olsen JC, Swanstrom R (1988) The avian retrovirus *env* gene family: Molecular analysis of host range and antigenic variants. J Virol 62: 75–83

Chattopadhyay SK, Cloyd MW, Linemeyer DL, Lander MR, Rands E, Lowy DR (1982) Cellular origin and role of mink cell focus-forming viruses in murine thymic lymphomas. Nature 295: 25–31

Chattopadhyay SK, Baroudy BM, Holmes KL, Frederickson TN, Lander MR, Hartley HCM III, Hartley JW (1989) Biological and molecular genetic characteristics of a unique MCF virus that is highly leukemogenic in ecotropic virus-negative mice. Virology 168: 90–100

Coffin JM (1979) Structure, replication, and recombination of retrovirus genomes: some unifying hypotheses. J Gen Virol 42: 1–26

Coffin JM (1986) Genetic variation in AIDS viruses. Cell 46: 1–14

Coffin JM (1990) Genetic variation in retroviruses. In: Kurstak E, Marusyk RG, Murphy FA, Van Regenmortel MHV (eds) Applied Virology Research. Volume 2: Virus Variability, Epidemiology, and Control, Plenum, New York, pp 11–33

Coffin JM (1990b) Retroviridae and their replication. In: Fields B, Knipe D, Chanock R (eds) Virology, 2nd ed. Raven, New York, pp 1437–1500

Coffin JM, Tsichlis PN, Barker CS, Voynow S (1980) Variation in avian retrovirus genomes. Ann NY Acad Sci 354: 410–425

Colicelli J, Goff SP (1987) Identification of endogenous retroviral sequences as potential donors for recombinational repair of mutant retroviruses: Positions of crossover points. Virology 160: 518–522

Cordonnier A, Montagnier L, Emerman M (1989) Single amino-acid changes in HIV envelope affect viral tropism and receptor binding. Nature 340: 571–574

Danos O, Mulligan RC (1988) Safe and efficient generation of recombinant retroviruses with amphotropic and ecotropic host ranges. Proc Natl Acad Sci USA 85: 6460–6464

Delassus S, Cheynier R, Wain-Hobson S (1991) Evolution of human immunodeficiency virus type 1 nef and long terminal repeat sequences over 4 years in vivo and in vitro. J Virol 65: 225–231

Doggett DL, Drake AL, Hirsch V, Rowe ME, Stallard V, Mullins JI (1989) Structure, origin and transforming activity of feline leukemia virus-myc recombinant provirus FTT. J Virol 63: 2108–2117

Doolittle RF, Feng D-F, Johnson MS, McClure MA (1989) Origins and evolutionary relationships of retroviruses. Q Rev Biol 64: 1–30

Doolittle RF, Feng DF, McClure MA, Johnson MS (1990) Retrovirus phylogeny and evolution. In: Swanstrom R, Vogt PK (eds) Retroviruses. Strategies of replication. Springer, Berlin Heidelberg New York, pp 1–18

Dorner AJ, Coffin JM (1986) Determinants for receptor interaction and cell killing on the avian retrovirus glycoprotein gp85. Cell 45: 365–374

Dorner AJ, Stoye JP, Coffin JM (1985) Molecular basis of host range variation in avian retroviruses. J Virol 53: 32–39

Dougherty JP, Temin HM (1988) Determination of the rate of base-pair substitution and insertion mutations in retrovirus replication. J Virol 62: 2817–2822

Dougherty JP, Wisniewski R, Yang S, Rhode BW, Temin HM (1989) New retrovirus helper cells with almost no nucleotide sequence homology to retrovirus vectors. J Virol 63: 3209–3212

Freed EO, Myers DJ, Risser R (1991) Identification of the principal neutralizing determinant of human immunodeficiency virus type 1 as a fusion domain. J Virol 65: 190–194

Goldfarb MP, Weinberg RA (1981) Generation of novel, biologically active Harvey sarcoma viruses via apparent illegitimate recombination. J Virol 38: 136–150

Golemis EA, Speck NA, Hopkins N (1990) Alignment of U3 region sequences of mammalian type C viruses: identification of highly conserved motifs and implications for enhancer design. J Virol 64: 534–542

Goodrich DW, Duesberg PH (1990) Evidence that retroviral transduction is mediated by DNA, not by RNA. Proc Natl Acad Sci USA 87: 3604–3608

Gopinathan KP, Weymouth LA, Kunkel TA, Loeb LA (1979) Mutagenesis in vitro by DNA polymerase from an RNA tumor virus. Nature 278: 857–859

Griffiths JC, Berrie EL, Holdsworth LN, Moore JP, Harris SJ, Senior JM, Kingsman SM, Kingsman AJ, Adams SE (1991) Induction of high-titer neutralizing antibodies, using hybrid human immunodeficiency virus V3-Ty viruslike particles in a clinically relevant adjuvant. J Virol 65: 450–456

Gross L (1951) "Spontaneous" leukemia developing in C3H mice following inoculation, in infancy, with AK-leukemic-cell extracts, or AK-embryos. Proc Soc Exp Biol Med 76: 27–32

Hahn BH, Gonda MA, Shaw GM, Popovic M, Hoxie JA, Gallo RC, Wong-Staal F (1985) Genomic diversity of the acquired immune deficiency syndrome virus HTLV-III: different viruses exhibit greatest divergence in their envelope genes. Proc Natl Acad Sci USA 82: 4813–4817

Hahn BH, Shaw GM, Taylor ME, Redfield RR, Markham PD, Salahuddin SZ, Wong-Staal F, Gallo RC, Parks ES, Parks WP (1986) Genetic variation in HTLV-III/LAV over time in patients with AIDS or at risk for AIDS. Science 232: 1548–1553

Hartley JW, Wolford NK, Old LJ, Rowe WP (1977) A new class of murine leukemia virus associated with the development of spontaneous lymphomas. Proc Natl Acad Sci USA 74: 789–792

Helseth E, Oshevsky U, Gabuzda D, Ardman B, Haseltine W, Sodroski J (1990) Changes in the transmembrane region of the human immunodeficiency virus type 1 gp41 envelope glycoprotein affect membrane fusion. J Virol 64: 6314–6318

Herman SA, Coffin JM (1986) Differential transcription from the long terminal repeats of integrated avian leukosis virus DNA. J Virol 60: 497–505

Herman SA, Coffin JM (1987) Efficient packaging of readthrough RNA in ALV: Implications for oncogene transduction. Science 236: 845–848

Hirsch VM, Edmondson P, Murphey-Corb M, Arbeille B, Johnson PR, Mullins JI (1989) SIV adaptation to human cells. Nature 341: 573–574

Hoggan MD, O'Neill RR, Kozak CA (1986) Nonecotropic murine leukemia viruses in BALB/c and NFS/N mice: Characterization of the BALB/c Bxv-1 provirus and the single NFS endogenous xenotrope. J Virol 60: 980–986

Holland CA, Thomas CY, Chattopadhyay SK, Koehne C, O'Donnell PV (1989) Influence of enhancer sequences of thymotropism and leukemogenicity of mink cell focus-forming viruses. J Virol 63: 1284–1292

Holland JJ, de la Torre JC, Steinhauer DA, Clark D, Duarte E, Domingo E (1989) Virus mutation frequencies can be greatly underestimated by monoclonal antibody neutralization of virions. J Virol 63: 5030–5036

Holland JJ, Domingo E, de la Torre JC, Steinhauer DA (1990) Mutation frequencies at defined single codon sites in vesicular stomatitis virus and poliovirus can be increased only slightly by chemical mutagenesis. J Virol 64: 3960–3962

Hu WS, Temin HM (1990a) Retroviral recombination and reverse transcription. Science 250: 1227–1233

Hu WS, Temin HM (1990b) Genetic consequences of packaging two RNA genomes in one retroviral particle: pseudodiploidy and high rate of genetic recombination. Proc Natl Acad Sci USA 87: 1556–1560

Huet T, Cheynier R, Meyerhans A, Roelants G, Wain-Hobson S (1990) Genetic organization of a chimpanzee lentivirus related to HIV-1. Nature 345: 356–359

Japour AJ, Chatis PA, Eigenrauch HA, Crumpacker CS (1991) Detection of human immunodeficiency virus type 1 clinical isolates with reduced sensitivity to zidovudine and dideoxyinosine by RNA-RNA hybridization. Proc Natl Acad Sci USA 88: 3092–3096

Junghans RP, Boone LR, Skalka AM (1982) Retroviral DNA H structures: Displacement-assimilation model of recombination. Cell 30: 53–62

Kodama T, Wooley DP, Naidu YM, Kestler HWI, Daniel MD, Li Y, Desrosiers RC (1989) Significance of premature stop codons in env of simian immunodeficiency virus. J Virol 63: 4709–4714

Larder BA, Kemp SD (1989) Multiple mutations in HIV-1 reverse transcriptase confer high-level resistance to zidovudine (AZT). Science 246: 1155–1158

Larder BA, Darby G, Richman DD (1989) HIV with reduced sensitivity to zidovudine (AZT) isolated during prolonged therapy. Science 243: 1731–1734

Lee YMH, Coffin JM (1990) Efficient autointegration of avian retrovirus DNA in vitro. J Virol 64: 5958–5965

Leider JM, Palese P, Smith FI (1988) Determination of the mutation rate of a retrovirus. J Virol 62: 3084–3091

Li J-P, Baltimore D (1991) Mechanism of leukemogenesis induced by mink cell focus-forming murine leukemia viruses. J Virol 65: 2408–2414

Li Y, Golemis E, Hartley JW, Hopkins N (1987) Disease specificity of nondefective Friend and Moloney murine leukemia viruses is controlled by a small number of nucleotides. J Virol 61: 693–700

Linial ML, Miller AD (1990) Retroviral RNA packaging: Sequence requirements and implications. In: Swanstrom R, Vogt PK (eds) Retroviruses. Strategies of replication. Springer, Berlin Heidelberg New York, pp 125–152

Massey AC, Coppola MA, Thomas CY (1990) Origin of pathogenic determinants of recombinant murine leukemia viruses: analysis of Bxv-1-related xenotropic viruses from CWD mice. J Virol 64: 5491–5499

McClure MA (1991) Sequence analysis of eukaryotic retroid proteins. Adv Math Comp Med (in press)

McClure MA, Johnson MS, Feng D-F, Doolittle RF (1988) Sequence comparisons of retroviral proteins: relative rates of change and general phylogeny. Proc Natl Acad Sci USA 85: 2469–2473

Meyerhans A, Cheynier R, Albert J, Seth M, Kwok S, Sninsky J, Morfeldt-Manson L, Asjo B, Wain-Hobson S (1989) Temporal fluctuations in HIV quasispecies in vivo are not reflected by sequential HIV isolations. Cell 58: 901–910

Miller AD, Buttimore C (1986) Redesign of retrovirus packaging cell lines to avoid recombination leading to helper virus production. Mol Cell Biol 6: 2895–2902

Myers G, Rabson AB, Josephs SF, Smith TF, Berzofsky JA, Wong-Staal F (1990) Human retroviruses and AIDS 1990. Los Alamos National Laboratory, Los Alamos

Nara PL, Smit L, Dunlop N, Hatch W, Merges M, Waters D, Kelliher J, Gallo RC, Fischinger PJ, Goudsmit J (1990) Emergence of viruses resistant to neutralization by V3-specific antibodies in experimental human immunodeficiency virus type 1 IIIB infection of chimpanzees. J Virol 64: 3779–3791

O'Brien WA, Koyanagi Y, Namazie A, Zhao J-Q, Dagne A, Idler K, Zack JA, Chen ISY (1990) HIV-1 tropism for mononuclear phagocytes can be determined by regions of gp120 outside the CD4-binding domain. Nature 348: 69–73

Olsen JC, Bova-Hill C, Grandgenett DP, Quinn TP, Manfredi JP, Swanstrom R (1990) Rearrangements in unintegrated retroviral DNA are complex and are the result of multiple genetic determinants. J Virol 64: 5475–5484

Parvin JD, Moscona A, Pan WT, Leider JM, Palese P (1986) Measurement of the mutation rates of animal viruses: influenza A and poliovirus type 1. J Virol 59: 377–383

Pathak VK, Temin HM (1990a) Broad spectrum of in vivo forward mutations, hypermutations and mutational hotspots in a retroviral shuttle vector after a single replication cycle: Deletions and deletions with insertions. Proc Natl Acad Sci USA 87: 6024–6028

Pathak VK, Temin HM (1990b) Broad spectrum of in vivo forward mutations, hypermutations, and mutational hotspots in a retroviral shuttle vector after a single replication cycle: Substitutions, frameshifts and hypermutations. Proc Natl Acad Sci USA 87: 6019–6023

Preston BD, Poiesz BJ, Loeb LA (1988) Fidelity of HIV-1 reverse transcriptase. Science 242: 1168–1171

Rein A (1982) Interference grouping of murine leukemia viruses: A distinct receptor for MCF-recombinant viruses in mouse cells. Virology 120: 251–257

Repaske R, Steele PE, O'Neill RR, Rabson AB, Martin MA (1985) Nucleotide sequence of a full-length human endogenous retroviral segment. J Virol 54: 764–772

Roberts JD, Bebenek K, Kunkel TA (1988) The accuracy of reverse transcriptase from HIV-1. Science 242: 1171–1173

Roberts JD, Preston BD, Johnston LA, Soni A, Loeb LA, Kunkel T (1989) Fidelity of two retroviral reverse transcriptases during DNA-dependent DNA synthesis in vitro. Mol Cell Biol 9: 469–476

Shioda T, Levy JA, Cheng-Mayer C (1991) Macrophage and T cell-line tropisms of HIV-1 are determined by specific regions of the envelope gp120 gene. Nature 349: 167–169

Shoemaker CS, Goff S, Gilboa E, Paskind M, Mitra SW, Baltimore D (1980) Structure of a cloned circular Moloney murine leukemia virus molecule containing an inverted segment: Implications for retrovirus integration. Proc Natl Acad Sci USA 77: 3932–3936

Smith DB, Inglis SC (1987) The mutation rate and variability of eukaryotic viruses: An analytical review. J Gen Virol 68: 2729–2740

Smith TF, Srinivasan A, Schochetman G, Marcus M, Myers G (1988) The phylogenetic history of immunodeficiency viruses. Nature 333: 573–575

Speck NA, Baltimore D (1987) Six distinct nuclear factors interact with the 75-base-pair repeat of the Moloney murine leukemia virus enhancer. Mol Cell Biol 7: 1101–1110

Speck NA, Renjifo B, Hopkins N (1990) Point mutations in the Moloney murine leukemia virus enhancer identify a lymphoid-specific viral core motif and 1,3-phorbol myristate acetate-inducible element. J Virol 64: 543–550

Stoye JP, Coffin JM (1987) The four classes of endogenous murine leukemia virus: Structural relationships and potential for recombination. J Virol 61: 2659–2669

Stoye JP, Moroni C, Coffin J (1991a) Virological events leading to spontaneous AKR thymomas. J Virol 65: 1273–1285
Swain A, Coffin JM (1989) Polyadenylation at correct sites in genome RNA is not required for retrovirus replication or genome encapsidation. J Virol 63: 3301–3306
Swain A, Coffin JM (1991) Mechanism of oncogene transduction by retroviruses. Science (in press)
Swanstrom R, Parker RC, Varmus HE, Bishop JM (1983) Transduction of a cellular oncogene: The genesis of Rous sarcoma virus. Proc Natl Acad Sci USA 80: 2519–2523
Taylor BA, Rowe L, Jenkins NA, Copeland NG (1985) Chromosomal assignment of two endogenous ecotropic murine leukemia virus proviruses of AKR/J mouse strains. J Virol 56: 172–175
Thomas CY, Coffin JM (1982) Genetic alteration of RNA leukemia viruses associated with development of spontaneous thymic lymphoma in AKR/J mice. J Virol 50: 397–407
Varmus HE (1987) Reverse transcription. Sci Am 257: 56–66
Varmus H (1988) Retroviruses. Science 240: 1427–1435
Varmus HE, Swanstrom R (1984) Replication of retroviruses. In: Weiss R, Teich N, Varmus H, Coffin J (eds) RNA tumor viruses, 2nd ed, pt 1. Cold Spring Harbor Laboratory, Cold Spring Harbor, pp 369–512
Varmus HE, Swanstrom R (1985) Replication of retroviruses. In: Weiss R, Teich N, Varmus H, Coffin J (eds) RNA tumor viruses. Cold Spring Harbor Laboratory, Cold Spring Harbor, pp 74–134
Vartanian J-P, Meyerhans A, Asjo B, Wain-Hobson S (1991) Selection, recombination, and G-A hypermutation of human immunodeficiency virus type 1 genomes. J Virol 65: 1779–1788
Voynow SL, Coffin JM (1985a) Evolutionary variants of Rous sarcoma virus: Large deletion mutants do not result from homologous recombination. J Virol 55: 67–78
Voynow SL, Coffin JM (1985b) Truncated gag-related proteins are produced by large deletion mutants of Rous sarcoma virus and form virus particles. J Virol 55: 79–85
Weiss RA (1982) Experimental biology and assay of RNA tumor viruses. In: Weiss R, Teich N, Varmus H, Coffin J (eds) RNA tumor viruses. Cold Spring Harbor Laboratory, Cold Spring Harbor, pp 209–260
Wong-Staal F, Shaw GM, Hahn BH, Salahuddin SZ, Popovic M, Markham P, Redfield R, Gallo RC (1985) Genomic diversity of human T-lymphotropic virus type II (HTLV-III). Science 229: 759–762
Xiong Y, Eickbush TH (1990) Origin and evolution of retroelements based on their reverse transcriptase sequences. EMBO J 9: 3353–3362

Retroviral Reverse Transcriptases: Error Frequencies and Mutagenesis

K. J. WILLIAMS and L. A. LOEB

1 Introduction

For most organisms the fidelity of genomic replication is an exceptionally accurate process. This accuracy must be high enough to guarantee that the nucleotide sequence of the parent is transmitted to subsequent generations with few if any errors. Infrequent errors are required, however, to produce mutations that drive the evolution of species through selection. Survival within a hostile environment is governed by the selection of variants, generating new organisms best able to survive in the environment that surrounds them. Survival within an exceptionally hostile environment might be favored by populations containing a wide spectrum of pre-existing mutants that provide a diverse repertoire for selection.

The Joseph Gottstein Memorial Cancer Research Laboratory, Department of Pathology SM-30, University of Washington, Seattle, WA 98195, USA

Current Topics in Microbiology and Immunology, Vol. 176

2 RNA Viruses as a Quasispecies

The exceptionally high mutation rate of RNA viruses provides unusual insights into evolutionary processes. The mutation rate of RNA tumor viruses is so great that within a population of virions there is no single sequence; the nucleotide sequence of each daughter virion is different from that of its parent. As a result, these viruses evolve as a "quasispecies," i.e., a distribution of mutants, rather than unique genomes that identify clonal populations (EIGEN et al. 1981). In essence, survival of an RNA virus could be dependent upon the mutational distributions within each quasispecies, rather than the presence of rare mutants with selective advantages within a predominantly homogeneous population.

Retroviruses constitute a quasispecies of particular interest for several reasons. First, they have the ability to interconvert their genomes from RNA single-stranded molecules contained within infectious particles to a DNA double-stranded provirus integrated within host chromosomal DNA. This genomic plasticity may be a manifestation of a parasitic existence within a hostile cellular environment. Second, the genomic variation of surviving retroviral particles infecting a host organism has now become recognized as perhaps the most intricate and rapidly paced ongoing evolutionary process available to research. Finally, the wide range of pathological processes resulting from retroviral infection are of major concern in both human and animal populations.

3 Human Immunodeficiency Virus

The most studied example of successful retroviral evolution observed today is human immune deficiency virus 1 (HIV-1), associated with acquired immune deficiency syndrome (AIDS) (for review see FAUCI 1988; COFFIN 1986). The ability of HIV-1 to survive one of the most highly evolved, self-protective environments on the evolutionary scale is ultimately derived from a continuous evolution of its own genome through mutagenic events. The ability of HIV-1 to survive could depend on both the diversity of genotypes within a quasispecies and on the high rate of genomic evolution. While it is possible that host DNA or RNA polymerases may play a role in HIV-1 adaptive mutational processes during the course of an infection, recent investigations have demonstrated that HIV-1 reverse transcriptase (RT) is highly error prone when compared to mammalian DNA replicating enzymes and enzyme complexes.

This chapter will consider the evidence implicating HIV-1 RT as the primary replicative component responsible for the high frequency of mutation leading to heterogeneity between different isolates of the HIV-1. We will consider the role of different polymerases in the life cycle of RNA tumor viruses. Results from several recent investigations, comparing the mechanism of catalysis and the fidelity of the RT to that of cellular polymerases, reveal the error proneness of the reverse transcriptase during the copying of DNA and RNA templates in vitro. HIV-1 genomic sequence variations between different isolates, especially within the envelope region, will be analyzed. A computer analysis by this laboratory comparing specific variations among several published isolates will be presented and discussed in regard to pause sites and replication errors by the HIV RT.

3.1 HIV-1 Components and Life Cycle

HIV-1 is a member of the lentivirus ("slow" virus) subfamily of the *Retroviridae* (retrovirus). HIV-1 genomic RNA is approximately 10 kb in length and, similar to other retroviruses, contains: (a) flanking long terminal repeat (LTR) sequences that encode the regulatory regions for HIV replication, (b) the *gag* gene, the main structural protein of the virus capsid, (c) the *pol* gene that codes for the RT, RNase H, and the integration protein, and (d) the *env* gene, that codes for the virus envelope glycoprotein(s). Each of these are essential for viral replication and viability. HIV-1 also contains at least five additional genes whose functions are not as well known (FAUCI 1988).

The HIV-1 virion contains two complete plus strand copies of the RNA genome that, upon entering the host cell cytoplasm, serve as templates for DNA synthesis by the viral RT (Fig. 1). Double-stranded DNA is synthesized by a multistep process; the single-stranded genomic RNA is copied by the RT to produce the initial (minus) DNA strand, with the RNA template subsequently hydrolyzed by RT RNase H activity. The minus DNA strand is then copied by the RT to produce the second (plus) DNA strand, resulting in a double-stranded DNA copy of the viral RNA genome. The viral DNA is transported to the nucleus and is integrated into the host cell chromosome, forming a provirus. Proviral DNA replication is primarily dependent on host cell enzymes and occurs concomitantly with host chromosomal DNA replication. Transcription of viral genomic RNA is catalyzed by the host cell RNA polymerase II. A portion of the viral genomic RNA is spliced, translated and modified to produce proteins that constitute viral particles and that encapsulate two molecules of genomic RNA. This cycle is completed by the budding of viral particles from the host cell cytoplasmic membrane generating infective progeny.

Evolution of retroviruses occurs so rapidly that individual genomes of a continuously replicating viral particle can be considered to exist in a dynamic equilibrium (quasispecies). The high degree of genomic polymorphism observed for HIV-1 epitomizes this phenomenon (for review see KATZ and SKALKA 1990). Many explanations can be invoked for this exceptionally rapid evolution (for review see STEINHAUER and HOLLAND 1987). Prior to adsorption onto host cells, retroviruses can be inactivated by the hosts immune system; mutations in the viral *env* gene might alter the antigenicity of the envelope protein and enable the virus to evade immune surveillance. Since viruses are obligate parasites, survival is also dictated by their capacity to infect different hosts and different cell types. HIV-1 has an especially strong tropism for the T4 lymphocyte, probably due to a

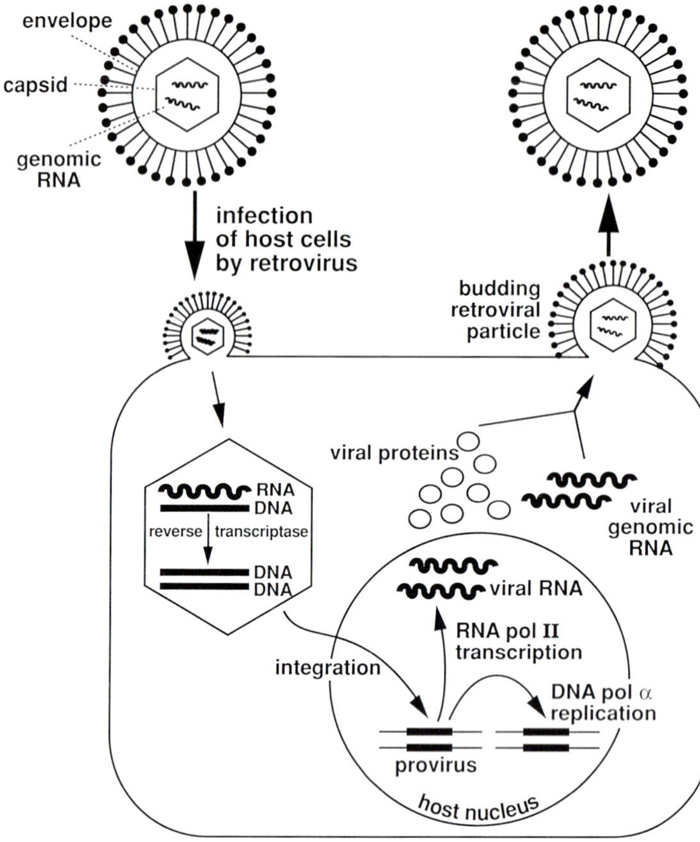

Fig. 1. Retroviral life cycle

high affinity for the T4 cell CD4 receptor molecule by the AIDS virus. The virus may exist in a latent stage, or produce infectious particles after lymphocyte activation. HIV-1 exhibits specific tropism for monocytes/macrophages where it appears to exist in a latent state, at a later stage infecting different organs in the body such as the lung and the brain (FAUCI 1988). In addition, recent evidence indicates that specific mutations in the coding region for RT are responsible for AIDS patients' reduced sensitivity after long-term therapy with zidovudine (3′-azido-3′-deoxythymidine, AZT), a chain-terminating nucleotide analogue (LARDER and KEMP 1989). This resistance to a synthetic drug may indicate an additional genomic "plasticity" of HIV-1 lacking in other retroviruses.

Mechanisms contributing to the high evolutionary rate of retroviruses, in general, and HIV, in particular, can be considered as only conjectural at this time. Presumably, the high rate of evolution is linked to specific events within the retroviral life cycle. Two interrelated biosynthetic events appear to be most important for the production of mutant retroviruses; retroviral recombination and error prone reverse transcription.

3.2 Involvement of RT in Viral Mutagenesis

Similar to all other retroviruses, HIV-1 encodes its own polymerase, the HIV-1 RT. HIV-1 RT is a dimeric protein composed of two polypeptide subunits, 66-kDA and 51-kDA that are present in a 1:1 stoichiometry. HIV-1 RT is a trifunctional enzyme: it synthesizes a DNA molecule from its genomic RNA template, then generates double-stranded DNA, and degrades the RNA template through its RNase H activity (HUBER et al. 1989). Similar to other RTs, HIV-1 RT lacks a $3' \rightarrow 5'$ DNA proofreading exonuclease activity. We know of no evidence that retroviral RT utilizes accessory host cell DNA replication factors which, although yet to be fully characterized, undoubtedly contribute to the high fidelity ascribed to mammalian DNA polymerases in vivo. This lack of utilization of host cell DNA replication components could be based on localization of RT polymerization activity within the virion particle in the cytoplasm rather than the host cell nucleus. Another consideration is that the RNA to DNA reverse transcription step may preclude the use of highly evolved mammalian DNA or RNA polymerase components.

In addition, HIV-1 RT may contribute to the observed high mutation rates through a role in retroviral recombination. Retroviral recombination requires a virion containing a dimeric RNA genome from different daughter particles (heterodimeric RNA molecules). Recent evidence indicates that retroviral recombination occurs during minus strand and plus strand DNA synthesis by inter- and intramolecular recombination (HU and TEMIN 1990). This recombination is mediated by more than one mechanism, each of which requires retroviral RT activity.

4 Viral RTs with RNA Templates

It is now apparent that all retroviral RTs so far studied, in particular HIV-1 RT (BEBENEK et al. 1989; PERRINO et al. 1989; PRESTON et al. 1988; ROBERTS et al. 1988; WEBER and GROSSE 1989) have a lower replicative fidelity than mammalian DNA polymerase complexes (LOEB and REYLAND 1987). This low fidelity undoubtedly contributes to the high retroviral in vivo mutation rates.

Virtually all experimental investigations on RT error frequency opposite RNA templates have been carried out with ribohomopolymers as template (BATTULA and LOEB 1974; TAKEUCHI et al. 1988). In these studies the template consists of a single nucleotide species and one measures the frequencies of incorporation of a radioactive nucleoside triphosphate that is noncomplementary to the template nucleotide. The earliest results indicated that RTs were error prone in the copying of homopolymers, and that the error rates of copying ribo and deoxyribo templates were similar (BATTULA and LOEB 1974). More recently, TAKEUCHI et al. (1988), using a polyadenylic acid template, compared the fidelity of purified HIV-1 RT from two independent isolates with that of purified AMV RT, M-MuLV RT and Rous-associated virus 2 (RAV-2) RT. The error rates of the HIV-1 RTs ranged from 1/17 400 to 1/38 300. The error rates of the three other RTs were much lower, ranging from 1/60 000 (AMV RT) to 1/152 000 (RAV-2 RT). These results indicate that the fidelity of the HIV-1 RTs was two to five times lower than that of the other RTs on this synthetic ribopolymer template. These studies are difficult to evaluate due to inherent problems of template purity and strand slippage during catalysis that occurs on a homopolymer template. Nevertheless, they point out that RTs are as likely to be error prone on RNA templates as they have been demonstrated to be in copying of a variety of DNA templates (BEBENEK et al. 1989; PERRINO et al. 1989; PRESTON et al. 1988, ROBERTS et al. 1988; WEBER and GROSSE 1989).

4.1 Fidelity of Viral RTs with DNA Templates

The fidelity of DNA synthesis by purified HIV RT has been studied extensively (BEBENEK et al. 1989; PERRINO et al. 1989; PRESTON et al. 1988; ROBERTS et al. 1988; TAKEUCHI et al. 1988; WEBER and GROSSE 1989). Although each group of investigators has used different in vitro assays, the consensus of results indicate that HIV-1 RT has a lower fidelity than most other polymerases thus far investigated (Table 1). Of the cellular DNA polymerases that have been investigated with natural DNA templates, only DNA polymerase-β, the enzyme involved in DNA repair, and the *Thermus aquaticus* (*Taq* polymerase, the enzyme obtained from bacteria that grow at high temperatures, have error rates that are consistently similar to that of HIV. However, from the wide range of reported results one can not conclude that HIV-1 RT is more error prone than RTs from other retroviruses. The low fidelity of RTs as a group is particularly notable

Table 1. Error rates of viral RTs and DNA polymerases

Assay	Enzyme	Error rate	Reference
ϕX174 DNA reversion assay	HIV-1 RT	1/4000	PRESTON et al. (1988)
	AMV RT	1/9000	PRESTON et al. (1988)
	DNA polymerase-β	1/8000	KUNKEL and LOEB (1981)
	DNA polymerase-α	1/30 000	LOEB and PERRINO (1990)
	DNA polymerase-α-primase	1/460 000	REYLAND and LOEB (1987)
M13mp2 DNA forward mutation assay	HIV-1 RT	1/4800	BEBENEK et al. (1989)
	AMV RT	1/17 000	ROBERTS et al. (1988)
	M-MuLV	1/30 000	ROBERTS et al. (1988)
	Taq DNA polymerase	1/9000	TINDALL and KUNKEL (1988)
	DNA polymerase-β	1/14 000	ROBERTS et al. (1988)
	DNA polymerase-α-primase	1/5000	ROBERTS and KUNKEL (1988)
	SV40 DNA polymerase complex	1/150 000	ROBERTS and KUNKEL (1988)

when one considers that most cellular DNA polymerases are components of a replicating complex and are likely to be associated with $3' \rightarrow 5'$ proofreading exonucleolytic activities (LOEB and REYLAND 1987).

PRESTON et al. (1988) used the ϕX174*am*3 DNA template in three different assays to evaluate the fidelity of DNA synthesis by HIV-1 RT purified from both virions and *Escherichia coli* expressing the recombinant enzyme. There were no differences found between the two sources of HIV-1 RT indicating the authenticity of the recombinant RT and the lack of any posttranslation modification that might affect the fidelity of DNA synthesis. A qualitative assessment of misincorporation was made by measuring the ability of HIV-1 RT to extend oligonucleotide primers using reaction mixtures lacking one of the four dNTPs. The extent of copying past template nucleotides that are complementary to the missing nucleotide implicates misincorporation by the RT at that template site. This "minus" sequencing gel assay revealed that the relative frequencies of misinsertion were HIV-1 RT > DNA polymerase-α > AMV RT > M-MuLV. In addition the relative abilities of different polymerases to extend terminal mismatches were HIV-1 RT > AMV RT > DNA polymerase-α. Thus, by primer extension, HIV-1 RT consistently surpassed all of the other polymerases in its ability to both insert and extend nucleotide mispairs. In a second type of assay, the fidelity of site-specific nucleotide misincorporation was quantitated by measuring the ratio of V_{max}/K_m for the single addition of incorrect and correct nucleotide (BOOSALIS et al. (1987). Although HIV-1 RT and AMV RT incorporated noncomplementary nucleotides opposite a dA residue in a single-stranded ϕX174 DNA template with similar relative preferences, A:C ≫ A:G > A:A; HIV-1 RT was approximately ten times more error prone than AMV RT. A third assay that measured reversion of a single base mutation in ϕX174*am*3 DNA during in vitro synthesis was performed to determine the fidelity of HIV-1 RT in reaction with all four dNTPs. In this fidelity assay, the estimated error rates were approximately 1/4000 for HIV-1 RT and 1/9000 for AMV RT (Table 1). A compilation of data from all three assays indicates that during DNA polymerization, HIV-1 RT introduces base substitution errors at frequencies ranging between 1/2000 and 1/4000.

In a subsequent study, PERRINO et al. (1989) showed that the efficient addition of a complementary nucleotide onto a 3′ terminal mismatch is a major determinant of the infidelity of HIV-1 RT. They measured separately the two bond-forming steps that result in base substitution mutagenesis: nucleotide misinsertion and elongation from 3′ terminal DNA mispairs, and compared the results with HIV-1 RT to that obtained with DNA polymerase-α. To measure the misinsertion step, they used a correctly paired 15-mer DNA primer hybridized to a 30-mer oligonucleotide in a reaction mixture containing only dATP, that is noncomplementary to the first template nucleotide and complementary to the second. The kinetic constants for the formation of the first A:A mispair were measured by the primer extension gel assay and found to be similar for HIV-1 RT and DNA polymerase-α. However, further extension by correct insertion of dATP opposite the second template nucleotide, thymidine, revealed significant differences between the two polymerases. Whereas HIV-1 RT extended more than 95% of all A:A mispairs, DNA polymerase-α extended less than 5%. The efficiency of mispair extension by HIV-1 RT was analyzed using a series of 16-mer primers that formed 3′ terminal A:A, A:C, or A:G mismatches. Estimates of substrate efficiencies (i.e., V_{max}/K_m) in this assay indicated that the A:C mispair and the A:A mispair were extended 8- to 16-fold more efficiently than the A:G mispair by HIV-1 RT. Moreover, HIV-1 RT extended an A:C mispair 25-fold more efficiently than DNA polymerase-α. The A:C mispair was, in fact, the only mispair that DNA polymerase-α detectably extended, whereas every mispair was readily extended by HIV-1 RT.

In studies that complement the results with the ϕX fidelity assay, ROBERTS et al. (1988) used a bacteriophage DNA M13mp2 nonsense codon-based reversion assay to compare the error rate of HIV-1 RT to the error rates of five other polymerases. HIV-1 RT and AMV RT generated revertants at fifty times above the spontaneous background reversion frequency of uncopied M13mp2 DNA. In contrast, the error rates of DNA polymerase-γ and -δ, both of which contain an associated proofreading exonuclease activity, were severalfold lower. A further expansion of this approach is feasible with ϕX174*am*16 DNA, as a number of substitutions at the amber codon can be scored. WEBER and GROSSE (1989) copied ϕX174*am*16 with HIV-1 RT and reported that the overall error rate ranged between 1/5000 and 1/7000. In comparison, a control experiment revealed the overall fidelity of human lymphoblast DNA polymerase-α to be approximately $1/10^6$. Estimated error rates (interpolated from pool-bias experiments) of individual nucleotide mispairs by HIV-1 RT at the ϕX174*am*16 codon ranged from 1/8000 to $< 1/300\,000$ (limit of assay) with $T_{(template)}$:G > A:G > G:A > T:C > A:C > G:G > T:T.

RICCHETTI and BUC (1990) used the approach pioneered by BOOSALIS et al. (1987) to measure the rate of incorporation of correct and incorrect dNTP by purified HIV-1 RT, AMV RT, and M-MuLV RT into a series of DNA templates—including part of the HIV-1 *gag* DNA minus strand. In these experiments, the rates of incorporation of correct and incorrect nucleotides were determined in reaction mixtures with limiting enzyme concentrations. The overall frequency of misincorporation by HIV-1 RT was found to be similar to the other two RTs with an average of 1.9×10^{-4} for HIV-1 RT, 4.9×10^{-4} for AMV RT, and $\sim 10^{-3}$ for M-MuLV RT. Further, the relative occurrences of the twelve possible types of mismatches were similar for the three RTs, with the exception that $A_{(template)}$:G mismatches were found to be significantly more abundant for HIV-1 RT than for the other two RTs. In agreement with others (PERRINO et al. 1989), the ability of HIV-1 RT to further elongate a mismatch was clearly demonstrated using an oligonucleotide template that coded for a portion of the HIV-1 *gag* gene. Amazingly, the lack of fidelity was so great that at specific positions, HIV-1 RT not only extended terminal mismatches, but incorporated as many as four mismatches in a row.

5 Mutational Spectrum of HIV RT

In order to determine the spectrum of nucleotides that were misincorporated by HIV-1 RT, ROBERTS et al. (1988), utilized a forward mutation assay that scores for a wide spectrum of errors during copying of β-galactosidase, a nonessential gene. Using this type of assay, their data indicates that HIV-1 RT is highly inaccurate, with overall polymerization errors ten times greater than AMV or M-MuLV RTs. Examination of the spectrum of mutations in this assay yielded three classes of errors: single base substitutions, −1 errors and +1 errors, all of which were dramatically nonrandom in their distribution. The positions for the mutational hot spots that were found with HIV-1 RT were not found with other DNA polymerases analyzed. HIV-1 RT single base substitution errors at one site occurred at a frequency of 1/70 and −1 frameshift errors occurred at another site with a frequency of 1/250. The dichotomy between the average error rate of 1/4000 (Table 1) and the high error rates at hot spots demonstrates the effect of sequence context on misincorporation.

6 Relationship of Misincorporation to Processivity

The high frequency of errors by HIV-1 RT at specific nucleotide sequences could be the result of differences in enzyme-template interactions that occur during the course of polymerization. To investigate this process, BEBENEK et al. (1989) compared the frequency and specificity of base substitution and −1 frameshift errors to the processivity of DNA synthesis by HIV-1 RT, i.e., the number of nucleotides incorporated by the polymerase prior to dissociation from the template primer. No significant correlation was discerned between hot spots for base substitution errors and sites of termination (sequences that slowed the progression of DNA synthesis). There was, however, a significant correlation between −1 frameshift mutations and the termination of DNA synthesis in runs of three or more identical nucleotides. Each major frameshift site was at a polymerase pause site and at a stretch of three to five identical template nucleotides. Thus, homopolymer runs with high termination probability also induced −1 frameshifts. A Streisinger strand slippage mechanism (STREISINGER et al. 1966) was given as a likely explanation for this type of misincorporation. Even though the base substitution hot spots did not correlate with termination sites by HIV-1 RT, every base substitution hot spot was located within or at the boundaries of stretches of identical nucleotides. The authors suggested that these base substitution hot spots could result from transient template-primer misalignments and termed this "mechanism dislocation" (KUNKEL and ALEXANDER 1986).

To precisely explore the relationship between stretches of identical template nucleotides and pausing by HIV-1 RT, we inserted homonucleotide sequences at a specific position within M13 DNA (WILLIAMS et al. 1990). In general, these sequences are pause sites during catalysis by DNA polymerases and RTs; different nucleotide sequences have different effects on different polymerases and RTs (WEISMAN-SHOMER et al. 1989; WILLIAMS et al. 1990). HIV-1 RT is potently inhibited opposite a $(dA)_{16}$ insert, and this inhibition cannot be abnegated by alterations in reaction conditions or by prolonged incubation. Furthermore, this inhibition is observed with both recombinant and virion-purified HIV-1 RT. Competition experiments reveal that the striking inhibition of progression opposite the $(dA)_{16}$ homopolymeric stretch by HIV-1 RT was not due to irreversible enzyme-template binding, nor did it appear to be caused by increased enzyme-template disassociation at this site. Preincubation of HIV-1 RT with M13 $(dA)_{16}$ template with increasing molar ratios of radioactively labeled wild-type M13 template did not inhibit or *enhance* the ability of HIV-1 RT to copy the wild-type M13 DNA when compared to the same preincubation studies with an M13 $(dG)_{16}$ template that does not block the progression of HIV-1 RT. These studies indicate the HIV-1 RT slows down, but does not preferentially dissociate opposite homonucleotide sequences in DNA.

7 Relationship of Errors by RTs to Evolution of RNA Viruses

The high error rates for viral RTs provide a direct but not compelling explanation for the high frequency of mutagenesis exhibited by these viruses in vivo. The above in vitro studies of HIV-1 RT indicate this polymerase may have an in vivo error frequency as high as $2–5 \times 10^{-3}$ per nucleotide per replication cycle (PRESTON et al. 1988; ROBERTS et al. 1988; PERRINO et al. 1989). An in vivo base pair substitution rate of 2×10^{-5} per nucleotide per replication cycle was determined for avian spleen necrosis virus by DOUGHERTY and TEMIN (1986), and a rate of 1.4×10^{-5} mutations per nucleotide per replication cycle was obtained for Rous sarcoma virus by LEIDER et al. (1988). These results indicate that HIV-1 RT may be ten fold more error prone than other retroviral RTs and are in accord with estimates of the rate of evolution of the HIV genome.

Proviral DNA replication catalyzed by the host's DNA replicating enzymes is likely to be very accurate. Although estimates on the in vitro error frequencies of purified mammalian replicating DNA polymerases have varied widely—depending on the source of the polymerase, its mode of purification, and assay of its fidelity (Table 1)—these enzymes are invariably more accurate than RTs. The highest accuracies of mammalian DNA polymerases are obtained when the polymerase contains or is associated with a proofreading exonuclease. For example, DNA polymerase-α-primase complex is highly accurate as is the endogenous complex that is able to copy simian virus 40 (SV40) DNA in vitro. It should be noted that the results on DNA polymerase-α-primase are not the same in the reversion and forward mutation assays, and this difference could be the result of DNA sequence or enzyme purification. Most importantly, the spontaneous mutation rate in eukaryotic cells is about 10^{-9}–10^{-11} mutations per nucleotide per cell division, and the overall error rate of DNA replication cannot be greater. As a result it is unlikely that proviral replication by host polymerases is a major source of viral mutagenesis. Evidence for the disparity between viral mutagenesis and the high fidelity of proviral replication is dramatically illustrated by studies on the *mos* oncogene. The rate of evolution of the v-*mos* gene of Moloney murine sarcoma virus has been estimated at 1.31×10^{-3} nucleotide substitutions per site per year while that of the c-*mos* is 1.71×10^{-9}, a millionfold difference in mutagenic rates between retroviral and mammalian genomes (GOJOBORI and YOKOYAMA 1985).

A partial explanation for the consistently high error frequencies observed for RT enzymes may be the lack of cooperative interactions with cellular auxiliary proteins (such as $3' \rightarrow 5'$ exonuclease proofreading activity and numerous others not yet characterized) associated with the most highly accurate mammalian DNA polymerases.

Viewed as a whole, HIV-1 RT is certainly as inaccurate as other retroviral RTs, and may be as much as an order of magnitude more inaccurate when traversing specific template sequences, such as within its own *env* gene in which error frequencies have been estimated to be as high as 1×10^{-2} nucleotide substitutions per site per year (MYERS et al. 1989).

7.1 HIV-1 RT In Vivo

The high in vitro error rates of HIV-1 RT and other retroviral polymerases strongly implicate these enzymes as major contributors to the high rate of mutagenesis observed in vivo. However, the studies demonstrating a high rate of in vitro mutagenesis have been mainly limited to DNA templates. Additional fidelity studies with natural RNA templates are now clearly necessary to determine at which stage of the HIV life cycle the HIV-1 RT contributes to the high in vivo rate of mutagenic evolution.

Evidence obtained by cell culture technique indicates that the RT is primarily responsible for the hypervariability of the viral genome. Virus that has been harvested from repeatedly passaged latently infected cells and therefore has been replicated primarily by cellular DNA polymerases appear quite stable. In contrast, virus grown by rapid passage from one cell culture to another can be highly variable (for review see STEINHAUER and HOLLAND 1987; COFFIN 1986). However, this type of analysis cannot exclude cell culture selectivity for specific viral variants, nor can it distinguish RT replication from RNA polymerase II transcription events, for which the error rate is not yet known.

Genomic clones obtained from isolates of different HIV-1 infected individuals (ALIZON et al. 1986; SAAG et al. 1988; STARCHIC et al. 1986; WILLEY et al. 1986), from the same individual over time (HAHN et al. 1986; SAAG et al. 1988; TERSMETTE et al.

1989), and even separate isolates from one infected individual at the same time (FISHER et al. 1988; WILLEY et al. 1986) demonstrate a high degree of sequence variation within the HIV genome and the clustering of mutations at specific sites. The *env* gene is the most variable part of the HIV-1 genome, within which hypervariable stretches are located primarily in sequences coding for the external envelope glycoprotein (WILLEY et al. 1986; STARCHIC et al. 1986). Selection for hypervariability at specific genomic locations is not unique to HIV-1. A monoclonal antibody selective for a single RNA viral antigenic determinant will result in rapid selection (10^{-4}–10^{-5} mutations per replication) of viral mutants resistant to that monoclonal antibody.

The mechanism for primary localization of sequence hypervariability to regions of the envelope gene remains to be determined. Two interrelated explanations are experimentally testable—the hypervariability is coded for by the nucleotide sequence within this gene, or the hypervariability is the direct result of selection of immunologically resistant clones. Evidence obtained by several investigators which demonstrates unique mutational "hot spots" by HIV-1 RT (BEBENEK et al. 1989; ROBERTS et al. 1988; RICCHETTI and BUC 1990) gives credence to the possibility that genomic sequence can be a major determinant for the fidelity of replication.

We have observed strong pausing of HIV RT opposite homo-oligomeric (dA) stretches in vitro (WILLIAMS et al. 1990), and such sequences have been associated with increased errors (BEBENEK et al. 1989). Furthermore, it has been demonstrated that HIV-1 RT has decreased fidelity in comparison to other RTs while copying poly (rA) in vitro (TAKEUCHI et al. 1988). If HIV-1 RT also copies homo-oligomeric (rA) stretches with decreased fidelity in vivo, it could be manifested by a decreased homology within these stretches amongst HIV genomic isolates.

An analysis of the variability of different repetitive sequences within the HIV genome is shown in Table 2 (unpublished data). Locations of homo-oligomeric tracts of $\geqq 5$ nucleotides were identified in aligned sequences of complete and partial variant HIV genomes (MYERS et al. 1989) by computer search. This computer analysis reveals an increased number of oligoadenylyl tracts relative to all other repetitive sequences throughout the HIV genome. The total number of locations of oligoadenylyl stretches of five or more was 161, and this is more than five times greater than that of any other homo-oligomeric stretch. In addition, the fraction of oligoadenylyl tracts located within the *env* gene (0.41) is disproportionately high in relation to the size of the *env* gene fraction compared to the total size of the HIV genome (0.27). Therefore, oligoadenylyl tracts outnumber all other homo-oligomers examined throughout the HIV genome, with the *env* gene containing a significantly higher proportion of this tract than its size warrants. Physiological reasons for this are unknown. One possibility might be due to sequences within the *env* gene coding for particular amino acids or peptides most successfully used by HIV-1 to escape host immune surveillance. Most importantly, the variability of nucleotide sequence homology within oligoadenylyl tracts in the *env* gene is 1.5- to 2.2-fold higher than the variance of sequence

Table 2. Analysis of variant HIV sequence homology[1]

Nucleotide	No. of 'other' analyzed[2]	'Other'[3] (%)	No. of env analyzed[2]	Env[3] (%)
≧AAAAA	85 (114)	56	21 (47)	34
≧TTTTT	13 (14)	70	5 (6)	51
≧CCCCC	12 (20)	40	2 (4)	75
≧GGGGG	15 (23)	63	3 (8)	70
rndm[4]	40	69	16	46.5

[1] Locations of homo-oligomeric sequences of ≧5 nucleotides were identified by computer search in all aligned HIV genomes. Average number of aligned genomes analyzed within the envelope gene and within the rest of the genome was 26.6 and 18.5 respectively

[2] Only those homo-oligomeric sequences which were found in at least two of all aligned genomes at each location were analyzed for percent homology. 'Other' indicates all genomic locations outside of envelope sequences. 'Env' is only locations within envelope sequences. Number in parenthesis is actual total number of locations of repetitive sequences identified, including unique sequences is alignment not analyzed for percent homology

[3] Locations of all sequences identified outside the envelope gene ('Other'), or within the envelope gene (Env) were compared for percent homology with all other sequences in alignment, except for unique sequences as noted above

[4] Two random sequences were generated to determine average percent homology among all aligned isolates: GACAT and GCTGC. The percent homology of all consensus sequences at all locations of each random sequence was determined individually. Results were not significantly different between the two random sequence locations, therefore the combined average is presented

within other repetitive (rT), (rC), and (rG) runs. The extent of degeneracy of oligo (rA) tracts (34% homology) is also higher than the average degeneracy of consensus sequences (46.5% homology) in the *env* gene. Moreover, the variability of oligoadenylyl tracts located within the *env* gene is much higher than the extent of change of oligoadenylyl tracts within the rest of the genome (56% homology). These combined observations suggest a very high rate of mutational change of oligoadenylyl tracts within the *env* gene.

It can be argued that the presence and the sequence variation of poly (rA) tracts are the result of selective pressures, and need not be connected with errors by the HIV RT. However, the high degree of sequence variation in poly (rA) tracts is in accord with in vitro results on the error prone nature of poly (dA) tracts and on pausing by RTs at poly (dA) tracts (Takeuchi et al. 1988; Bebenek et al. 1989; Williams et al. 1990).

From this analysis it is possible to conjecture a mechanism which involves template localization of error by HIV-1 RT resulting in localized genomic variability. Increased errors at oligoadenylyl stretches within the HIV genome could be a manifestation of such a mechanism. Thus the cooperative interaction between HIV-1 RT and specific genetic sequences provides a mechanism for increased hypervariability at specific locations within the *env* gene. Experiments focused on the interaction of HIV-1 RT and its own template, particularly the *env* gene, should provide more definitive conclusions regarding template-directed infidelity of replication within the HIV genome.

8 Conclusion

It is not known whether errors in vivo occur predominantly at the level of DNA replication or RNA reverse transcription. In addition, the template sequence itself (whether composed of DNA or RNA polynucleotides) may be a primary determinant in error frequency as indicated by increasing evidence of unique patterns of mutational hot spots by each different polymerase investigated, using the same template and the same in vitro reaction conditions (BEBENEK et al. 1989; ROBERTS et al. 1988; RICCHETTI and BUC 1990). Despite inherent problems associated with in vitro analytical methodology, specific phenomena and mechanisms of action by HIV-1 RT, in comparison to other polymerases, have been discovered. These investigative procedures have contributed significantly to the ongoing quest to determine the extent to which HIV-1 RT contributes to the high in vivo variability of this organism. There are still several important questions that require answers before a comprehensive understanding of the underlying mechanisms of HIV-1 genomic mutation is obtained. The error rate of mammalian RNA polymerase II is a primary question not yet answered. Is the error rate of RNA polymerase II significantly higher than mammalian DNA polymerases? If so, HIV-1 transcription should be carefully examined as a possible contributor toward the observed high in vivo mutation rate. A more direct, but perhaps more difficult question would be to ask at which stage of the retroviral life cycle viable mutations predominantly occur.

All information gathered to date leaves little doubt that HIV-1 RT plays a significant role in producing viable mutations during the course of the HIV-1 pathogenic evolution. HIV-1 has hypervariable regions within its own genomic sequences, and HIV-1 RT replication of other DNA templates results in unique mutational hot spots. A first step towards possible correlation of these two facts in regard to HIV-1 RT mechanism(s) of action would be to ask if the high in vitro error rates observed during DNA template replication by HIV-1 RT are also observed during RNA template replication. More specifically, do the mutational hot spots observed using DNA templates correlate with any mutational hot spots yet to be observed using similar RNA templates and, more importantly, do these "mutational profiles" correlate with the hypervariable regions identified within the HIV-1 genomic template?

Additional information obtained using DNA templates and in vitro methodology indicates that one of the predominant types of mutations produced by

HIV-1 RT is single base substitution (Bebenek et al. 1989). This correlates well with the observed ability of HIV-1 and other retroviral particles to escape host immune surveillance by single amino acid changes within the envelope glycoprotein (Holland et al. 1982). A predominance of frameshift mutations would not be likely to produce specifically altered virions.

It is known that retroviral particles consist of two heterodimeric single-stranded RNA genomes which undergo significant recombination during RNA → DNA and DNA → DNA replication by the RT (Hu and Temin 1990). Could base substitution mutations occurring before or during reverse transcription also play a second role of initiating recombination events? This would increase heterogeneity in retroviral progeny to an even greater extent than would be possible by single base substitution events alone.

It is apparent that many important questions remain unanswered before an understanding of retroviral replication and evolution can be achieved. It is however, equally important to realize that answers to these questions are obtainable by molecular biological techniques available today.

Acknowledgments. We thank Dr. G. Myers at Los Alamos National Laboratory, New Mexico for generously providing all of the aligned HIV genomic sequences, and Michael Fry and Dan Feig for generous counsel.

References

Alizon M, Wain-Hobson S, Montagnier L, Sonigo P (1986) Genetic variability of the AIDS virus: nucleotide sequence analysis of two isolates from African patients. Cell 46: 63–74

Battula N, Loeb LA (1974) The infidelity of avian myeloblastosis virus deoxyribonucleic acid polymerase in polynucleotide replication. J Biol Chem 249: 4086–4093

Bebenek K, Abbotts J, Roberts JD, Wilson SH, Kunkel TA (1989) Specificity and mechanism of error-prone replication by human immunodeficiency virus-1 reverse transcriptase. J Biol Chem 264: 16948–16956

Boosalis MS, Petruska J, Goodman MF (1987) DNA polymerase insertion fidelity. J Biol Chem 262: 14689–14696

Coffin JM (1986) Genetic variation in AIDS viruses. Cell 46: 1–4

Dougherty JP, Temin HM (1986) High mutation rate of a spleen necrosis virus-based retrovirus vector. Mol Cell Biol 168: 4387–4395

Eckert KA, Kunkel TA (1990) High fidelity DNA synthesis by the *Thermus aquaticus* DNA polymerase. Nucleic Acids Res 18: 3739–3744

Eigen M, Gardiner W, Schuster P, Winkler-Oswatitsch R (1981) The origin of genetic information. Sci Am 244 (4): 88–118

Fauci AS (1988) The human immunodeficiency virus: infectivity and mechanisms of pathogenesis. Science 239: 617–622

Fisher AG, Ensoli B, Looney D, Rose A, Gallo RC, Saag MS, Shaw GM, Hahn BH, Wong-Staal F (1988) Biologically diverse molecular variants within a single HIV-1 isolate. Nature 334: 444–447

Gojobori T, Yokoyama S (1985) Rates of evolution of the retroviral oncogene of Moloney murine sarcoma virus and of its cellular homologues. Proc Natl Acad Sci USA 82: 4198–4201

Hahn BH, Shaw GM, Taylor ME, Redfield RR, Markham PD, Salahuddin SZ, Wong-Staal F, Gallo RC, Parks ES, Parks WP (1986) Genetic variation in HTLV-III/LAV over time in patients with AIDS or at risk for AIDS. Science 232: 1548–1553

Holland J, Spindler K, Horodyski F, Grabau E, Nichol S, VandePol S (1982) Rapid evolution of RNA genomes. Science 215: 1577–1585

Hu W-S, Temin HM (1990) Retroviral recombination and reverse transcription. Science 250: 1227–1233

Huber HE, McCoy JM, Seehra JS, Richardson CC (1989) Human immunodeficiency virus 1 reverse transcriptase. J Biol Chem 264: 4669–4678

Katz RA, Skalka AM (1990) Generation of diversity in retroviruses. Annu Rev Genet 24: 409–445

Kunkel TA, Alexander PS (1986) The base substitution fidelity of eucaryotic DNA polymerase. J Biol Chem 261: 160–166

Kunkel TA, Loeb LA (1981) Fidelity of mammalian DNA polymerases. Science 213: 765–767

Larder BA, Kemp SD (1989) Multiple mutations in HIV-1 reverse transcriptase confer high-level resistance to zidovudine (AZT). Science 246: 1155–1158

Leider JM, Palese P, Smith FI (1988) Determination of the mutation rate of a retrovirus. J Virol 62: 3084–3091

Loeb LA, Reyland ME (1987) Fidelity of DNA synthesis. In: Eckstein T, Lilley DM (eds) Nucleic acids and molecular biology, vol 1. Springer, Berlin Heidelberg New York

Myers G, Rabson AB, Josephs SF, Smith TF, Wong-Staal F, Berzofsky JA (1989) Human retroviruses and AIDS. Los Alamos National Laboratory, Los Alamos

Perrino FW, Preston BD, Sandell LL, Loeb LA (1989) Extension of mismatched 3′ termini of DNA is a major determinant of the infidelity of human immunodeficiency virus type 1 reverse transcriptase. Proc Natl Acad Sci USA 86: 8343–8347

Preston BD, Poiesz BJ, Loeb LA (1988) Fidelity of HIV-1 reverse transcriptase. Science 242: 1168–1171

Reyland ME, Loeb LA (1987) On the fidelity of DNA replication. J Biol Chem 262: 10824–10830

Ricchetti M, Buc H (1990) Reverse transcriptases and genomic variability: the accuracy of DNA replication is enzyme specific and sequence dependent. EMBO J 9: 1583–1593

Roberts JD, Kunkel TA (1988) Fidelity of a human cell DNA replication complex. Proc Natl Acad Sci USA 85: 7064–7068

Roberts JD, Bebenek K, Kunkel TA (1988) The accuracy of reverse transcriptase from HIV-1. Science 242: 1171–1173

Saag MS, Hahn BH, Gibbons J, Li Y, Parks ES, Parks WP, Shaw GM (1988) Extensive variation of human immunodeficiency virus type-1 in vivo. Nature 334: 440–444

Starchic BR, Hahn BH, Shaw GM, McNeely PD, Modrow S, Wolf H, Parks ES, Parks WP, Josephs SF, Gallo RC, Wong-Staal F (1986) Identification and characterization of conserved and variable regions in the envelope gene of HTLV-III/LAV, the retrovirus of AIDS. Cell 45: 637–648

Steinhauer DA, Holland JJ (1987) Rapid Evolution of RNA viruses. Annu Rev Microbiol 41: 409–433

Streisinger G, Okada Y, Emrich J, Newton J, Tsugita A, Terzaghi E, Inouye M (1966) Frameshift mutations and the genetic code. Cold Spring Harbor Symp Quant Biol 31: 77–84

Takeuchi Y, Nagumo T, Hoshing H (1988) Low fidelity of cell-free DNA synthesis by reverse transcriptase of human immunodeficiency virus. J Virol 62: 3900–3902

Tersmette M, Gruters RA, DeWolf F, DeGoede REY, Lange JMA, Schellekens PTA, Goudsmit J, Huisman HG, Miedema F (1989) Evidence for a role of virulent human immunodeficiency virus (HIV) variants in the pathogenesis of acquired immunodeficiency syndrome: studies on sequential HIV isolates. J Virol 63: 2118–2125

Tindall KR, Kunkel TA (1988) The fidelity of DNA synthesis by the *Thermus aquaticus* DNA polymerase. Biochemistry 27: 6008–6013

Weber J, Grosse F (1989) Fidelity of human immunodeficiency virus type 1 reverse transcriptase in copying natural DNA. Nucleic Acids Res 17: 1379–1393

Weisman-Shomer P, Dube DK, Perrino FW, Stokes K, Loeb LA, Fry M (1989) Sequence specificity of pausing by DNA polymerases. Biochem Biophys Res Commun 164: 1149–1159

Willey RL, Rutledge RA, Dias S, Folks T, Theodore T, Buckler CE, Martin MM (1986) Identification of conserved and divergent domains within the envelope gene of the acquired immunodeficiency syndrome retrovirus. Proc Natl Acad Sci USA 83: 5038–5042

Williams KJ, Loeb LA, Fry A (1990) synthesis of DNA by human immunodeficiency virus reverse transcriptase is preferentially blocked at template oligo (deoxyadenosine) tracts. J Biol Chem 265: 18682–18689

Human Immunodeficiency Virus Type 1 Quasispecies In Vivo and Ex Vivo

S. WAIN-HOBSON

This chapter will cover the extensive data now available for human immunodeficiency virus type 1 (HIV-1) and attempt to point out the particular aspects associated with HIV-1 quasispecies. It should not come as any surprise to realise that much work remains to be done. Nonetheless there are many features of HIV-1 which render it unique. A discussion of HIV-1 genetic variation and quasispecies in order to be meaningful must bear in mind the biology of the virus. Accordingly a brief outline is included so as to make subsequent discussion more fruitful.

1 Human Immunodeficiency Virus Type 1 in Brief

Human immunodeficiency virus (HIV) belongs to the lentivirus subfamily of retroviruses. The HIV virion may enter CD4+ lymphocytes via the CD4 molecule as its cell surface receptor. When it comes to natural infection it is probable that the "second," as opposed to the "familiar," HIV-1 virion is every bit as important, if not more so. This "second" virion is the latently infected lymphocyte where the infectious nucleic acid is DNA, the nucleocapsid is the cell nucleus, and the viral membrane is the cytoplasmic membrane. Upon transmission the number of cells passed harboring HIV-1 proviruses will be very low—except in the case of blood transfusion. A mixed lymphocyte reaction ensues resulting in the activation of all latent proviruses and the production of virions which may go on to infect other lymphocytes (McCUNE 1991). It is generally agreed that lymphocytes need to be

Laboratoire de Rétrovirologie Moléculaire, Institut Pasteur, 28 Rue de Dr. Roux, 75724 Paris Cedex 15, France

Current Topics in Microbiology and Immunology, Vol. 176

activated, by antigens in vivo or mitogens ex vitro, in order to become infected by HIV (GOWDA et al. 1989). A few reports suggest that resting lymphocytes may be infected (STEVENSON et al. 1990b; ZACK et al. 1990). However this could only be shown by recourse to highly sensitive polymerase chain reaction (PCR) techniques, which must indicate that ony a very few cells may be so infected. Given the protocols used it is not known whether these few cells are really quiescent lymphocytes.

In vivo very few lymphocytes support active replication (HARPER et al. 1986). Recent PCR studies have shown that more lymphocytes harbor HIV-1 proviruses suggesting that most of the peripheral blood lymphocytes were latently infected (SCHNITTMAN et al. 1989). The proportion of cells harboring HIV-1 proviral DNA increased with a decline in clinical status. However even in acquired immunodeficiency syndrome (AIDS) cases not all CD4+ lymphocytes harbored virus. A greater proportion of CD4+ memory cells as opposed to CD4+ naive cells harbor HIV-1 proviruses (SCHNITTMAN et al. 1990)

In terms of nucleic acids the replication of HIV, or of any retrovirus for that matter, involves three distinct steps. If the familiar virion is taken as reference then the first step involves reverse transcription of the RNA (+) genome into a (−) DNA strand, followed by (+) DNA strand synthesis. Both these steps occur within the cytoplasm. These two steps are not equivalent by any means. Firstly, the templates are respectively RNA and DNA. The RNA–DNA hybrids can only adopt an A DNA configuration while the DNA–DNA hybrids will generally adopt a B DNA configuration. Nucleotide misincorporation goes unchecked as reverse transcriptase does not encode an exonuclease activity. Errors made during the (−) DNA synthesis are immortalized following degradation of the RNA strand in the RNA–DNA hybrid by the RNase H function associated with reverse transcriptase. The fate of any nucleotide misincorporation during (+) DNA strand synthesis is more variable. Upon migration of the double-stranded provirus to the nucleus cellular proofreading systems will come into play and repair some of the mismatches. In the case of G-T mismatches correction to G-C is extremely efficient (BROWN and JIRICNY 1987). Other mismatches are resolved differently (BROWN and JIRICNY 1988).

To complete the replication cycle full length genomic RNA is derived from the provirus by the host cell RNA polymerase II. Any errors made during transcription are not believed to be subject to proofreading. The relative contribution of each of these three steps to nucleotide misincorporation has been very hard to assess. Consequently nucleotide misincorporation rates for a single site per replication cycle have been defined. These values come out to be of the order of 1.4×10^{-4}–2×10^{-5} for spleen necrosis virus (SNV) and Rous sarcoma virus (RSV) (DOUGHERTY and TEMIN 1988; LEIDER et al. 1988; PATHAK and TEMIN 1990); neither are lentiviruses. As their proviruses are approximately 8 kb long, 0.2–1 substitutions per cycle may be expected on average. No comparable values are yet available for HIV or any lentivirus. Interestingly the few studies on transcription error rates yielded values which also fell into the same order (10^{-4}–10^{-5}) (BLANK et al. 1986; FERSHT 1980; SPRINGATE and LOEB 1975). This raises the interesting idea that genetic diversity among retroviruses may be as much due to a cellular as to the viral polymerase. However, these estimations are very difficult to realise. In vitro studies using purified reverse transcriptase and DNA templates and primers have shown that, averaged out over many sites, the fidelity of HIV, MoMLV, and AMV reverse transcriptases were all of the same order of 10^{-4} per base (PRESTON et al. 1988; ROBERTS et al. 1988; BEBENEK et al. 1989; MENDELMAN et al. 1990; RICHETTI and BUC 1990). In these studies the term "fidelity" is used to describe the proportion of misincorporated nucleotide at a given site. Some mismatches were more frequent than others, notably the G:T mismatch leading to the G to A transition (MENDELMAN et al. 1989). The kinetics of misincorporation were influenced by the two bases 5′ to the mismatch in the primer strand (MENDELMAN et al. 1989; RICHETTI and BUC 1990). However the ability of the HIV-1 reverse transcriptase to elongate beyond mismatches was particularly striking—as though the enzyme could more easily forget its errors. This was much more pronounced for the HIV enzyme than for the other two (RICCHETTI and BUC 1990). Some mismatches may make it so difficult for the enzyme to continue elongation that they effectively function as chain terminators. Consequently the error rate per cycle for HIV-1 might be expected to be greater than for the SNV and RSV systems already studied. Finally it should be pointed out that no published in vitro data yet exists for RNA-dependent DNA synthesis.

Initial genetic studies on HIV-1 strains showed that of all the orfs, the envelope orf was the most variable. Variation was most important in the gp120 sequences (the glycosylated gp160 precursor is cleaved into the surface glycoprotein, gp120, which recognizes the CD4 receptor, and the gp41 transmembrane protein). The gp120 sequence could be described in terms of hypervariable and constant regions, much like influenza A or the immunoglobulin V regions. With the accumulation of huge quantities of sequence data perhaps the most striking feature is just how conserved the constant regions are. There are five hypervariable regions, three of which are heavily glycosylated. In fact primary sequence variation results in the creation and loss of N-linked glycosylation sites. These regions most probably represent loops on the surface of the molecule which are tied down by a complex system of disulfide bridges (LEONARD et al. 1990). While it is impossible to compare HIV-1 and influenza A it might help to appreciate the extent of HIV variation by adding that the degree of sequence variation already described for gp120 is approximately twice the genetic drift encountered for the HA1 glycoprotein of flu H1 strains during the last 20 years.

Again comparison between influenza A and HIV is useful in appreciating the particularities of HIV. HIV can be sequestered away either as in integrated provirus in a nonproducing cell or within privileged sites like the brain where immune surveillance is less efficient. Consequently clearance of HIV infection is highly improbable, resulting in a lifelong infection. Thus many HIV variants may be accumulated during the infection. These options are not available to influenza A. This helps explain the observation that among any population of HIV positive individuals there is a degree of strain variation on a par with the number of infected individuals.

2 HIV Quasispecies

After the description of the extent of sequence variation among independent isolates from different groups and locations, attention was turned to the intrinsic variation within an isolate that was to be expected. The first study (SAAG et al. 1988) described the restriction maps of complete proviruses from different isolates as well as sequential isolates from the same individual. Clearly intraisolate variation was less than interisolate variation. Yet the degree of intraisolate variation, supported by the functional studies following up this work (FISHER et al. 1988), was sufficient to caution against describing the properties of an isolate using a single molecular clone. Other studies went on to show that different full length molecular clones derived from the same isolate had significantly different properties (SAKAI et al. 1988; GOLUB et al. 1990; STEVENSON et al. 1990a; GROENINK et al. 1991).

Another approach embraced PCR. This offered speed, and sequence data for the small fragments readily amplified were easily clonable in M13. Its drawbacks, Taq polymerase error, choice of primers, and the analysis of only small regions, proved not to be too restrictive. However recombination during PCR must be borne in mind (MEYERHANS et al. 1990); it has, nevertheless, now become the technique of choice. The initial study confined itself to a small segment of the p25 *gag* sequence and the first and second hypervariable regions of the gp120 sequence (GOODENOW et al. 1989). Invariably a single sequence was accompained by a plethora of minor forms. Analysis of 20 molecular clones proved to be sufficient to reliably and reproducibly describe the population of amplified sequences. Each HIV isolate was an entity unto itself. Thus no correlation could be found between the structure or complexity of a sequence population and disease progression; isolates derived from AIDS patients were as complex or as homogeneous as isolates from asymptomatic individuals. It is clearly an overwhelming task to define the complete sequence of a large number of molecular clones for several isolates. Therefore the word "quasispecies" will be used to describe a population of cloned and sequenced PCR products derived from a given sample. Thus a "tat quasispecies" will refer to a collection of *tat* gene sequences, etc.

A striking feature of HIV infection during the asymptomatic phase is the high frequency of HIV-specific, human leukocyte antigen (HLA)-restricted cytotoxic T lymphocytes (CTLs) (HOFFENBACH et al. 1989; MILLS et al. 1989; WALKER and PLATA 1990). The role of CTLs in HIV infection has been the subject of much discussion. The isolation of HIV is therefore somewhat special in that the ex vivo culture of infected CD4 cells takes place in the presence of HIV antigen-specific CTLs.

Certainly the CD8+ population can greatly restrict and even abolish HIV replication ex vivo (KANNAGI et al. 1990; WALKER et al. 1986; WALKER and LEVY 1989). Whether this is due to direct lysis of the target cells or inhibition of HIV replication is not clear. Other data suggest that a soluble factor secreted by the CD8+ population from infected individuals (BRINCHMANN et al. 1990; WALKER et al. 1986; WALKER and LEVY 1989) or even from uninfected (BRINCHMANN et al. 1990) lymphocytes may restrict viral replication ex vivo. Thus there is a distinct possibility that the ex vivo culture of HIV may result in the selection of certain variants. The selection of adapted variants in tissue culture in nothing new—live attenuated vaccines were developed this way.

In the context of RNA viruses little can be done to study this problem. Only for retroviruses is an in vivo/ex vivo comparison possible without recourse to an initial reverse transcription step, which would itself introduce errors. The exquisite sensitivity of PCR enables direct amplification of the DNA provirus (OU et al. 1988). This allowed the undertaking of a sequential in vivo/ex vivo comparison of HIV-1 *tat* gene quasispecies (MEYERHANS et al. 1989). The structures of the quasispecies fluctuated between sequential in vivo samples in as little as 3 months. Equally, sequential ex vivo quasispecies differed. The structures of the quasispecies in vivo were always more complex than those ex vivo, a finding confirmed in all subsequent studies. Most importantly there was no correlation between the two. Invariably a minor species in vivo dominated the culture ex vivo. Subsequent work showed that passage of HIV in donor peripheral blood mononuclear cells (PBMCs) and especially passage to established cell lines resulted in extensive selection (VARTANIAN et al. 1991). Until ways are found to culture HIV-1 resulting in minimal deformation of the initial quasispecies then the appropriateness of data derived from ex vivo culture must always be borne in mind.

The factors involved may be multiple. Firstly the influence of patient CD8+ cells as well as donor PBMCs as mentioned above must be addressed. Secondly chance may be an important factor. Isolation of HIV, especially from the PBMCs of an asymptomatic individual, must be made from as many cells as possible. In these individuals sometimes as few as 1/80000 cells may be infected. If only 2×10^5 cells were put in culture then the structure of the ensuing quasispecies may have as much to do with sampling as with anything else. Inversely, when analysing HIV directly from blood the largest possible number of PBMCs is desirable. Thus the recent observation that isolation of HIV from limiting dilutions of PBMCs resulted in isolates manifesting different biological properties should not be surprising (GROENINK et al. 1991). Isolation or amplification of HIV from patients with AIDS-rlated complex (ARC) or AIDS should not be fraught with this problem as the proportion of infected cells is considerably greater (SCHNITTMAN et al. 1989).

Finally there is the possibility that the particular environment favors the outgrowth of a particular variant. It the case of the study of virus passage to established cell lines this latter possibility clearly must pertain. The use of established cell lines as a means of isolating HIV or to describe the properties of an isolate is simply erroneous, resulting in the selection of those variants from the plethora present which are best adapted to the cell line.

The transmission of HIV in vivo and ex vivo differ. Unless the moi is very low, it may be expected that the best adapted (fittest) variants will dominate. In vivo, however, transmission bottlenecks occur due to the small size of the innoculum. In such circumstances it is not a foregone conclusion that the fittest variant, if this notion is at all meaningful, is passed. Indeed a study of the low dilution passage of P2 phage has made this point most elegantly (CHAO 1990). It is perhaps not surprising that a longitudinal analysis of the HIV proviruses in vivo showed no selection for variants with enhanced *tat* gene or long terminal repeat (LTR) activities (DELASSUS et al., unpublished data).

Most studies have confined themselves to small regions of 300 bp or so (GOODENOW et al. 1989; HUET et al. 1989; MEYERHANS et al. 1989; BALFE et al. 1990; SIMMONDS et al. 1990; EPSTEIN et al. 1991; PEDROZA MARTINS et al. 1991). One, however, described the evolution of the nef and LTR sequences (approximately 850 bp) over 4 years (DELASSUS et al. 1991). In fact little evolution was easily discernible due to the extraordinary diversity manifested. This was so profound that the actual meaning of a "HIV sequence" was discussed. Extrapolating from these data it was estimated that any two proviruses in peripheral blood may differ by between 10–20 substitutions. Even at the amino acid level most of the nef sequences were unique. However as these sequences were derived from PBMCs these data cannot be used to derive a nucleotide substitution rate for HIV-1.

Analysis of samples from the same Swedish patient has been extented to cover the second *rev* coding exon, which overlaps with that part of the env orf encoding the gp 41 sequences. The structure of the populations of rev protein sequences increased in complexity with disease, while those of the corresponding env sequences derived from the same nucleotide sequence remained complex. This suggests that the rev and env populations evolved differently probably reflecting differential selection pressures. Only two out of eighty second rev exon sequences were functionally defective. These results do not parallel those of the first *rev* coding exon where up to 30% of sequences were *rev*$^-$. After analysing three HIV loci (15% of the genome) from the same individual over 4 years, it is clear that no two loci evolved similarly, indicating the difficulties in comparing data from different loci.

The magnitude of the HIV provirus population in an individual will vary according to the disease stage (SCHNITTMAN et al. 1989). Assuming a single provirus/PBMC then one may calculate that for asymptomatic carriers the number of infected CD4+ cells ranges between 6×10^6 and 2×10^8. This calculation ignores all infected immobilized lymphocytes and antigen-presenting cells. It is therefore possible that for an individual these numbers may be a factor of 10^2 or even greater. Even given the little that is known for the HIV-1 misincorporation rate/replication cycle, it is most probable that the number of distinct genomes will be within a factor of ten of the number of infected cells.

Efficient recombination between retroviral genomes has been described for a number of years. Using the SNV system it was possible to show that recombination required a heterozygous virion. The frequency of recombination was shown to be of the order of 0.2 per cycle (Hu and Temin 1990). Relatively few examples of recombination among HIV-1 genomes have been described (Clavel et al. 1989). In the above nef and LTR study it was noted that motifs in the nef and LTR sequences were uncoupled, as though recombination were responsible (Delassus et al. 1991). Another study demonstrated recombinant genomes derived from two distinct strains that were passaged together (Vartanian et al. 1991). Certainly with frequencies as high as 0.2 per cycle it is likely that the there can be few cis constraints on the genome. Thus while the HIV-1 genome is colinear it may be more correct to envisage it as effectively a linear series of segments.

All this makes molecular biology particularly difficult where the infectious full length molecular clone is the gold standard. An additional level of complexity was afforded upon functional analysis of the amplified genes and LTR sequences. Thus the proportion of functionally defective genomes varied from 5%–15% per quasispecies (20 sequences). Yet these loci represented only a fraction of the genome. Possibly a substantial proportion of HIV-1 proviruses in PBMCs may be functionally defective. As ever, it is hard to generalize about HIV isolates and quasispecies. More recently it has been shown that the PBMCs of two asymptomatics, as evidenced by limiting dilution followed by PCR and viral isolation, harbored very few proviruses (Brinchmann et al. 1991). Others also saw little evidence of defective genomes (Balfe et al. 1990). This feature would seem therefore to be a variable. Whether or not it may play a role in virus spread in vivo is unknown.

All the major forms tested, whether the gene be *rev* or *tat*, or the sequences be U3 or R, had activities comparable to that of the corresponding HIV-1 *Lai* gene or sequence. However it is possible that our experimental approaches, i.e., transfection of mammalian cells and transient expression of reporter genes such as chloramphenicol acetyltransferase (CAT) or secreted alkaline phosphatase (SEAP), may not be sufficiently sensitive to detect subtle differences in gene function. Therefore it is difficult to decide whether or not a natural amino acid substitution is important. This could be overcome by cloning back the variants into an infectious molecular clone. Any subtle fitness advantage of a particular variant with respect to its parent might be evident after multiple rounds of replication. Here a problem arises. Which infectious molecular clone should be used? Should it be one of the molecular clones derived from continuously passaged virus? Recently it has been shown that continuous passage of an HIV-1 isolate on PBMCs ow even a single passage to an established cell line constitutes a very strong selection pressure (Vartanian et al. 1991). Given the high frequency of retroviral recombination (Hu and Temin 1990) as well as the intrinsic nucleotide misincorporation error rate associated with the reverse transcriptase, is it indeed possible to isolate, or define, a representative provirus?

The major forms of any quasispecies differed usually by 1–4 residues in the regulatory genes studied (Meyerhans et al. 1989; Delassus et al. 1991; Pedroza Martins et al. 1991). Are such differences sufficiently important to confer a selective advantage? Most variants endowed with a selective advantage must be derived from small genetic differences. Let's assume that the average nucleotide misincorporation rate per replication cycle for HIV-1 reverse transcriptase is on the order of 10^{-4} per genome per cycle. If ten substitutions were necessary for the production of a fitter variant, the probability of generating it would be of the order of 10^{-40}, safely excluding itself. Experimental observations (LOONEY et al. 1988; MCKEATING et al. 1989; REITZ et al. 1988) and theoretical considerations (NOWAK 1990) point to neutralizing antibody escape mutants being generated by a limited number of base substitutions. The inherent complexity of the RNA viral quasispecies may be seen, therefore, as necessary to ensure adaptation through the selection of novel variants.

3 G to A Hypermutation

One of the features of the quasispecies model is that there exists a replication error threshold beyond which there is a melting or total loss of information on the distribution in sequence space (EIGEN and BIEBRICHER 1988). Does such a situation really exist for an RNA virus and what in biochemical terms could this correspond to? The HIV genome is capable sometimes, for reasons unknown, of absorbing a startling proportion of G to A transitions. This phenomenon of monotonous base substitution has been referred to as "G to A hypermutation" (VARTANIAN et al. 1991). Up to 15% of genomes amplified were hypermutated. Unpublished work shows that this figure may be $\geqq 65\%$ (HENRY et al. 1991, unpublished data). Within a given sequence up to 40% of Gs could be substituted. A strong dinucleotide preference accompanied these transitions being GpA > GpG > GpT ~ GpC. This predilection for G to A transitions within the GpA dinucleotide may be explained by a mechanism termed "dislocation mutagenesis" (KUNKEL and ALEXANDER 1986). This mechanism emphasizes the fact that uncoordinated displacement of the primer and template may occur. Accordingly the G is not copied; rather, the preceding A is copied twice. Only during reverse transcription of RNA into DNA would the A residue to copied before the G and thus be able to influence its substitution by dislocation mutagenesis.

Why does hypermutation occur? Two possibilities are suggested: the first proposes a mutant polymerase which has problems in translocating through GpA dinucleotides. The second demands the local environmental conditions, anion or nucleotide concentrations perhaps, are such that polymerization is slow with respect to uncoordinated translocation of the primer and template. It is not yet possible to differentiate between the two. However as none of the sequences had all of their GpA dinucleotides substituted this partial or incomplete hypermutation would seem to argue against the mutant polymerase hypothesis. Furthermore the example of frequent G to A substitution at a single site in vitro was observed in the absence of dexoycytidine triphosphate (dCTP), again suggesting that latter of the two hypotheses. Why does G to A hypermutation, as opposed to any other monotonous substitution, occur? Again this is unclear. It could be the only efficient transition compatible with the stereochemistry and/or rigors inherent in repeated dislocation mutagenesis.

While most of the hypermutated genomes will presumably be defective, the possibility of recombination between a fragment of just such a genome and a replication competent genome would allow HIV genomes to evolve at extraordinary speeds. Indeed such a phenomenon may help explain the unusually elevated A composition of the HIV genome (i.e., 34%). Furthermore the high A content (34%–38%) is characteristic of all lentiviruses independent of host species. Virtually all other retroviruses have a lower A content, between 22%–30%. This would point to the lentiviral reverse transcriptase as being particularly susceptible to producing G to A transitions. Using the SNV system a single G to A hypermutated genome was noted (PATHAK and TEMIN 1990). Fifteen G to A transitions were noted within a 930-bp segment. While no mechanism was proposed, 8/15 transitions preceded an A residue. The data are particularly important as the sequence was derived without recourse to PCR, demonstrating once again that G to A hypermutation was not a result of Taq polymerase associated error. While the two experimental systems are not immediately comparable, it would appear that the probability is greater of finding a hypermutated genome within a HIV (3/20 in these instances), rather than a SNV (1/8000), quasispecies.

Does G to A hypermutation represent the excursion of HIV replication beyond the error threshold and into the catastrophe zone? Certainly it would seem this is the closest instance of a "melting of information" predicted by the quasispecies model.

4 Black Holes

As this field is only in its infancy there remain, as usual, more questions than answers. Thus there is no adequate data to explain why HIV quasispecies fluctuate in as little as 3 months. Methods for growing HIV with the least perturbation possible to the initial quasispecies are sorely lacking. Where do resting PBMCs become infected? How did resting memory cells get infected given that HIV infects for the most part activated lymphocytes? These are important questions as virtually all HIV virology is based on isolates derived from blood. Do HIV quasispecies differ between tissues as has been suggested (EPSTEIN et al. 1991)?

These are among the most prominant questions. Yet a number of very simple questions, all relating to sampling, need to be addressed. Does a blood sample split in two give the same HIV quasispecies when analyzed? Most work uses 1 μg of DNA, or 150 000 cell equivalents. For asymptomatic individuals a copy number of 1/50 000 is not unusual and thus the sampling problem is all too obvious. When working with samples from ARC or AIDS patients the problem should be much less. How similar are HIV quasispecies derived from say five different samples of the same organ? Until this is known it is not possible to attribute tissue-specific traits to data sets.

There are too few publications in which sequence data from uncultured PBMCs have been reported. Two of these described most complicated quasispecies in which perhaps two distinct sequences were discernible (Epstein et al. 1991; Wain-Hobson et al. 1991). In both cases the sequence data pertained to the V3 loop of the HIV gp120 molecule, in which 9/36 (25%) amino residues varied. The data is particularly intriguing as both cases had AIDS. More data over larger regions will be necessary before one can reliably conclude that infection by two different strains may occur.

5 Is the Quasispecies Description Applicable to HIV?

This question can be asked in general of RNA viruses. The quasispecies model treats an RNA virus as an infinite array of variants in equilibrium whereas quasispecies are, in fact, made up of only a discrete number of genomes that cannot be considered as being in equilibrium. Apart from this, there are a number of features that differentiate HIV and other RNA viruses. In considering HIV in vivo only a small fraction of lymphocytes express virus at any time. Given the nature of CD4+ lymphocytes, while not forgetting that the memory CD4+ lymphocytes are preferentially infected, these few cells were probably activated by antigen. Thus virus variants may be selected and amplified for reasons that have nothing to do with fitness of the variant but more with the probability of activating a latently infected lymphocyte with the appropriate antigen. This amplification will be exponential since antigen will also activate uninfected CD4+ lymphocytes. Yet these are most susceptible to subsequent infection by the virus progeny. This highly favorable situation, for the virus, will continue until the opportunistic infection starts to be cleared. Perhaps this scenario may help explain the fluctuating quasispecies.

A second particularity involves HIV transmission. As mentioned above except via blood transfusion only a small number of infected cells are transmitted. Thus only a few of the myriad of proviruses present. Thus it may be expected that the average sequence difference between a donor and a receiver may correspond to the intra-isolate divergence so long as the two could be analysed as close together as possible. Again chance, rather than fitness, comes into play.

Given these observations in which chance would appear to play a prominent role, the quasispecies, with its notion of a master sequence whose survival depends upon its fitness with respect to the mutant spectrum in a given environment, would seem not to be quite appropriate. Remaining replication competent is perhaps sufficient for this virus to wreak its havoc. It may simply be aided and abetted by the dense array of antigens which constitutes our world. The immune system could not do otherwise.

Acknowledgements. I would like to thank past and present numbers of my laboratory who all worked so well. This work was supported by grants from Institut Pasteur and l' Agence Nationale de Recherches sur le SIDA (ANRS).

References

Balfe P, Simmonds P, Ludlam CA, Bishop JO, Leigh Brown A (1990) Concurrent evolution of human immunodeficiency type 1 in patients infected from the same source: rate of sequence change and low frequency of inactivating mutations. J Virol 64: 6221–6233

Bebenek K, Abbotts J, Roberts JD, Wilson SH, Kunkel TA (1989) Specificity and mechanism of error prone replication by human immunodeficiency virus 1 reverse transciptase. J Biol Chem 264: 16948–16956

Blank A, Gallant JA, Burgess RR, Loeb LA (1986) An RNA polymerase mutant with reduced accuracy of chain elongation. Biochemistry 25: 5920–5928

Brinchmann JE, Gaudernack G, Vartdal F (1990) CD8+ T cell inhibit HIV replication in naturally infected CD4+ T cells. J Immunol 144: 2961–2966

Brinchmann JE, Albert J, Vartdal F (1991) Few infected CD4+ T cells but a high proportion of replication competent provirus copies in asymptomatic human immunodeficiency virus type 1 infection. J Virol 65: 2019–2023

Brown TC, Jiricny J (1987) A specific mismatch repair event protects mammalian cells from loss of 5-methylcytosine. Cell 50: 945–950

Brown TC, Jiricny J (1988) Different base/base mispairs are corrected with different efficiencies and specificities in monkey kidney cells. Cell 54: 705–711

Chao L (1990) Fitness of RNA virus decreased by Muller's ratchet. Nature 348: 454–455

Clavel F, Hoggan MD, Willey RL, Strebel K, Martin MA, Repaske R (1989) Genetic recombination of human immunodeficiency virus. J Virol 63: 1455–1459

Delassus S, Cheynier R, Wain-Hobson S (1991) Evolution of human immunodeficiency type 1 nef and long terminal repeat sequences over four years in vivo and in vitro. J Virol 65: 225–231

Dougherty JP, Temin H (1988) Determination of the rate of base pair substitution and insertion mutations in retrovirus replication. J Virol 62: 2817–2822

Eigen M, Biebricher CK (1988) Sequence space and quasispecies distribution. In: Domingo E, Holland JJ, Ahlquist P (eds) RNA genetics. CRC, Boca Raton, pp 211–245

Epstein LG, Kuiken C, Blumberg BM, Hartman S, Sharer LR, Clement M, Goudsmit J (1991) HIV-1 V3 domain variation in brain and spleen of children with AIDS: tissue specific evolution within host determined quasispecies. Virology 180: 583–590

Fersht AR (1980) Enzymatic editing mechanisms in protein synthesis and DNA replication. Trends Biochem Sci 5: 262–265

Fisher AG, Ensoli B, Looney D, Rose A, Gallo RC, Saag MS, Shaw GM, Hahn BH, Wong-Staal F (1988) Biologically diverse molecular variants within a single HIV-1 isolate. Nature 334: 444–447

Golub EI, Li G, Volsky DJ (1990) Differences in the basal activity of the long terminal repeat determine the different replicative capacities of two closely related human immunodeficiency virus type 1 isolates. J Virol 64: 3654–3660

Goodenow M, Huet T, Saurin W, Kwok S, Sninsky J, Wain-Hobson S (1989) HIV-1 isolates are rapidly evolving quasispecies: evidence for viral mixtures and preferred nucleotide substitutions. J AIDS 2: 344–352

Gowda SD, Stein BS, Mohagheghpour N, Benike CJ, Engleman EG (1989) Evidence that T cell activation is required for HIV-1 entry in CD4+ lymphocytes. J Immunol 142: 773–780

Groenink M, Fouchier RAM, de Goede REY, de Wolf F, Gruters RA, Cuypers HTM, Huisman HG, Tersmette M (1991) Phenotypic heterogeneity in a panel of infectious molecular human immunodeficiency virus type 1 clones derived from a single individual. J Virol 65: 1968–1975

Harper ME, Marselle LM, Gallo RC, Wong-Staal F (1986) Detection of lymphocytes expressing human T-lymphotropic virus type III in lymph nodes and peripheral blood from infected individuals by in situ hybridization. Proc Natl Acad Sci USA 83: 772–776

Hoffenbach A, Langlade-Demoyen P, Dadaglio G, Vilmer E, Michel F, Mayaud C, Autran B, Plata F (1989) Unusually high frequencies of HIV-specific cytotoxic lymphocytes in humans. J Immunol 142: 452–462

Hu W-S, Temin H (1990) Genetic consequences of packaging two RNA genomes in one retroviral particle: pseudodiploidy and high rate of genetic recombination. Proc Natl Acad Sci USA 87: 1556–1560

Huet T, Dazza MC, Brun-Vézinet F, Roelants GE, Wain-Hobson S (1989) A highly defective HIV-1 strain isolated from a healthy Gabonese individual presenting an atypical Western blot. AIDS 3: 707–715

Kannagi M, Masuda T, Hattori T, Kanoh T, Nasu K, Yamamoto N, Harada S (1990) Suppression of simian immunodeficiency virus replication in vitro by CD8+ lymphocytes. J Virol 64: 3399–3406

Kunkel TA, Alexander PS (1986) The base substitution fidelity of eucaryotic DNA polymerases: mispairing frequencies, site preferences, insertion preferences and base substitution by dislocation. J Biol Chem 261: 160–166

Leider JM, Palese P, Smith FI (1988) Determination of the mutation rate of a retrovirus. J Virol 62: 3084–3091

Leonard CK, Spellman MW, Riddle L, Harris RJ, Thomas JN, Gregory TJ (1990) Assignment of intrachain disulfide bonds and characterization of potential glycosylation sites of the type 1 recombinant human immunodeficiency virus envelope glycoprotein (gp120) expressed in chinese hamster ovary cells. J Biol Chem 265: 10373–10382

Looney DJ, Fisher AG, Putney SD, Rusche JR, Redfield RR, Burke SD, Gallo RC, Wong-Staal F (1988) Type restricted molecular clones of HIV. Science 241: 357–359

McCune JM (1991) HIV-1: the infective process in vivo. Cell 64: 351–363

McKeating J, Gow J, Goudsmit J, Pearl L, Mulder C, Weiss RA (1989) Characterization of HIV-1 neutralization escape mutants. AIDS 3: 777–784

Mendelman LV, Boosalis MS, Petruska J, Goodman MF (1989) Nearest-neighbour influences on DNA polymerase insertion fidelity. J Biol Chem 264: 14414–14423

Mendelman LV, Petruska J, Goodman MF (1990) Base mispair extension kinetics: comparison of DNA polymerase α and reverse transcriptase. J Biol Chem 265: 2338–2346

Meyerhans AE, Cheynier R, Albert J, Seth M, Kwok S, Sninsky J, Morfeldt-Manson L, Asjö B, Wain-Hobson S (1989) Temporal fluctuations in HIV quasispecies in vivo are not reflected by sequential HIV isolations. Cell 58: 901–910

Meyerhans AF, Vartanian J-P, Wain-Hobson S (1990) DNA recombination during PCR. Nucleic Acids Res 18: 1687–1691

Mills KHG, Nixon DF, McMichael AJ (1989) T-cell strategies in AIDS vaccines: MHC-restricted T-cell responses to HIV proteins. AIDS 3: S101–S110

Nowak M (1990) HIV mutations rate. Nature 347: 522

Ou CY, Kwok S, Mitchell SW, Mack DH, Sninsky JJ, Krebs JW, Feorino P, Warfield D, Schochetman G (1988) DNA amplification for direct detection of HIV-1 in DNA of peripheral blood mononuclear cells. Science 239: 295–297

Pathak VK, Temin H (1990) Broad spectrum of in vitro forward mutations, hypermutations, and mutational hotspots in a retroviral shuttle vecto after a single replication cycle: substitutions, frameshifts, and hypermutations. Proc Natl Acad Sci USA 87: 6019–6023

Pedroza Matrins L, Chenciner N, Åsjö B, Meyerhans A, Wain-Hobson S (1991) Independent fluctuation of HIV-1 rev and gp41 quasispecies in vivo. J Virol 65: 4502–4507

Preston BD, Poiesz BJ, Loeb LA (1988) Fidelity of HIV-1 reverse transcriptase. Science 242: 1168–1171

Reitz MS, Wilson C, Naugle C, Gallo RC, Robert-Guroff M (1988) Generation of a neutralization resistant variant of HIV-1 is due to selection for a point mutation in the envelope gene. Cell 54: 57–63

Ricchetti M, Buc H (1990) Reverse transcriptases and genomic variability: the accuracy of DNA replication is enzyme specific and sequence dependent. EMBO J 9: 1583–1593

Roberts JD, Bebenek K, Kunkel TA (1988) The accuracy of reverse transcriptase from HIV-1. Science 242: 1171–1173

Saag MS, Hahn BH, Gibbons J, Li Y, Parks ES, Parks WP, Shaw GM (1988) Extensive variation of human immunodeficiency virus type 1 in vitro. Nature 334: 440–444

Sakai K, Dewhurst S, Ma X, Volsky D (1988) Differences in cytopathogenicity and host cell range among infectious molecular clones in human immunodeficiency virus type 1 simultaneously isolated from an individual. J Virol 62: 4078–4085

Schnittman SM, Psallidopoulos MC, Lane HC, Thompson L, Baselar M, Massari M, Fox CH, Salzman NP, Fauci AS (1989) The reservoir for HIV-1 in human peripheral blood is a T cell that maintains expression of CD4. Science 245: 305–308

Schnittman SM, Lane HC, Greenhouse J, Justement JS, Baselar M, Fauci AS (1990) Preferential infection of CD4+ memory T cells by human immunodeficiency virus type 1: evidence for a role in the selective T cell functional defects observed in infected individuals. Proc Natl Acad Sci USA 87: 6058–6062

Simmonds P, Balfe P, Ludlam CA, Bishop JO, Leigh Brown A (1990) Analysis of sequence diversity in hypervariable regions of the external glycoprotein of human immunodeficiency virus type 1. J Virol 64: 5840–5850

Springate CF, Loeb LA (1975) On the fidelity of transcription by Escherichia coli ribonucleic acid polymerase. J Mol Biol 97: 577–591

Stevenson M, Haggerty S, Lamonica C, Mann AM, Meier C, Wasiak A (1990a) Cloning and characterization of human immunodeficiency virus type 1 variants diminished in the ability to induce syncytium-independent cytolysis. J Virol 64: 3792–3803

Stevenson M, Stanwick TL, Dempsey MP, Lamonica CA (1990b) HIV-1 replication is controlled at the level of T cell activation and proviral integration. EMBO J 9: 1551–1560

Vartanian JP, Meyerhans A, Åsjö B, Wain-Hobson S (1991) Selection, recombination and G→A hypermutation of HIV-1 genomes. J Virol 65: 1779–1788

Wain-Hobson S, Vartanian J-P, Henry M, Chenciner N, Cheynier R, Delassus S, Pedroza Martins L, Sala M, Nugeyre M-T, Guétard D, Gluckman J-C, Klatzmann D, Rozenbaum W, Barré-Sinoussi F, Montagnier L (1991) LAV revisited: origins of the early HIV isolates from Institut Pasteur. Science 252: 961–965

Walker BD, Plata F (1990) Cytotoxic T lymphocytes against HIV. AIDS 4: 177–184

Walker CM, Levy JA (1989) A diffusable lymphokine produced by CD8+ T lymphocytes suppresses HIV replication. Immunology 66: 628–630

Walker CM, Moody DJ, Stites DP, Levy JA (1986) CD8+ lymphocytes can control HIV infection by suppressing virus replication. Science 234: 1563–1566

Zack JA, Arrigo SJ, Weitsman SR, Go AS, Haislip A, Chen ISY (1990) HIV-1 entry into quiescent primary lymphocytes: molecular analysis reveals a labile, latent viral structure. Cell 61: 213–222

Tracing the Origin of Retroviruses

R. F. DOOLITTLE and D.-F. FENG

1 Introduction

Retroviruses are so named because of their ability to transcribe their RNA genome into DNA by reverse transcription. The resulting double-stranded DNA is integrated into the nuclear DNA of the host cell, and host cell enzymes subsequently transcribe the integrated DNA back to RNA, either as transcripts that can be translated into precursors of the viral component proteins, or full-length transcripts destined to be the genetic material for newly assembled viruses. For the most part, this unusual life cycle is made possible by four virus-encoded enzymes and a few structural proteins. The enzymes are (a) the reverse transcriptase, (b) a ribonuclease H for the digestion of the RNA portion of the DNA–RNA heteroduplex so that the DNA second strand can be made, (c) an endonuclease (integrase) for cutting the host DNA as a part of the integration process, and (d) a protease for processing newly made polyprotein precursors. The structural proteins include an RNA-binding protein, capsid proteins, and envelope proteins. Ordinarily, all of the genetic information for these proteins is

Center for Molecular Genetics, University of California, San Diego, La Jolla, California 92093-0634, USA

Current Topics in Microbiology and Immunology, Vol. 176

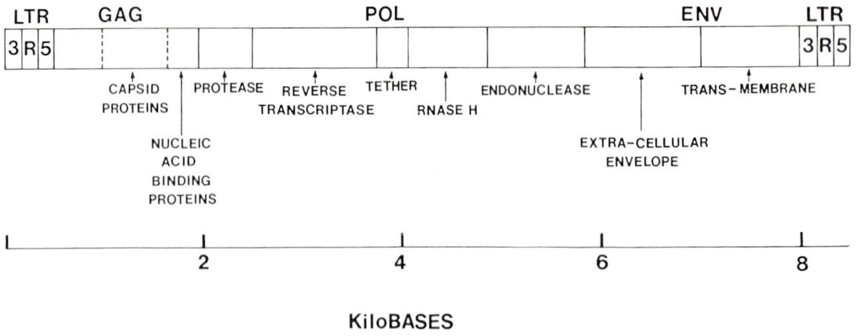

Fig. 1. Schematic depiction of typical retrovirus (DNA form). The *gag* region encodes structural proteins, and the *pol* region a protease, a reverse transcriptase, a ribonuclease and an endonuclease. The *env* gene encodes the envelope protein system. RNASE H, ribonuclease H; LTR, long terminal repeat. (From DOOLITTLE et al. 1989a)

encompassed in less than 8 kilobases (kb) of RNA (Fig. 1). Retroviruses also have untranslated RNA sequences at their 5′ and 3′ extremities, which in their DNA versions are reciprocally extended to yield perfectly repeated sequences—long terminal repeats (LTRs). The repeats are formed during the reverse transcription process and are an integral part of the mechanism that insures the entire genome is copied. These sequences contain transfer RNA (tRNA) primer binding sites, promoter sequences and polyadenylation signals. The standard equipment for an independent retrovirus thus comprises:

1. Reverse transcriptase
2. Ribonuclease H
3. Endonuclease
4. Protease
5. RNA-binding protein
6. Capsid protein(s)
7. Envelope protein
8. Long terminal repeat (LTR)

Some retroviruses also contain additional sequences that may act as enhancers or that encode unique proteins that may aid and abet replication.

How and when were these various sequences assembled into integrated units during evolution? As it happens, homologues of all four enzymes have been found in non-retrovirus settings, offering clues as to their individual origins. The structural proteins are more difficult to track, but, as we shall see, recognizably similar proteins do occur in certain transposable elements. In this chapter we review current thinking about the origins of retroviruses and transposable elements, the emphasis being on relationships inferred from the comparison of amino acid sequences. We begin by examining the phylogenetic relationships of the various groups of retroviruses.

2 Classification of Retroviruses

Until recently, retroviruses were classified according to their gross morphology in the electron microscope (TEICH 1984). Briefly, type A particles were described as being 60–90 nm in diameter and double shelled, whereas type B were larger and more doughnut shaped with spikes. Type C viruses were usually associated with budding of the host cell's plasma membrane and type D viruses had short spikes and other distinguishing features.

Retroviruses have also been classified according to their biological behavior, either by the nature and consequences of their action, or by the range of their host specificity. Thus, it is customary to divide them into three general groups: the oncoviruses, the slow viruses, and the foamy viruses (TEICH 1984).

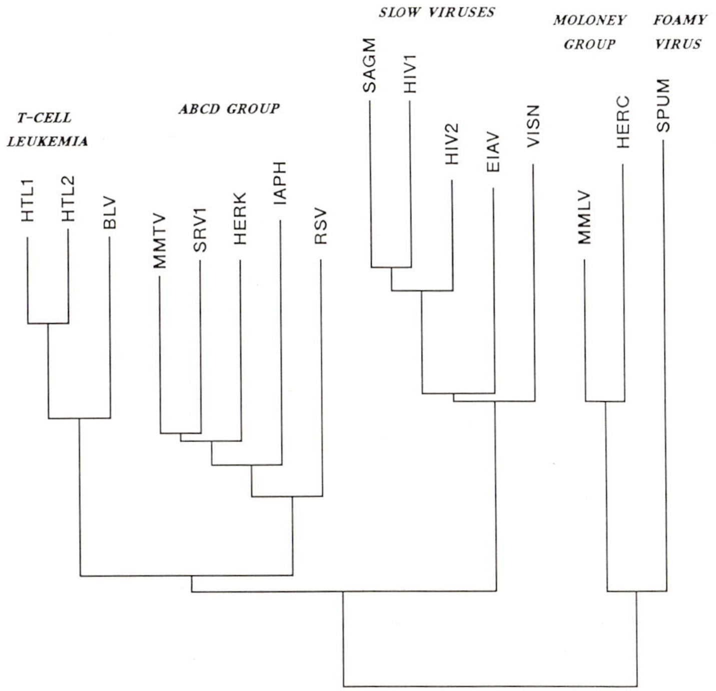

Fig. 2. Retrovirus phylogeny based on reverse transcriptase sequences. *HTL1,2,* human T-cell leukemia virus I and II; *BLV*, bovine leukemia virus; *SRV1*, simian retrovirus I; *MMTV*, mouse mammary tumor virus; *HERK*, human endogenous retrovirus (K); *IAPH*, Syrian hamster intracisternal particle; *RSV*, Rous sarcoma virus; *VISN*, visna lentivirus; *EIAV*, equine infectious anemia virus; *SAGM*, simian immunodeficiency virus, African green monkey; *HIV1,2*, human immunodeficiency virus 1 and 2; *MMLV*, Moloney mouse leukemia virus; *HERC*, human endogenous retrovirus (C); *SPUM*, human spumavirus. The Moloney mouse group also includes the feline leukemia virus, baboon endogenous virus, and avian retriculoendothelial virus (Adapted from DOOLITTLE et al. 1990)

With regard to host range, avian viruses are commonly discussed separately from murine viruses, which in turn are often considered apart from those infecting primates. Finally, exogenous viruses are usually distinguished from endogenous viruses. The latter, which are carried in the germline of the host, are ordinarily noninfectious and often defective in some key feature (COFFIN 1984).

The availability of genomic sequence data for a wide variety of retroviruses has rendered much of the earlier taxonomy moot. Thus, phylogenies derived from comparing the inferred amino acid sequences of any or all of the retrovirus enzymes delineate several major groups that are quite different from taxonomies based on gross morphology (Fig. 2). Indeed, one of the major subgroups includes all four morphological types: type A (Syrian hamster intracisternal particle 18), type B (mouse mammary tumor virus), type C (Rous sarcoma virus), and type D (simian retrovirus 1). The inadequacy of particle morphology as a taxonomic tool is underscored by the recent finding that a single amino acid substitution in a *gag* protein can change a type D retrovirus into a type C (RHEE and HUNTER 1990).

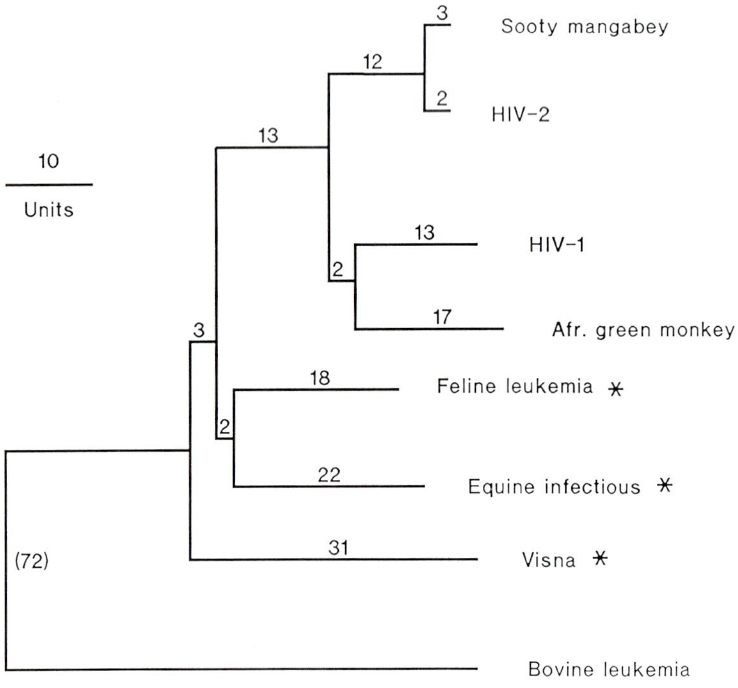

Fig. 3. Slow virus (lentivirus) phylogeny based on reverse transcriptase sequences. The bovine leukemia virus, which is not a slow virus (see Fig. 2), was used as an outgroup in order to root the other sequences. The viruses marked with *asterisks* have a captured host gene that has been identified by MCGEOCH (1990) as coding for deoxyuridine triphosphatase

Similarly, sequence-based phylogenies make little distinction on the basis of host specificity, avian and mammalian viruses being found together in the same subgroups, and the possibility of horizontal infections across class lines from mammals to birds cannot be excluded. This is not to say that host range boundaries are not observed; just that on their own such categorizations are unreliable. On the other hand, the fact that lentiviruses have yet to be reported among birds argues that this group of viruses evolved after the appearance of mammals. As a final point, phylogenies derived from sequences do not distinguish between endogenous and exogenous retroviruses, a point of major consequence in any consideration of their origins.

We don't mean to imply that sequence data have resolved all matters dealing with retrovirus phylogenies. Relationships can be confounded by recombination between divergent viruses as well as by horizontal transfers. Moreover, within any given subgroup some relationships are more secure than others, and the literature contains a number of disputed arrangements. These are not always trivial matters, dealing as they may with issues as important as the independent origins of HIV-1 and HIV-2 (Fig. 3). The interested reader will want to consult the excellent review by MYERS and PAVLAKIS (1991), which deals with "within group" relationships of the more complex retroviruses.

3 Evolutionary Rates

As is well known, retroviruses—and RNA viruses in general—mutate at vastly greater rates than DNA-based organisms (HOLLAND et al. 1982). This is at least partly due to RNA polymerases lacking the sophisticated editing machinery associated with DNA polymerases. By virtue of their life cycle, retroviruses actually have a twofold opportunity for experiencing this less faithful replication, the one instance involving the reverse transcriptase copying RNA to DNA on the way to integration in the host DNA, the second involving the host RNA polymerase transcribing new retrovirus genomes (MYERS and PAVLAKIS 1991). The inescapable consequence of this heightened mutation rate is a proportionately more rapid evolution, a fact reflected in the proteases of HIV and visna being as different to each other as the corresponding acid proteases of mammals and fungi, and the proteases of T-cell leukemia viruses and slow viruses being as different from each other as human pepsin and a hypothetical bacterial protease (DOOLITTLE et al. 1989a). If, as seems to be the case, the slow viruses first appeared after the evolution of mammals, they must have diverged as much in less than a hundred million years as the rest of the biological world has in a billion years.

Given this accelerated evolution, it is a wonder we are able to recognize the non-viral ancestors of *any* retrovirus proteins. That similarities are in fact observed is usually explained by noting that, whereas infectious retroviruses do change with extraordinary rapidity, endogenous retroviruses, which are transmitted vertically in the host germline, do not. There is more to this argument than meets the eye at first glance. First, infection and the opportunity for an increased number of replications must weigh heavily in the accelerated evolution of exogenous retroviruses. Second, even endogenous retroviruses ought to evolve faster than the host genome, so long as they continue to indulge in reverse transcription. Implicit in this argument is the realization that exogenous retroviruses must be extremely short lived in an evolutionary sense (DOOLITTLE et al. 1989a), the bulk of the history of any given lineage residing in quiet periods of endogenous existence and perhaps even quieter times not involving reverse transcription. Once integrated in the host germline, retroviruses must abide by

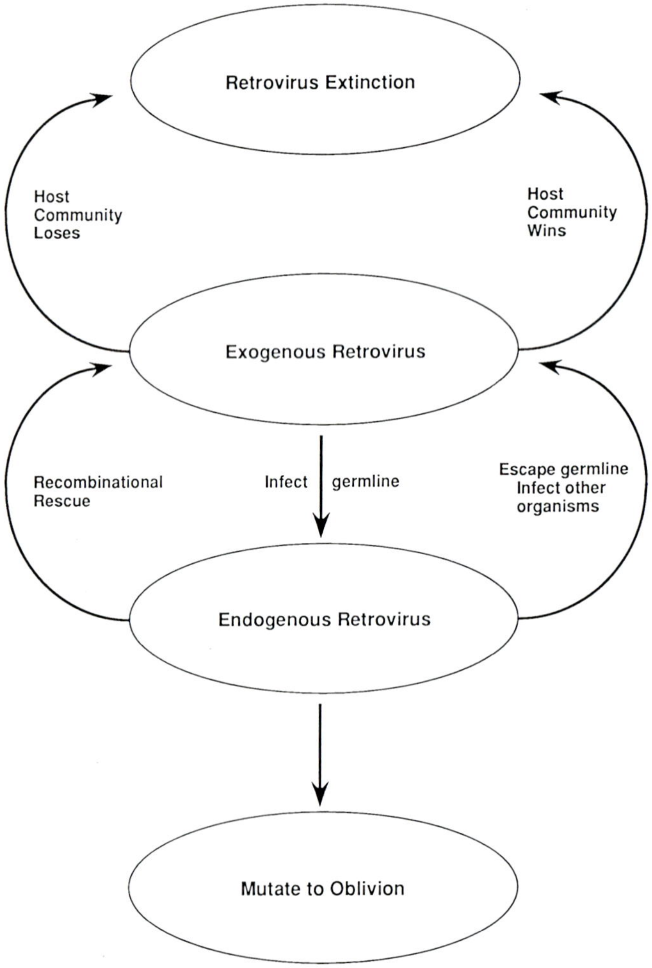

Fig. 4. Postulated natural history of exogenous and endogenous retroviruses

the evolutionary dictum of "use it or lose it," by which we mean that the particle must actively continue its reverse transcription-based life cycle or be doomed to becoming a mere array of pseudogenes. Pseudogenes, while changing faster than functional cellular genes, evolve much more slowly that those of infectious retroviruses. A simple schema describing a putative natural history for exogenous and endogenous retroviruses is depicted in Fig. 4.

Although the reverse transcriptase is the slowest changing of the eight to ten definable proteins common to all retroviruses, reliable in-group phylogenies can often be constructed with the sequences of the other retrovirus proteins as well. For the most part, the trees that emerge are congruent with the reverse transcriptase trees. Occasionally, however, significant differences are observed, and in at least one case the difference is best interpreted as due to a recombinational event between ancestors of different subgroups (McClure et al. 1988).

4 Distribution of Reverse Transcriptase

Although reverse transcriptase was initially thought to be unique to RNA tumor viruses (Baltimore 1970; Temin and Mizutani 1970), the enzyme has since been found in a wide variety of settings, both viral and nonviral including:

1. Retroviruses
2. Hepadnoviruses
3. Transposable elements (LTR type)
4. Caulimoviruses
5. Transposable elements (poly-A type)
6. Mitochondrial introns
7. Chloroplast introns
8. Mitochondrial plasmids
9. Bacterial elements
10. Telomerase

For example, it is the mainstay of hepatitis B virus (Summers and Mason 1982), and also the caulimoviruses of plants (Toh et al. 1983). Both of these are DNA viruses, but replication in each proceeds by way of an RNA intermediate. Reverse transcriptases are also found in numerous transposable elements that are widely distributed in the eukaryotic world, as well as in the repetitive elements known as LINEs (long interspersed nuclear elements) (Loeb et al. 1986). The enzyme is also found in organellar introns of some fungi (Michel and Lang 1985) and algae (Kuck 1989), as well as in certain mitochondrial plasmids (Nargang et al. 1984). Most recently, it has been found in diverse strains of some bacteria in association with unique single-strand DNA (Inouye et al. 1989; Lim and Mass 1989). Finally, there is evidence that telomerase, an enzyme presumably

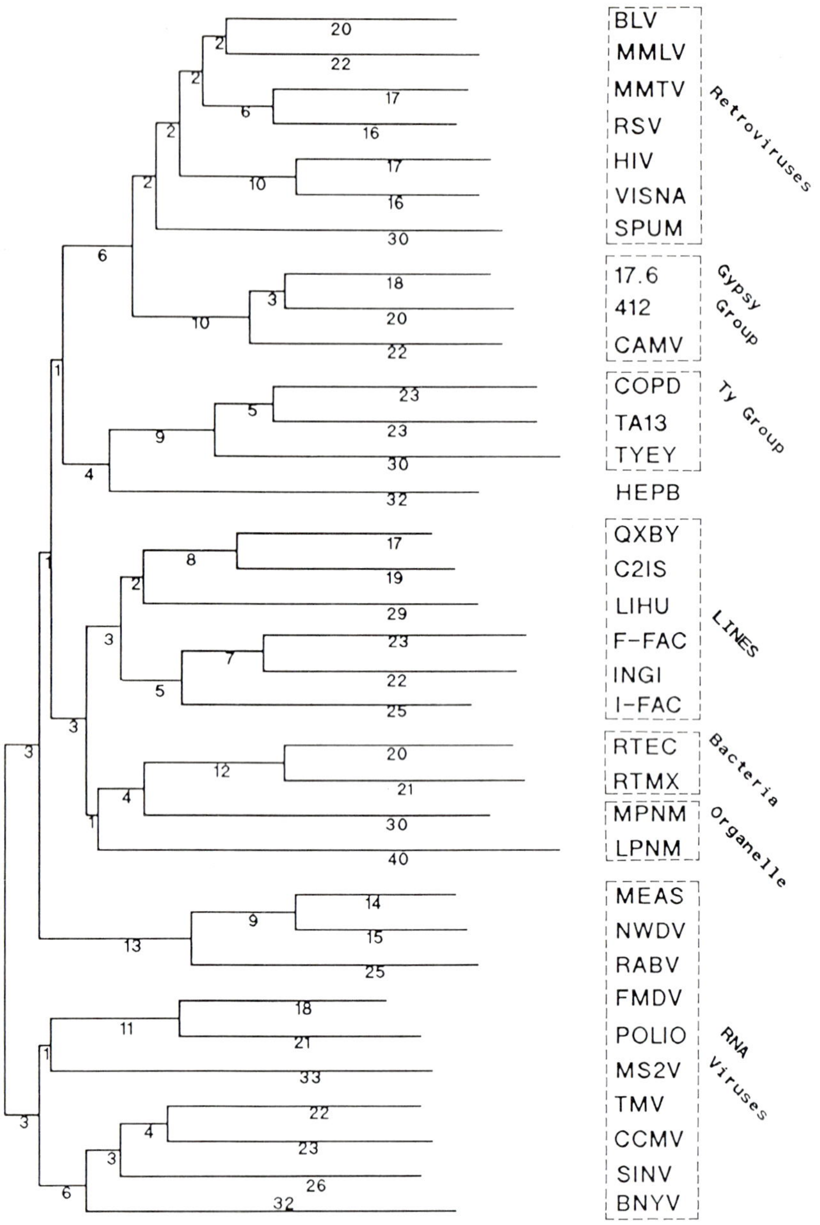

Fig. 5. A phylogeny of reverse trancriptase-containing entities. The tree was constructed with the program PAPA (DOOLITTLE and FENG 1990) and is based on the alignment of partial sequences of reverse transcriptases assembled by POCH et al. (1989); the corresponding segments of some recently published reverse transcriptases from a foamy virus (*SPUM*), a plant (*TA13*) and bacteria (*RTEC* and *RTMX*) have been added, as well as a DNA-dependent RNA polymerase from a mitochondrial plasmid (*LPNM*). Numbers are proportional to evolutionary distances. *BLV*, bovine leukemia virus; *MMLV*, Moloney mouse leukemia virus; *MMTV*, mouse mammary tumor virus; *RSV*,

ubiquitous to all eukaryotic cells, is a reverse transcriptase (LUNDBLAD and BLACKBURN 1990).

Reverse transcriptase is an RNA-dependent DNA polymerase. KAMER and ARGOS (1984) pointed out that there are weak but persistent similarities in retroviral reverse transcriptases to the RNA-dependent RNA polymerases of other RNA viruses, a point that was subsequently underscored by POCH et al. (1989) who aligned portions of polymerases from a large number of RNA viruses and transposable elements. ARGOS (1988) has defined a short sequence motif based on the well known "D–D" feature of reverse transcriptase that embraces RNA–RNA, DNA–DNA, and DNA–RNA polymerases as well. In aggregate, the data make it seem likely that all polymerases evolved from a common ancestor long before the divergence of prokaryotes and eukaryotes. At which juncture in history the reverse transcriptase diverged from the others remains unclear, a point we will return to momentarily.

In what may be an unusual and special case, SCHULTE and LAMBOWITZ (1991) have isolated a plasmid from neurospora mitochondria that contains a DNA-dependent RNA polymerase that is homologous with the reverse transcriptases found in similar plasmids in other strains (Fig. 5). In this case the highly conserved D–D sequence found in almost all reverse transcriptases has been changed to D–E, suggesting that this one amino acid replacement may be crucial to the changeover from an RNA template to a DNA template.

5 The Origin of Endogenous Retroviruses

In a prescient consideration made in the immediate wake of the discovery of reverse transcriptase in RNA tumor viruses, TEMIN (1970) suggested that RNA leukemia viruses might arise from protoviruses carried in the host genome by a "system that may be similar to modifying elements in maize." He came to this conclusion by reasoning that RNA sarcoma viruses seemed to arise spontaneously as the result of mutations in RNA leukemia viruses, both types of virus

Fig. 5. (*Continued*)
Rous sarcoma virus; *HIV*, human immunodeficiency virus 1; *VISNA*, visna virus of sheep; *SPUM*, foamy virus; *17.6* and *412* are both *Drosophila* elements; *CAMV*, cauliflower mosaic virus; *COPD*, *copia* element of *Drosophila*; *TA13*, *Arabidopsis* element; *TYEY*, TY912 of yeast; *HEPB*, hepatitis virus; *QXBY* and *C2IS* are from yeast mitochondrial introns; *LIHU*, human LINE element; *F-FAC*, and *I-FAC* are F and I factors of *Drosophila*; *INGI*, ING trypanosome element; *RTEC*, reverse transcriptase from *Escherichia coli*; *RTMX*, *Myxococcus xanthus*; *MPNM*, Mauriceville plasmid; *LPNM*, LaBelle plasmid; *MEAS*, measles virus; *NWDV*, Newcastle disease virus; *RABV*, rabies virus, *FMDV*, foot and mouth disease virus; *POLIO*, polio virus; *MS2V*, phase MS2; *TMV*, tobacco mosaic virus; *CCMV*, cucumber mosaic virus, *SINV*, Sindbis virus; *BNYV*, beet necrotic yellow vein virus. (The Ty group is referred to in the text and Fig. 6 as the *copia* group)

replicating through an RNA/DNA/RNA cycle. But where did leukemia viruses come from? He hypothesized that they may be the result of protoviruses modifying host genetic material by way of a DNA/RNA/DNA cycle. This was in contrast to the provirus hypothesis of HUEBNER and TODARO (1969), which asserted that RNA leukemia viruses originated from repressed proviruses or oncogenes. TEMIN further suggested that the protovirus, not being a true virus, would not have an envelope protein. It is now clear that this view is essentially correct. A number of transposable elements that have the same genetic equipment as retroviruses, except for envelope proteins, are now known to be widely distributed among eukaryotes (SHIBA and SAIGO 1983). The most retrovirus-like of these is a widespread group of transposable elements typified by the Gypsy element of *Drosophila*, close relatives of which are also found in plants and fungi (Fig. 5).

Transposable elements of this sort are carried in multiple copies in the germlines of their hosts; they ordinarily have reverse transcriptase, ribonuclease H, integrase and acid protease sequences, often in exactly the same order as occurs in a typical retrovirus (Fig. 1). They have an RNA-binding protein and capsid proteins, as well as typical LTRs with tRNA priming sites. Moreover, they have been shown to exist as intracellular particles (ADAMS et al. 1987) and replicate through an RNA intermediate (BOEKE et al. 1985). In the final analysis, the one thing that distinguishes this group of elements from a vertebrate retrovirus is the absence of envelope proteins. Indeed, one would be hardput to distinguish a typical mammalian A-type intracisternal particle (ONO et al. 1985) from a transposable element of the Gypsy type, by any criterion. Like so much else in the biological world, these gene clusters can be viewed as clusters of selfish genes, their survival depending on a balance of generating an occasionally advantageous new gene arrangement in the host, on the one hand, and the chance disruption of important host genes, on the other.

6 Classifying Transposable Elements

Not all transposable elements involve reverse transcription, of course. In fact, many prokaryotic and eukaryotic elements appear to depend exclusively on an endonuclease (transposase). Our trail backwards in search of retrovirus roots will follow only reverse transcriptase-bearing elements, however (Sect. 4). In this regard, the transposable elements described in the preceding section can be divided into two groups on the basis of their gene arrangement. Thus, the Gypsy group has its four key enzymes in exactly the same order as retroviruses: protease, reverse transcriptase, ribonuclease, endonuclease. Another related group, typified by the *Drosophila* element *copia*, has the endonuclease 5′ to the protease. Both groups have natural histories that are much the same as endogenous retroviruses. They occur in variable numbers of copies in the host genome, the result of sundry past episodic transposition events. Many of the copies in any particular instance are likely to be defective.

Another kind of element that occurs throughout most of the eukaryotic world, similar to but critically different from the transposable elements discussed above, is the LINEs group (BURTON et al. 1986). These elements also have reverse transcriptase sequences and open reading frames that may encode some other features found in retroviruses. LINEs sequences are typically degenerate, however, and it is usually necessary to piece together the information from a consensus rather than a single entity. As a result, the situation with regard to other genes like those for the protease or ribonuclease is still not fully understood. The mechanics of replication are still unclear, although recently evidence has been found for a translated LINEs protein (LEIBOLD et al. 1990). The LINEs family of elements seems more primitive than the *copia* and Gypsy groups of elements in that they lack tRNA priming and LTR generation as a part of their reverse transcription. This may partly explain why most mammalian LINE sequences are truncated to varying degrees at their 5′ ends.

The LINEs group includes elements found in plants (SCHWARZ-SOMMER et al. 1987), insects (FAWCETT et al. 1986), and protists (KIMMEL et al. 1987; GABRIEL et al. 1990). Although they occur in vast copy numbers in mammals, copy numbers in the other groups appear to be more moderate and the destinies more confined. An RNA intermediate has recently been reported in the case of *Drosophila* I factor (CHABOISSIER et al. 1990), and endonuclease activity has been demonstrated in the case of the R2Bm element of *Bombyx mori* (XIONG and EICKBUSH 1988b).

Evidence has been accumulating that the reverse transcriptase-bearing mitochondrial introns are also a kind of mobile element (LAMBOWITZ 1989). The mobility is apparently dependent on an accompanying endonuclease activity. Although the sequences surrounding the reverse transcriptases in these entities include additional open reading frames, it has not been possible to identify unequivocally other gene products that might be involved, whether the endonuclease, ribonuclease H, protease, or structural proteins.

Finally, the bacterial reverse transcriptase associated with the peculiar single-strand DNA appears to behave like a transposable element. Typical of selfish genes, these systems are sporadically distributed, some strains of a bacterial species having the sequences, others not (INOUYE et al. 1989; LIM and MAAS 1989).

7 Phylogenies Based on Reverse Transcriptases

If the reverse transcriptase is the hallmark of the retrovirus lineage, then a sequence-based tree should reflect the full retrovirus history, and attempts have been made in the past to establish the major connections (XIONG and EICKBUSH

1988a, 1990; DOOLITTLE et al. 1989b). The sequences are widely divergent, however, and as a result some of the most distant relationships remain equivocal. There is broad agreement on the principal point that vertebrate retroviruses form a distinct cluster of the most recently diverged sequences and that their closest nonretrovirus relatives are the LTR-containing transposable elements dubbed the "Gypsy" group (DOOLITTLE et al. 1989a). The uncertainties have to do with the relative relationships of the LINEs group, organellar introns, and the bacteria (Fig. 5). Thus, XIONG and EICKBUSH (1990), using only the most conserved portions of the reverse transcriptase sequences, constructed a tree from which they argue the LINEs group is more primitive than the bacteria sequences. It is their contention that the bacterial reverse transcriptases were likely acquired by horizontal transfer. The phylogenetic tree shown in Fig. 5 is based on an alignment scheme of POCH et al. (1989), although we used our own tree-growing program to construct it (DOOLITTLE and FENG 1990). Happily, the resulting topology is similar to that obtained by XIONG and EICKBUSH (1990). It is our position, nonetheless, that one cannot distinguish whether the LINEs or the bacterial sequences are the more primitive from such a tree.

8 An Evolutionary Scenario

The question arises, can we reconcile the reverse transcriptase-based phylogeny depicted in Fig. 5 with the occurrence of the other known features of retroviruses? The problem is that many of the other components evolve faster than the reverse transcriptase, and as a result we are unable to identify them in some of the primitive systems, if indeed they exist there (Table 1). Nonetheless, let us propose that the first step on the way to a future retrovirus was heralded by the juxtaposition of a reverse transcriptase and a prokaryotic transposase (Fig. 6). Let us further propose that the occasion of the juxtaposition coincided with the invasion of primitive eukaryotes by endosymbiotic prokaryotes about 1.5–2.0 billion year ago (DOOLITTLE et al. 1989b). In defense of these proposals, we may just note that endonucleases are as fundamental to the transposition of retroviruses as reverse transcriptases, and, as we have implied, also have deep prokaryotic roots—low-level sequence resemblances to bacterial transposases having been noted (YUKI et al. 1986; JOHNSON et al. 1986). At the same time, even though an impressive alignment of LTR-containing retroviruses and transposable elements can be made with bacterial insertion (IS) sequences (KHAN et al. 1991), it is somewhat disconcerting that it has not so far proved possible to do so with the organellar-type systems or any of the LINEs family of elements—trypanosomal, invertebrate or plant—even though endonuclease activity has been demonstrated in one of these systems (XIONG and EICKBUSH 1988b). Taken at face value, the data imply that the two different lineages acquired their endonucleases independently. The alternative is that an excessive rate of

Table 1. Distribution of other genes in reverse transcriptase-containing entities

	LTR	CA	NC	PR	RN	IN	ENV
Infectious retroviruses (birds, mammals)	+	+	+	+	+	+	+
Defective retroviruses (VL30s, IAPs, etc.)	+	v	+	+	+	+	v
Hepatitis B virus (birds, mammals)	–	–	–	?	+	–	+
LTR transposable elements (fungi, invertebrate animals, plants)	+	+	v	+	+	+	(–)
Plant DNA viruses (e.g., cauliflower mosaic)	+	+	+	+	+	–	–
LINEs (vertebrates)	–	(+)	–	+	?	?	–
LINE-like transposable elements (protists, plants, invertebrate animals)	–	(+)	v	?	+	v	–
Mitochondrial group II introns (fungi)	–	–	–	?	?	?	–
Mitochondrial plasmids (fungi)	–	–	–	?	–	?	–
ms DNA (assorted bacteria)	–	–	–	–	?	?	–

LTR, long terminal repeats; CA, capsid or *gag* core; NC, *gag* RNP; PR, protease; RN, ribonuclease H; IN, integrase; ENV, envelope; +, always present; –, always absent; v, variable; ?, not resolved at present

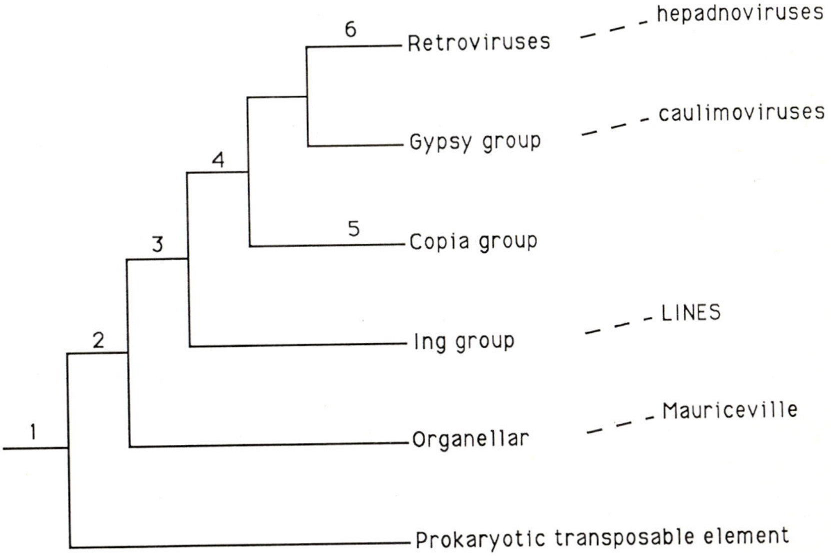

Fig. 6. A simple scenario marking the evolutionary progression to infectious retroviruses. *1*, Juxtaposition of prokaryotic transposase and reverse transcriptase; *2*, primitive retrotransposon active in organelles (prokaryotes) during early endosymbiotic period, aided by RNA-binding protein; *3*, acquisition of polyadenylation signal allows escape from organelle to host; *4*, introduction of LTR improves replication efficiency; *5*, rearrangement of endonuclease and reverse transcriptase regions; *6*, invention of spliced envelope protein allows escape from cell of manufacture

change in the LINEs group lineage has blurred the resemblances beyond recognition.

Which of the other accessory genes might have been recruited next is open to question. It is likely, however, that capsid and RNA-binding proteins were necessary before any egress from the organelle into the host would be possible. Further studies of mobile organellar introns may be revealing in this regard. In the meantime, the incidental acquisition of a polyadenylation signal by some ancestor of the LINEs lineage may have provided a kind of eukaryotic legitimacy that accommodated transcription from a host setting.

Although polyadenylation may have been a big step forward, the replication of LINEs elements appears to have been hobbled historically by incomplete reverse transcription. This limitation may have been overcome with the advent of tRNA priming and the introduction of the LTR. Consistent with this reasoning, the LINEs family of transposable elements is phylogenetically more primitive than the LTR-containing elements as reflected in their biological distribution, the latter not yet having been identified in any protist, whereas LINE-like elements, as noted above, have been found in trypanosomes (KIMMEL et al. 1987) and related organisms (GABRIEL et al. 1990). This assessment presumes that the distribution reflects a conventional history and is not the result of horizontal transfers. Similarly, we can place the origin of the LINEs family after the introduction of organelles into eukaryotes and anticipate that they will not be found in those primitive eukaryotes like giardia, creatures that diverged before the organellar invasion. These observations are consistent with the chronology afforded by the reverse transcriptase phylogenetic tree (Fig. 5).

The transposable element system made possible by tRNA priming and LTR generation is now much in evidence throughout the eukaryotic world. In cellular terms, this invention may have extended the territorial imperative to protracted stays in the cytoplasm, since safe reverse transcription was insured. It was the invention of the spliced envelope protein a billion years later, however, that was to allow the escape of these particles from the cell of their manufacture. The resulting retroviruses were able to realize even more distant horizons, cell to cell, individual to individual, and occasionally species to species. Selfish as they must be, these explorations are often ill-fated and destined for dead ends (Fig. 4). What may seem to be a great natural advantage at first—the capture of some host growth-promoting factor, for example—may prove self-defeating in the end if the host is overly compromised.

9 Summary and Conclusions

Reverse transcriptase sequences, which are fundamental to retrovirus existence, are widely distributed in the living world. Phylogenies based on their sequences set vertebrate retroviruses apart as relatively modern creations. Their nearest evolutionary relatives are a large group of transposable elements that have all the standard retrovirus equipment except spliced envelope proteins. The distribution of these elements suggests a long-standing presence predating the radiation of plants, fungi, and animals. There is another large group of elements, LINEs, that also contain recognizable reverse transcriptase sequences and which likely diverged even earlier, as evidenced by their presence in trypanosomes and other protists. They lack tRNA priming sites—which they could have lost—but they do exhibit characteristic eukaryotic polyadenylation. These elements are problematic in that the sequences are so degenerate in most instances that it is not possible to identify the accessory enzymes or structural proteins with any confidence, leaving major gaps in our reconstruction of events. Even with these gaps, however, the historical beginnings of retroviruses can be traced back to events coincident with the prokaryotic invasion of primitive eukaryotes.

References

Adams SE, Mellor J, Gull K, Sim RB, Tuite MF, Kingsman SM, Kingsman AJ (1987) The functions and relationships of Ty-VLP proteins in yeast reflect those of mammalian retroviral proteins. Cell 49: 111–119

Argos P (1988) A sequence motif in many polymerases. Nucleic Acids Res 16: 9909–9916

Baltimore D (1970) Viral RNA-dependent DNA polymerase. Nature 226: 1209–1211

Boeke JD, Garfinkel DJ, Styles CA, Fink GR (1985) Ty elements transpose through an RNA intermediate. Cell 40: 491–500

Burton FH, Loeb DD, Voliva CF, Martin SL, Edgell MH, Hutchinson CA III (1986) Conservation throughout mammalia and extensive protein-encoding capacity of the highly repeated DNA long interspersed sequence one. J Mol Biol 187: 291–304

Chaboissier M-C, Busseau I, Prosser J, Finnegan DJ, Bucheton A (1990) Identification of a potential RNA intermediate for transposition of the LINE-like element I factor in *Drosophila melanogaster*. EMBO J 9: 3557–3563

Coffin J (1984) Endogenous Retroviruses. In: Weiss R, et al. (eds) RNA tumor viruses, 2nd edn. Cold Spring Harbor Laboratory, Cold Spring Harbor, pp 1109–1203

Doolittle RF, Feng DF (1990) Nearest neighbor procedure for relating progressively aligned amino acid sequences. Methods Enzymol 183: 659–669

Doolittle RF, Feng DF, Johnson MS, McClure MA (1989a) Origins and evolutionary relationships of retroviruses. Q Rev Biol 64: 1–30

Doolittle RF, Anderson KL, Feng DF (1989b) Estimating the prokaryote-eukaryote divergence time from protein sequences. In: Fernholm F, Bremer K, Jornvall H (eds) The hierarchy of life. Excerpta Medica, Amsterdam

Doolittle RF, Feng DF, McClure MA, Johnson MS (1990) Retrovirus phylogeny and evolution. Curr Top Microbiol Immunol 157: 1–17

Fawcett DH, Lister CK, Kellett E, Finnegan DJ (1986) Transposable elements controlling I-R hybrid dysgenesis in *D. melanogaster* are similar to mammalian LINEs. Cell 47: 1007–1015

Gabriel A, Yen TJ, Schwartz DC, Smith CL, Boeke JD, Sollner-Webb B, Cleveland DW (1990) A rapidly rearranging retrotransposon within the miniexon gene locus of *Crithidia fasciculata*. Mol Cell Biol 10: 615–624

Holland J, Spindler K, Horodyski F, Grabau E, Nichol S, VandePol S (1982) Rapid evolution of RNA genomes. Science 215: 1577–1585

Huebner RJ, Todaro GJ (1969) Oncogenes of RNA tumor viruses as determinants of cancer. Proc Natl Acad Sci USA 64: 1087–1094

Inouye S, Hsu M-Y, Eagle S, Inouye M (1989) Reverse transcriptase associated with the biosynthesis of the branched RNA-linked msDNA in *Myxococcus xanthus*. Cell 56: 709–717

Johnson MS, McClure MA, Feng DF, Gray J, Doolittle RF (1986) Computer analysis of retroviral *pol* genes: assignment of enzymatic functions to specific sequences and homologies with nonviral enzymes. Proc Natl Acad Sci USA 83: 7648–7652

Kamer G, Argos P (1984) Primary structural comparison of RNA-dependent polymerases from plant, animal and bacterial viruses. Nucleic Acids Res 12: 7269–7282

Khan E, Mack JPG, Katz RA, Kulkosky J, Skalka AM (1991) Retroviral integrase domains: DNA binding and the recognition of LTR sequences. Nucleic Acids Res 19: 8651–8660

Kimmel BE, Ole-Moiyoi OK, Young JR (1987) Ingi, a 5.2-kb dispersed sequence element from *Trypanosoma brucei* that carries half of a smaller mobile element at either end and has homology with mammalian LINEs. Mol Cell Biol 7: 1465–1475

Kuck U (1989) The intron of a plastid gene from a green alga contains an open reading frame for a reverse transcriptase-like enzyme. Mol Gen Genet 218: 257–265

Lambowitz A (1989) Infectious introns. Cell 56: 323–326

Leibold DM, Swergold GD, Singer MF, Thayer RE, Dombroski BA, Fanning TG (1990) Translation of LINE-1 DNA elements in vitro and in human cells. Proc Natl Acad Sci USA 87: 6990–6994

Lim D, Maas WK (1989) Reverse transcriptase-dependent synthesis of a covalently linked, branched DNA–RNA compound in *E. coli* B. Cell 56: 891–904

Loeb DD, Padgett RW, Hardies SC, Shehee WR, Comer MB, Edgell MH, Hutchison CA III (1986) The sequence of a large L1Md element reveals a tandemly repeated 5′ end and several features found in retrotransposons. Mol Cell Biol 6: 168–182

Lundblad V, Blackburn EH (1990) RNA-dependent polymerase motifs in EST1: tentative identification of a protein component of an essential yeast telomerase. Cell 60: 529–530

McClure MA, Johnson MS, Feng DF, Doolittle RF (1988) Sequence comparisons of retroviral proteins: relative rates of change and general phylogeny. Proc Natl Acad Sci USA 85: 2469–2473

McGeoch DJ (1990) Protein sequence comparisons show that "pseudoproteases" encoded by poxviruses and certain retroviruses belong to the deoxyuridine triphosphatase family. Nucleic Acids Res 18: 4105–4110

Michel F, Lang BF (1985) Mitochondrial class II introns encode proteins related to the reverse transcriptases of retroviruses. Nature 316: 641–643

Myers G, Pavlakis GN (1991) Evolutionary potential of complex retroviruses. In: Wagner RR, Fraenkel-Conral H (eds) The viruses: the retroviridiae. Plenum, New York

Nargang FE, Bell JB, Stohl LL, Lambowitz AM (1984) The DNA sequence and genetic organization of a neurospora mitochondrial plasmid suggest a relationship to introns and mobile elements. Cell 38: 441–453

Ono M, Toh H, Miyata T, Awaya T (1985) Nucleotide sequence of the Syrian hamster intracisternal A-particle gene: close evolutionary relationship of type A particle gene to types B and D oncovirus genes. J Virol 55: 387–394

Poch O, Sauvaget I, Delarue M, Tordo N (1989) Identification of four conserved motifs among the RNA-dependent polymerase encoding elements. EMBO J 8: 3867–3874

Rhee SS, Hunter E (1990) A single amino acid substitution within the matrix protein of a type D retrovirus converts its morphogenesis to that of a type C retrovirus. Cell 63: 77–86

Schulte U, Lambowitz AM (1991) The LaBelle mitochondrial plasmid of Neurospora intermedia encodes a novel DNA polymerase that may be derived from a reverse transcriptase. Mol Cell Biol 11: 1696–1706

Schwarz-Sommer Z, Leclercq L, Gobel E, Saedler H (1987) Cin4, an insert altering the structure of the *A1* gene in *Zea mays*, exhibits properties of nonviral retrotransposons. EMBO J 6: 3873–3880

Shiba T, Saigo K (1983) Retrovirus-like particles containing RNA homologous to the transposable element *copia* in *Drosophila melanogaster*. Nature 302: 119–124

Summers J, Mason WS (1982) Replication of the genome of a hepatitis B-like virus by reverse transcription of an RNA intermediate. Cell 29: 403–415

Teich N (1984) Taxonomy of retroviruses. In: Weiss R et al. (eds) RNA tumor viruses, 2nd edn. Cold Spring Harbor Laboratory, Cold Spring Harbor, pp 25–207

Temin HM (1970) Malignant transformation of cells by viruses. Perspect Biol Med 14: 11–26

Temin HM, Mizutani S (1970) RNA-dependent DNA polymerase in virions of Rous Sarcoma Virus. Nature 226: 1211–1213

Toh H, Hayashida H, Miyata T (1983) Homology of reverse transcriptase of retrovirus with putative polymerase gene products of hepatitis B virus and Cauliflower mosaic virus. Nature 305: 827–829

Xiong Y, Eickbush TH (1988a) Similarity of reverse transcriptase-like sequences of viruses, transposable elements, and mitochondrial introns. Mol Biol Evol 5: 675–690

Xiong Y, Eickbush TH (1988b) Functional expression of a sequence-specific endonuclease encoded by the retrotransposon R2Bm. Cell 55: 235–246

Xiong Y, Eickbush TH (1990) Origin and evolution of retroelements based upon their reverse transcriptase sequences. EMBO J 9: 3353–3362

Yuki S, Ishimaru S, Inouye S, Saigo K (1986) Identification of genes for reverse transcriptase-like enzymes in two *Drosophila* retrotransposons, *412* and *gypsy*; a rapid detection method of reverse transcriptase genes using YXDD box probes. Nucleic Acids Res 14: 3017–3030

Replication and Evolution of Viroid-Like Pathogens

H. D. ROBERTSON

1 Introduction

1.1 Viroid-Like RNAs and Circular RNA Replication

It is becoming increasingly evident that certain basic processes of macromolecular biology require RNA. Whether as a key component of ribosomes in the translation process, or as small nuclear RNAs in particles carrying out eukaryotic messenger RNA (mRNA) splicing, RNA—perhaps because of its historical role in molecular evolution—occupies a central position. Another class of RNA molecules—the pathogenic viroid-like RNAs—are also providing new insights into the role of RNA in gene expression. Until recently, these circular, self-replicating RNAs—250–400 bases in length—were found only in plants. Beginning in 1986, however, several reports have confirmed that the causative agent for delta hepatitis in mammals contains a circular, viroid-like RNA (WANG et al. 1986; KOS et al.1986; CHEN et al. 1986; TAYLOR et al. 1987). This delta RNA is about four times the size of plant viroid RNAs. Knowledge that such RNAs can proliferate within cells has come at the same time as an increasing interest in the

Department of Biochemistry, Cornell University Medical College, 1300 York Avenue, New York, N.Y., USA

Current Topics in Microbiology and Immunology, Vol. 176

role of RNA in the evolution of primitive self-replicating systems. Several proposals based on RNA—a material with both template and enzymatic properties—as the initial genetic substance have appeared (GILBERT 1986; SHARP 1985). So far, none of these has taken into account the potential for RNA circles to simplify the tasks required for replication in a primitive environment. Furthermore, key steps involving cleavage and ligation, which are required for successful replication of RNA circles (BRANCH and ROBERTSON 1984), may also help to provide explanations for the way in which RNA molecules were able to assort and reassort themselves. We will first list several hypotheses about early RNAs and their properties. Then we will consider how our knowledge of present-day viroid replication steps could help our understanding of these properties. Next we will consider how delta agent RNA appears to be the result of RNA conjunction between a viroid-like replication entity and an mRNA coding segment, yielding two characteristic domains in one molecule. Finally, we will suggest ways in which the organization of modern eukaryotic genomes into coding stretches and intervening sequences may have come about as a consequence of a previous genomic system involving such conjoined RNAs.

2 Early RNA Genomes

Our first hypothesis is that the properties of early RNA-dependent systems may be ascertainable from an examination of RNA molecules surviving today. We also assume that RNA molecules evolved self-replication first, then the property of protein coding, and finally an information storage system using DNA copies. This idea leads to the prediction that todays genetic systems will contain features reflecting this particular history, and that intermediates in the development of protein coding sequences in the context of self-replicating RNAs may still exist in recognizable form.

One way to test the above assumptions is to consider the way todays viroid-like RNAs, including that of the delta agent, are thought to replicate. We have proposed in earlier publications (BRANCH and ROBERTSON 1984) a rolling circle pathway for the replication of these RNAs, in which multimeric copies of one or both RNA strands are synthesized and then processed to yield monomeric progeny molecules. This pathway has now been successfully demonstrated for a number of viroid-like pathogens, including the delta agent (CHEN et al. 1986). It has been assumed that protein enzymes provided by the host cell are required for the RNA synthetic steps of this pathway, although these enzymes have yet to be identified. These appear to be the only proteins absolutely required for the replication of todays viroid-like RNAs, as can be seen from the well-documented cases of self-cleavage and self-ligation.

2.1 Self-Copying of Circular RNA Templates

Some reports (reviewed in Cech 1989) have begun to demonstrate how RNA may have first begun to copy itself. A consideration of such RNA-catalyzed self-copying reveals several potential problems, e.g., how to copy accurately (and protect from breakdown) the ends of such molecules; how to unwind the newly synthesized RNA strand from a stable duplex with its template so that the next round of copying can proceed; and how to initiate synthesis without a preexisting set of initiation factors. A circular template simplifies all of these problems. Since it has no ends, its structure is stabilized in a way not possible with linear molecules. Furthermore, a circular template, once undergoing synthesis, will lead directly to greater than unit length copies, so that the first copy is automatically displaced from the replication complex by the second, overcoming the unwinding dilemma. Finally, initiation anywhere on a circular template leads to a complete copy with no risk of losing ends or other regions. Given a primitive environment in which circular, self-replicating RNAs could proliferate, what clues can be found relating to the transition from that state to the one prevailing today? A key development in the history of RNA—the advent of protein-coding sequences—must have occurred within a reasonable time after the emergence of the self-replicating elements described above. Given the emergence of self-replicating RNA entities ("RNA replicons") on the one hand, and the potential for protein coding on the other, how did these two capabilities become harmoniously conjoined into the primitive genetic material of the RNA protein (RNP) world, a proposed stage on the way from the RNA world to that of DNA (GILBERT 1986)?

2.2 Self-Cleavage and Religation of Circular RNAs

In considering the conjunction of RNAs of such different function, we were struck by two points emerging from studies of viroid-like RNAs in general, and delta RNA in particular. First, it is evident that the rolling circle pathway (BRANCH and ROBERTSON 1984) has as an absolute requirement the efficient ability of the RNA molecules involved to cleave at specific sites (to reduce multimeric precursors to monomeric progeny RNAs), and to ligate at these same sites (to convert linear monomers to circular, mature RNA). These same properties—if applied at some frequency to exogenous RNA moleclues—could also serve as a primitive system of RNA reassortment. Such a development would allow the viroid-like RNA replicons to pick up different segments of RNA, including primitive protein-coding sequences. If we assume, therefore, that a circular RNA has a single self-cleavage site which can open and religate with a certain frequency, then it is easy to imagine (even if specific terminal sequences are required) a low but significant rate at which outside RNAs would be ligated into the RNA replicon's cleavage/ligation site.

3 Delta Agent RNA

There is one property of delta RNA sufficiently striking to provide further insight into the process of RNA conjunction. In reviewing the properties of delta agent RNA (BRANCH et al. 1989), we were impressed not only by its greater size than other viroid-like RNAs and its possession of a template segment encoding an mRNA for a protein called the delta antigen (WANG et al. 1986), but also by several ways in which its properties appear to segregate into domains. Figure 1 shows the delta RNA genome presented in the collapsed rod configuration first proposed by WANG et al. (1986). Three properties characteristic of viroids are clustered in the left-hand quarter of the RNA: regions of conserved sequence; an element of local tertiary structure which can undergo ultraviolet light-induced cross-linking; and sites able to undergo RNA-catalyzed self-cleavage. Meanwhile, the protein-coding segment has little or no overlap with this region, occupying most of the upper strand of the right-hand three-quarters of the map in Fig. 1.

3.1 Central Conserved Regions of Viroids and Delta RNA

A number of studies of plant viroids have led to the proposal of a central conserved region (CCR) in which about 50 bases are retained, presumably

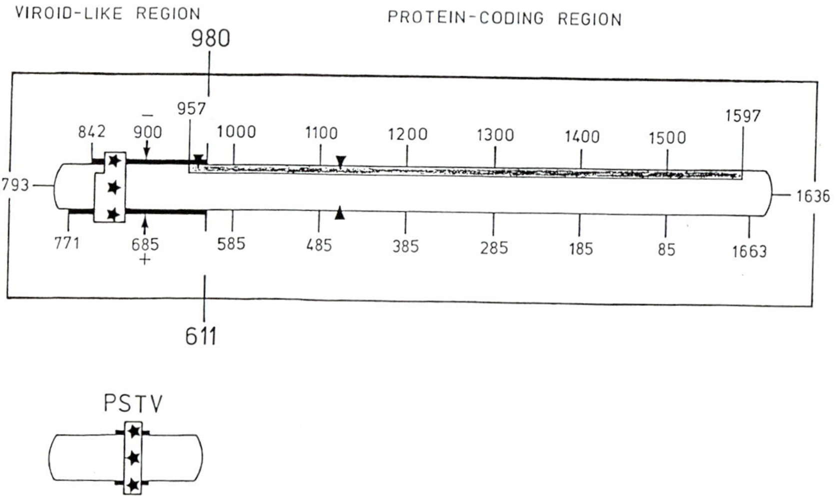

Fig. 1 Map of the genomic RNA of the delta agent. *Light-shaded region*, Region encoding a delta-specified protein (delta antigen); *stars*, a novel UV-sensitive structural element; *dark shaded region*, sequences conserved either between delta isolates (WANG et al. 1986; MAKINO et al. 1987) or among the PSTV group of viroids (see KEESE and SYMONS 1985). *Insert*, this viroid RNA is drawn to scale with the RNA of the delta agent.

because of some critical function involved in replication (KEESE and SYMONS 1985). In comparing the strains of delta agent so far sequenced in full, there is an average of 10%–15% variation, but it is nonrandomly placed. In particular, two extensive regions of exact homology (the ony two in the entire delta RNA molecule) are present, both occurring inside the 379-base left-hand quarter of the RNA, including residues 611–771 and 842–957. These two conserved regions are also situated across from each other in the map (see Fig. 1) in a fashion analogous to the viroid CCR (KEESE and SYMONS 1985).

An additional property of the viroid CCR which we have previously reported is the presence of a characteristic region of local tertiary structure which can be identified by ultraviolet light-induced cross-linking (BRANCH et al. 1985). We have described the discovery of a similar structural element, also susceptible to ultraviolet light-induced cross-linking, within the conserved region of delta RNA (BRANCH et al. 1989). Finally, several reports have described efficient self-cleavage of RNA from this domain of the delta genomic and antigenomic RNA (SHARMEEN et al. 1988; WU and LAI 1989). A number of viroid-like RNAs of plants are known to undergo self-cleavage in an analogous manner. We believe that these three properties of the region encompassing residues 611–989 of the delta agent RNA are sufficiently singular and striking as to define a viroid-like domain of this RNA molecule.

3.2 Two Domains of the Delta RNA Genome

The presence of such a viroid-like domain has caused us to take a closer look at the entire genomic delta RNA molecule. As shown in Fig. 1, the delta antigen protein is encoded by the complement to the RNA in the region of residues 1597–957. Thus there is at most a seven amino acid overlap (at the carboxy terminus) between the coding region and the viroid-like domain. Furthermore, with respect to variation, MAKINO et al. (1987) point out that certain parts of this protein-coding domain have up to 20% variability in two strains whose sequences have been completely determined and compared.

The differences described here between the two domains of delta agent RNA suggest to us that the viroid-like and protein-coding regions originated separately and were then combined by a process of RNA conjunction like that described in hypothetical terms above. If this were the case, it would be the first evidence for the existence of a class of molecules—conjoined RNAs—which could assist our understanding not only of RNA's evolution but also of its present-day function. These conclusions would remain in effect regardless of whether delta RNA itself actually is a primitive molecule—a "missing link" in the chain of molecular evolution—or whether it represents a recent reoccurrence of processes which have a constant potential to occur among informational RNA molecules which are active in present-day cells.

4 Evolution to DNA Systems

Possible ways should also be considered by which RNA conjunction could have influenced present-day genomes, and how conjoined RNAs—if they were the precursors to a DNA storage system—might have shaped the properties of that system in ways which are evident today. We would hypothesize that a transition from self-replicating circular RNAs, as the major component of primitive molecular life, to an RNP-based system in which conjoined RNAs—circular elements containing both viroid-like domains for replication with protein-coding segments attached—were the genetic material took place resulting in a population of molecules not unlike delta RNA in many respects. Furthermore, as long as the viroid-like RNA replicons remained in control of RNA replication, it would be reasonable to assume that they, as in delta RNA, would be more highly conserved than their protein-coding counterparts. If we now assume that a DNA storage system emerged, which copied faithfully the conjoined RNAs presented to it, then we would expect DNA genomes to be a mosaic of coding segments interspersed with elements formerly capable of replication and circularization—the viroid-like replicons. These elements would thus become, at the DNA level, intervening sequences whose survival as replicons could endanger the new stability of the DNA-level system, and whose removal at the RNA level would be needed to allow the most efficient use and assortment of the mRNA coding segments.

Present-day eukaryotic DNA genomes demonstrate some of the above properties, as if they actually might have originated as copies of conjoined RNAs. Since replication functions would now occur at the DNA level, strong pressure would be exerted favoring drift in these intervening sequences. However, certain functions, according to this reasoning, would be retained. In particular, as mentioned above, a critical factor favoring the process of RNA conjunction in the first place was the precise cleavage and ligation capability manifested by conjoined RNAs and their precursors. If this same ability were retained in RNA transcripts of the early DNA genomic storage system, then a close relative of the present-day mRNA splicing process would be built in from the start. At the borders between the former DNA replicons (now intervening sequences) and the mRNA coding segments, cleavage would occur; furthermore, the property of ligation between the ends so produced would confer the ability of neighboring mRNA segments to combine, allowing new protein combinations without further genomic variation. Present mRNA molecules, containing multiple coding and intervening sequences, could reflect the results of such a process.

4.1 DNA Mosaics Encoding Conjoined RNAs

What we see, then, is a system in which a DNA mosaic encoding conjoined RNAs emerges, with a ready-made RNA splicing system, to liberate the coding segments for mRNA function. This early emergence of RNA splicing may explain why it has been retained by eukaryotic genomes despite the puzzle of its awkward and energy-consuming logistics. Furthermore, the potential for intervening sequences to retain at least those functions required for cleavage and ligation steps in RNA splicing suggests that they may be less inert than previously suspected. One of the ideas suggested here—that intervening sequences began as viroid-like RNA replicons—carries with it the possibility that self-replicating RNAs may reemerge from transcripts of DNA, combine with other RNA segments, and give rise to new combinations of genetic material. In this regard, it is possible to imagine directed versions of such a process leading to a new class of RNA-level vectors capable of changing the genetic expression of the cells to which they are added. It is also possible that naturally occurring conjoined RNAs with pathogenic potential continue to arise with some regularity in vivo. Whether the delta agent RNA arose in this way, or whether it represents an ancestral intermediate in molecular evolution, remains to be determined. We conclude, however, that its status as a prototype for RNA conjunction is sufficiently striking to justify (a) comparative sequencing analysis of various additional delta agent RNA strains; (b) directed mutagenesis of test the prediction that abolishing mRNA activity in the delta coding segment could still, under certain conditions, allow replication controlled by the viroid-like domain; and (c) a careful search among other present-day RNAs (including populations of intervening sequences) for additional evidence of RNA conjunction.

References

Branch AD, Robertson HD (1984) A replication cycle for viroids and other small infectious RNAs. Science 223: 450–455

Branch AD, Benenfeld BJ, Robertson HD (1985) Ultraviolet light-induced cross-linking reveals a unique region of local tertiary structure in potato spindle tuber viroid and HeLa 5S RNA. Proc Natl Acad Sci USA 82: 6590–6594

Branch AD, Benenfeld BJ, Baroudy BM, Wells FV, Gerin JL, Robertson HD (1989) An ultraviolet-sensitive RNA structural element in a viroid-like domain of the hepatitis delta virus. Science 243: 649–652

Cech TR (1989) RNA enzymes. Adv Enzymol 62: 1–36

Chen PJ, Kalpana G, Goldberg J, Mason W, Werner B, Gerin J, Taylor J (1986) Structure and replication of the genome of the hepatitis delta virus. Proc Natl Acad Sci USA 83: 8774–8778

Gilbert W (1986) The RNA world. Nature 319: 618

Keese P, Symons RH (1985) Domains in viroids: evidence of intermolecular RNA rearrangements and their contribution to viroid evolution. Proc Natl Acad Sci USA 82: 4582–4586

Kos A, Kijkema R, Arnberg AC, van der Meide PH, Schellekens H (1986) The hepatitis delta virus possesses a circular RNA. Nature 323: 558–560

Makino S, Chang MF, Shieh CK, Kamahora T, Vannier DM, Govindarajan S, Lai MMC (1987) Molecular cloning and sequencing of a human hepatitis delta virus RNA. Nature 329: 343–346

Sharmeen L, Kuo MYP, Dinter-Gottlieb G, Taylor J (1988) Antigenomic RNA of human hepatitis delta virus can undergo self-cleavage. J Virol 62: 2674–2679

Sharp PA (1985) On the origin of RNA splicing and introns. Cell 42: 397–400

Taylor J, Mason W, Summers J, Goldberg J, Aldrich C, Coates L, Gerin J, Gowans E (1987) Replication of human hepatitis delta virus in primary cultures of woodchuck hepatocytes. J Virol 61: 2891–2895

Wang KS, Choo QL, Weiner AJ, Ou JH, Najarian RC, Thayer RM, Mullenbach GT, Denniston KJ, Gerin JL Houghton M (1986) Structure, sequence and expression of the hepatitis delta viral genome. Nature 323: 508–514

Wu HN, Lai MMC (1989) Reversible cleavage ligation of hepatitis delta virus RNA. Science 243: 652–654

Subject Index

Current Topics in Microbiology and Immunology

Volumes published since 1986 (and still available)

Vol. 132: **Melchers, Fritz; Potter, Michael (Ed.):** Mechanisms in B-Cell Neoplasia. Workshop at the National Cancer, Institute, National Institutes of Health, Bethesda, MD, USA, March 24–26, 1986. 1986. 156 figs. XII, 374 pp. ISBN 3-540-17048-0

Vol. 133: **Oldstone, Michael B. (Ed.):** Arenaviruses. Genes, Proteins, and Expression. 1987. 39 figs. VII, 116 pp. ISBN 3-540-17246-7

Vol. 134: **Oldstone, Michael B. (Ed.):** Arenaviruses. Biology and Imminotherapy. 1987. 33 figs. VII, 242 pp. ISBN 3-540-14322-6

Vol. 135: **Paige, Christopher J.; Gisler, Roland H. (Ed.):** Differentiation of B Lymphocytes. 1987. 25 figs. IX, 150 pp. ISBN 3-540-17470-2

Vol. 136: **Hobom, Gerd; Rott, Rudolf (Ed.):** The Molecular Biology of Bacterial Virus Systems. 1988. 20 figs. VII, 90 pp. ISBN 3-540-18513-5

Vol. 137: **Mock, Beverly; Potter, Michael (Ed.):** Genetics of Immunological Diseases. 1988. 88 figs. XI, 335 pp. ISBN 3-540-19253-0

Vol. 138: **Goebel, Werner (Ed.):** Intracellular Bacteria. 1988. 18 figs. IX, 179 pp. ISBN 3-540-50001-4

Vol. 139: **Clarke, Adrienne E.; Wilson, Ian A. (Ed.):** Carbohydrate-Protein Interaction. 1988. 35 figs. IX, 152 pp. ISBN 3-540-19378-2

Vol. 140: **Podack, Eckhard R. (Ed.):** Cytotoxic Effector Mechanisms. 1989. 24 figs. VIII, 126 pp. ISBN 3-540-50057-X

Vol. 141: **Potter, Michael; Melchers, Fritz (Ed.):** Mechanisms in B-Cell Neoplasia 1988. Workshop at the National Cancer Institute, National Institutes of Health, Bethesda, MD, USA, March 23–25, 1988. 1988. 122 figs. XIV, 340 pp. ISBN 3-540-50212-2

Vol. 142: **Schüpach, Jörg:** Human Retrovirology. Facts and Concepts. 1989. 24 figs. 115 pp. ISBN 3-540-50455-9

Vol. 143: **Haase, Ashley T.; Oldstone Michael B. A. (Ed.):** In Situ Hybridization 1989. 22 figs. XII, 90 pp. ISBN 3-540-50761-2

Vol. 144: **Knippers, Rolf; Levine, A. J. (Ed.):** Transforming. Proteins of DNA Tumor Viruses. 1989. 85 figs. XIV, 300 pp. ISBN 3-540-50909-7

Vol. 145: **Oldstone, Michael B. A. (Ed.):** Molecular Mimicry. Cross-Reactivity between Microbes and Host Proteins as a Cause of Autoimmunity. 1989. 28 figs. VII, 141 pp. ISBN 3-540-50929-1

Vol. 146: **Mestecky, Jiri; McGhee, Jerry (Ed.):** New Strategies for Oral Immunization. International Symposium at the University of Alabama at Birmingham and Molecular Engineering Associates, Inc. Birmingham, AL, USA, March 21–22, 1988. 1989. 22 figs. IX, 237 pp. ISBN 3-540-50841-4

Vol. 147: **Vogt, Peter K. (Ed.):** Oncogenes. Selected Reviews. 1989. 8 figs. VII, 172 pp. ISBN 3-540-51050-8

Vol. 148: **Vogt, Peter K. (Ed.):** Oncogenes and Retroviruses. Selected Reviews. 1989. XII, 134 pp. ISBN 3-540-51051-6

Vol. 149: **Shen-Ong, Grace L. C.; Potter, Michael; Copeland, Neal G. (Ed.):** Mechanisms in Myeloid Tumorigenesis. Workshop at the National Cancer Institute, National Institutes of Health, Bethesda, MD, USA, March 22, 1988. 1989. 42 figs. X, 172 pp. ISBN 3-540-50968-2

Vol. 150: **Jann, Klaus; Jann, Barbara (Ed.):** Bacterial Capsules. 1989. 33 figs. XII, 176 pp. ISBN 3-540-51049-4

Vol. 151: **Jann, Klaus; Jann, Barbara (Ed.):** Bacterial Adhesins. 1990. 23 figs. XII, 192 pp. ISBN 3-540-51052-4

Vol. 152: **Bosma, Melvin J.; Phillips, Robert A.; Schuler, Walter (Ed.):** The Scid Mouse. Characterization and Potential Uses. EMBO Workshop held at the Basel Institute for Immunology, Basel, Switzerland, February 20–22, 1989. 1989. 72 figs. XII, 263 pp. ISBN 3-540-51512-7

Vol. 153: **Lambris, John D. (Ed.):** The Third Component of Complement. Chemistry and Biology. 1989. 38 figs. X, 251 pp. ISBN 3-540-51513-5

Vol. 154: **McDougall, James K. (Ed.):** Cytomegaloviruses. 1990. 58 figs. IX, 286 pp. ISBN 3-540-51514-3

Vol. 155: **Kaufmann, Stefan H. E. (Ed.):** T-Cell Paradigms in Parasitic and Bacterial Infections. 1990. 24 figs. IX, 162 pp. ISBN 3-540-51515-1

Vol. 156: **Dyrberg, Thomas (Ed.):** The Role of Viruses and the Immune System in Diabetes Mellitus. 1990. 15 figs. XI, 142 pp. ISBN 3-540-51918-1

Vol. 157: **Swanstrom, Ronald; Vogt, Peter K. (Ed.):** Retroviruses. Strategies of Replication. 1990. 40 figs. XII, 260 pp. ISBN 3-540-51895-9

Vol. 158: **Muzyczka, Nicholas (Ed.):** Viral Expression Vectors. 1992. 20 figs. IX, 176 pp. ISBN 3-540-52431-2

Vol. 159: **Gray, David; Sprent, Jonathan (Ed.):** Immunological Memory. 1990. 38 figs. XII, 156 pp. ISBN 3-540-51921-1

Vol. 160: **Oldstone, Michael B. A.; Koprowski, Hilary (Ed.):** Retrovirus Infections of the Nervous System. 1990. 16 figs. XII, 176 pp. ISBN 3-540-51939-4

Vol. 161: **Racaniello, Vincent R. (Ed.):** Picornaviruses. 1990. 12 figs. X, 194 pp. ISBN 3-540-52429-0

Vol. 162: **Roy, Polly; Gorman, Barry M. (Ed.):** Bluetongue Viruses. 1990. 37 figs. X, 200 pp. ISBN 3-540-51922-X

Vol. 163: **Turner, Peter C.; Moyer, Richard W. (Ed.):** Poxviruses. 1990. 23 figs. X, 210 pp. ISBN 3-540-52430-4

Vol. 164: **Bækkeskov, Steinnun; Hansen, Bruno (Ed.):** Human Diabetes. 1990. 9 figs. X, 198 pp. ISBN 3-540-52652-8

Vol. 165: **Bothwell, Mark (Ed.):** Neuronal Growth Factors. 1991. 14 figs. IX, 173 pp. ISBN 3-540-52654-4

Vol. 166: **Potter, Michael; Melchers, Fritz (Ed.):** Mechanisms in B-Cell Neoplasia 1990. 143 figs. XIX, 380 pp. ISBN 3-540-52886-5

Vol. 167: **Kaufmann, Stefan H. E. (Ed.):** Heat Shock Proteins and Immune Response. 1991. 18 figs. IX, 214 pp. ISBN 3-540-52857-1

Vol. 168: **Mason, William S.; Seeger, Christoph (Ed.):** Hepadnaviruses. Molecular Biology and Pathogenesis. 1991. 21 figs. X, 206 pp. ISBN 3-540-53060-6

Vol. 169: **Kolakofsky, Daniel (Ed.):** Bunyaviridae. 1991. 34 figs. X, 256 pp. ISBN 3-540-53061-4

Vol. 170: **Compans, Richard W. (Ed.):** Protein Traffic in Eukaryotic Cells. Selected Reviews. 1991. 14 figs. X, 186 pp. ISBN 3-540-53631-0

Vol. 171: **Kung, Hsing-Jien; Vogt, Peter K. (Eds.):** Retroviral Insertion and Oncogene Activation. 1991. 18 figs. X, 179 pp. ISBN 3-540-53857-7

Vol. 172: **Chesebro, Bruce W. (Ed.):** Transmissible Spongiform Encephalopathies. 1991. 48 figs. X, 288 pp. ISBN 3-540-53883-6

Vol. 173: **Pfeffer, Klaus; Heeg, Klaus; Wagner, Hermann; Riethmüller, Gert (Ed.):** Function and Specificity of γ/δ T Cells. 1991. 41 figs. XII, 296 pp. ISBN 3-540-53781-3

Vol. 174: **Fleischer, Bernhard; Sjögren, Hans Olov (Eds.):** Superantigens. 1991. 13 figs. IX, 137 pp. ISBN 3-540-54205-1

Vol. 175: **Aktories, Klaus (Ed.):** ADP-Ribosylating Toxins. 1992. 23 figs. IX, 148 pp. ISBN 3-540-54598-0